4 WEEKS

W9-BXY-938

WITHDRAWN

Teen Health Series

Gastrointestinal
Diseases and Disorders
SOURCEBOOK

Second Edition

Health Reference Series

Second Edition

Gastrointestinal
Diseases and Disorders
SOURCEBOOK

*Basic Consumer Health Information about the Upper
and Lower Gastrointestinal (GI) Tract, Including the
Esophagus, Stomach, Intestines, Rectum, Liver, and
Pancreas, with Facts about Gastroesophageal Reflux
Disease, Gastritis, Hernias, Ulcers, Celiac Disease,
Diverticulitis, Irritable Bowel Syndrome, Hemorrhoids,
Gastrointestinal Cancers, and Other Diseases and
Disorders Related to the Digestive Process*

*Along with Information about Commonly Used
Diagnostic and Surgical Procedures, Statistics, Reports
on Current Research Initiatives and Clinical Trials,
a Glossary, and Resources for Additional Help
and Information*

Edited by
Sandra J. Judd

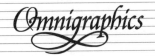

615 Griswold Street • Detroit, MI 48226

Bibliographic Note

Because this page cannot legibly accommodate all the copyright notices, the Bibliographic Note portion of the Preface constitutes an extension of the copyright notice.

Edited by Sandra J. Judd

Health Reference Series

Karen Bellenir, *Managing Editor*
David A. Cooke, M.D., *Medical Consultant*
Elizabeth Barbour, *Research and Permissions Coordinator*
Cherry Stockdale, *Permissions Assistant*
Dawn Matthews, *Verification Assistant*
Laura Pleva Nielsen, *Index Editor*
EdIndex, Services for Publishers, *Indexers*

* * *

Omnigraphics, Inc.

Matthew P. Barbour, *Senior Vice President*
Kay Gill, *Vice President—Directories*
Kevin Hayes, *Operations Manager*
Leif Gruenberg, *Development Manager*
David P. Bianco, *Marketing Director*

* * *

Peter E. Ruffner, *Publisher*

Frederick G. Ruffner, Jr., *Chairman*

Copyright © 2006 Omnigraphics, Inc.

ISBN 0-7808-0798-7

Library of Congress Cataloging-in-Publication Data

Gastrointestinal diseases and disorders sourcebook : basic consumer health information about the upper and lower gastrointestinal (GI) tract, including the esophagus, stomach, intestines, rectum, liver, and pancreas, with facts about gastroesophageal reflux disease, gastritis, hernias, ulcers, celiac disease, diverticulitis, irritable bowel syndrome, hemorrhoids, gastrointestinal cancers, and other diseases and disorders related to the digestive process; along with information about commonly used diagnostic and surgical procedures, statistics, reports on current research initiatives and clinical trials, a glossary, and resources for additional help and information / edited by Sandra J. Judd.-- 2nd ed.
    p. cm. -- (Health reference series)
  Summary: "Provides basic consumer health information about digestive diseases and disorders of the gastrointestinal tract. Includes index, glossary of related terms, and other resources"--Provided by publisher.
  Includes bibliographical references and index.
  ISBN 0-7808-0798-7 (hardcover : alk. paper)
  1. Gastrointestinal system--Diseases--Popular works. I. Judd, Sandra J. II. Health reference series (Unnumbered)
  RC806.G37 2006
  616.3--dc22
                                                                    2005029568

Table of Contents

Visit www.healthreferenceseries.com to view *A Contents Guide to the Health Reference Series*, a listing of more than 10,000 topics and the volumes in which they are covered.

Part II: Diagnostic and Surgical Procedures Used for Gastrointestinal Disorders

Part III: Disorders of the Upper Gastrointestinal Tract

Part IV: Disorders of the Lower Gastrointestinal Tract

Part V: Disorders of the Digestive System's Solid Organs: The Liver and Pancreas

Part VI: Cancers of the Gastrointestinal Tract

Preface

About This Book

The gastrointestinal tract includes the stomach, intestines, and other organs related to digestion—the process by which food and drink are changed into molecules of nutrients that can be carried to the body's cells. Disorders that interfere with this process affect an estimated 60 to 70 million Americans and account for more than 35 million doctor visits every year. According to the National Institute of Diabetes and Digestive and Kidney Diseases, researchers have only recently begun to understand many gastrointestinal diseases and disorders. As a result, the process of helping people set aside common misconceptions about the causes of symptoms and turn to scientifically based treatments instead of folkloric remedies is progressing only gradually.

Gastrointestinal Diseases and Disorders Sourcebook, Second Edition provides readers with updated health information about the causes, symptoms, diagnosis, and treatment of diseases and disorders affecting the esophagus, stomach, intestines, appendix, gall bladder, liver, and pancreas. It also describes how the gastrointestinal tract can be affected by food intolerances, infectious diseases, and various cancers. The structure and function of the digestive system, common diagnostic methods, medical treatments, surgical procedures, and current research initiatives are described. The book concludes with a glossary of related terms and directory of resources for further help and information.

How to Use This Book

This book is divided into parts and chapters. Parts focus on broad areas of interest. Chapters are devoted to single topics within a part.

Part I: Introduction to the Digestive System begins with a look at the anatomy and physiology of the digestive system. It describes commonly experienced symptoms and discusses how the gastrointestinal tract can be impacted by tobacco use or by frequently used medications.

Part II: Diagnostic and Surgical Procedures Used for Gastrointestinal Disorders provides a detailed look at endoscopic procedures and other types of tests used to diagnose gastrointestinal disorders. It also explains ostomy, colostomy, ileostomy, and other surgical procedures.

Part III: Disorders of the Upper Gastrointestinal Tract looks at disorders of the esophagus and the stomach. It describes the risk factors, symptoms, and treatment options for each of the disorders covered.

Part IV: Disorders of the Lower Gastrointestinal Tract describes the risk factors, symptoms, and treatment options for disorders affecting the large and small intestines, appendix, gall bladder, anus, and rectum.

Part V: Disorders of the Digestive System's Solid Organs: The Liver and the Pancreas offers current information about the risk factors, symptoms, and treatment options for pancreatitis, hepatitis, cirrhosis of the liver, and other liver disorders.

Part VI: Cancers of the Gastrointestinal Tract provides a detailed look at the different cancers that affect the gastrointestinal tract. Each chapter reports on risk factors, symptoms, diagnostic methods, staging information, treatment options, and clinical trials.

Part VII: Food Intolerances and Infectious Disorders of the Gastrointestinal Tract discusses lactose intolerance, celiac disease, and diseases transmitted by viral, bacterial, or parasitic contamination of food or drinking water.

Part VIII: Additional Help and Information provides a glossary of gastrointestinal terms and a directory of organizations that can provide further information.

Bibliographic Note

This volume contains documents and excerpts from publications issued by the following U.S. government agencies: Centers for Disease Control and Prevention (CDC); National Cancer Institute (NCI); National Institute of Diabetes and Digestive and Kidney Diseases (NIDDK); National Institutes of Health (NIH); National Women's Health Information Center (NWHIC); and the U.S. Food and Drug Administration (FDA).

In addition, this volume contains copyrighted documents from the following organizations: A.D.A.M., Inc.; American Academy of Family Physicians; American Association for Clinical Chemistry; American Liver Foundation; American Society of Gastrointestinal Endoscopy; American Urogynecologic Society; Case Nutrition Consulting; Cedars-Sinai Health System; Cincinnati Children's Hospital Medical Center; Cleveland Clinic; Colorectal Surgical Society of Australasia; Crohn's and Colitis Foundation of America; J-Pouch Group; Nemours Foundation; North American Society for Pediatric Gastroenterology, Hepatology and Nutrition; Texas Pediatric Surgical Associates; United Ostomy Association; and the Wisconsin Department of Health and Family Services.

Full citation information is provided on the first page of each chapter. Every effort has been made to secure all necessary rights to reprint the copyrighted material. If any omissions have been made, please contact Omnigraphics to make corrections for future editions.

Acknowledgements

Thanks go to the many organizations, agencies, and individuals who have contributed materials for this *Sourcebook* and to medical consultant Dr. David Cooke, verification assistant Dawn Matthews, and document engineer Bruce Bellenir. Special thanks go to managing editor Karen Bellenir and permissions coordinator Liz Barbour for their help and support.

About the Health Reference Series

The *Health Reference Series* is designed to provide basic medical information for patients, families, caregivers, and the general public. Each volume takes a particular topic and provides comprehensive coverage. This is especially important for people who may be dealing with a newly diagnosed disease or a chronic disorder in themselves or in a family member. People looking for preventive guidance, information about disease warning signs, medical statistics, and risk factors for health problems will also find answers to their questions in the *Health Reference Series*. The *Series*, however, is not intended to serve as a tool for diagnosing illness, in prescribing treatments, or as a substitute for the physician/patient relationship. All people concerned about medical symptoms or the possibility of disease are encouraged to seek professional care from an appropriate health care provider.

Locating Information within the Health Reference Series

The *Health Reference Series* contains a wealth of information about a wide variety of medical topics. Ensuring easy access to all the fact sheets, research reports, in-depth discussions, and other material contained within the individual books of the series remains one of our highest priorities. As the *Series* continues to grow in size and scope, however, locating the precise information needed by a reader may become more challenging.

A *Contents Guide to the Health Reference Series* was developed to direct readers to the specific volumes that address their concerns. It presents an extensive list of diseases, treatments, and other topics of general interest compiled from the Tables of Contents and major index headings. To access *A Contents Guide to the Health Reference Series*, visit www.healthreferenceseries.com.

Medical Consultant

Medical consultation services are provided to the *Health Reference Series* editors by David A. Cooke, M.D. Dr. Cooke is a graduate of Brandeis University, and he received his M.D. degree from the University of Michigan. He completed residency training at the University of Wisconsin Hospital and Clinics. He is board-certified in Internal Medicine. Dr. Cooke currently works as part of the University of Michigan Health System and practices in Ann Arbor, MI. In his free time, he enjoys writing, science fiction, and spending time with his family.

Our Advisory Board

We would like to thank the following board members for providing guidance to the development of this series:

Dr. Lynda Baker,
Associate Professor of Library and Information Science,
Wayne State University, Detroit, MI

Nancy Bulgarelli,
William Beaumont Hospital Library, Royal Oak, MI

Karen Imarisio,
Bloomfield Township Public Library, Bloomfield Township, MI

Karen Morgan,
Mardigian Library, University of Michigan-Dearborn,
Dearborn, MI

Rosemary Orlando,
St. Clair Shores Public Library, St. Clair Shores, MI

Health Reference Series *Update Policy*

The inaugural book in the *Health Reference Series* was the first edition of *Cancer Sourcebook* published in 1989. Since then, the *Series* has been enthusiastically received by librarians and in the medical community. In order to maintain the standard of providing high-quality health information for the layperson the editorial staff at Omnigraphics felt it was necessary to implement a policy of updating volumes when warranted.

Medical researchers have been making tremendous strides, and it is the purpose of the *Health Reference Series* to stay current with the most recent advances. Each decision to update a volume is made on an individual basis. Some of the considerations include how much new information is available and the feedback we receive from people who use the books. If there is a topic you would like to see added to the update list, or an area of medical concern you feel has not been adequately addressed, please write to:

Editor
Health Reference Series
Omnigraphics, Inc.
615 Griswold Street
Detroit, MI 48226
E-mail: editorial@omnigraphics.com

Part One

Introduction to the Digestive System

Chapter 1

Your Digestive System and How It Works

The digestive system is a series of hollow organs joined in a long, twisting tube from the mouth to the anus (see Figure 1.1). Inside this tube is a lining called the mucosa. In the mouth, stomach, and small intestine, the mucosa contains tiny glands that produce juices to help digest food.

Two solid organs, the liver and the pancreas, produce digestive juices that reach the intestine through small tubes. In addition, parts of other organ systems (for instance, nerves and blood) play a major role in the digestive system.

Why is digestion important?

When we eat such things as bread, meat, and vegetables, they are not in a form that the body can use as nourishment. Our food and drink must be changed into smaller molecules of nutrients before they can be absorbed into the blood and carried to cells throughout the body. Digestion is the process by which food and drink are broken down into their smallest parts so that the body can use them to build and nourish cells and to provide energy.

How is food digested?

Digestion involves the mixing of food, its movement through the digestive tract, and the chemical breakdown of the large molecules

Reprinted from "Your Digestive System and How It Works," National Institute of Diabetes and Digestive and Kidney Diseases, National Institutes of Health, NIH Publication No. 04-2681, May 2004.

of food into smaller molecules. Digestion begins in the mouth, when we chew and swallow, and is completed in the small intestine. The chemical process varies somewhat for different kinds of food.

Movement of Food through the System

The large, hollow organs of the digestive system contain muscle that enables their walls to move. The movement of organ walls can propel food and liquid and also can mix the contents within each organ. Typical movement of the esophagus, stomach, and intestine is

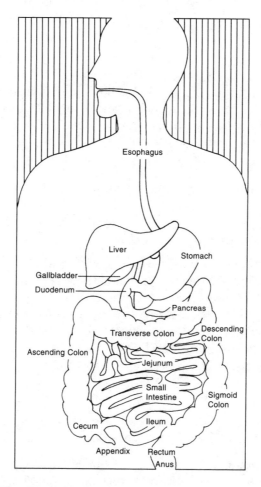

Figure 1.1. The Digestive System

4

called peristalsis. The action of peristalsis looks like an ocean wave moving through the muscle. The muscle of the organ produces a narrowing and then propels the narrowed portion slowly down the length of the organ. These waves of narrowing push the food and fluid in front of them through each hollow organ.

The first major muscle movement occurs when food or liquid is swallowed. Although we are able to start swallowing by choice, once the swallow begins, it becomes involuntary and proceeds under the control of the nerves.

The esophagus is the organ into which the swallowed food is pushed. It connects the throat above with the stomach below. At the junction of the esophagus and stomach, there is a ringlike valve closing the passage between the two organs. However, as the food approaches the closed ring, the surrounding muscles relax and allow the food to pass.

The food then enters the stomach, which has three mechanical tasks to do. First, the stomach must store the swallowed food and liquid. This requires the muscle of the upper part of the stomach to relax and accept large volumes of swallowed material. The second job is to mix up the food, liquid, and digestive juice produced by the stomach. The lower part of the stomach mixes these materials by its muscle action. The third task of the stomach is to empty its contents slowly into the small intestine.

Several factors affect emptying of the stomach, including the nature of the food (mainly its fat and protein content) and the degree of muscle action of the emptying stomach and the next organ to receive the contents (the small intestine). As the food is digested in the small intestine and dissolved into the juices from the pancreas, liver, and intestine, the contents of the intestine are mixed and pushed forward to allow further digestion.

Finally, all of the digested nutrients are absorbed through the intestinal walls. The waste products of this process include undigested parts of the food, known as fiber, and older cells that have been shed from the mucosa. These materials are propelled into the colon, where they remain, usually for a day or two, until the feces are expelled by a bowel movement.

Production of Digestive Juices

The glands that act first are in the mouth—the salivary glands. Saliva produced by these glands contains an enzyme that begins to digest the starch from food into smaller molecules.

The next set of digestive glands is in the stomach lining. They produce stomach acid and an enzyme that digests protein. One of the unsolved puzzles of the digestive system is why the acid juice of the stomach does not dissolve the tissue of the stomach itself. In most people, the stomach mucosa is able to resist the juice, although food and other tissues of the body cannot.

After the stomach empties the food and juice mixture into the small intestine, the juices of two other digestive organs mix with the food to continue the process of digestion. One of these organs is the pancreas. It produces a juice that contains a wide array of enzymes to break down the carbohydrate, fat, and protein in food. Other enzymes that are active in the process come from glands in the wall of the intestine or even a part of that wall.

The liver produces yet another digestive juice—bile. The bile is stored between meals in the gallbladder. At mealtime, it is squeezed out of the gallbladder into the bile ducts to reach the intestine and mix with the fat in our food. The bile acids dissolve the fat into the watery contents of the intestine, much like detergents that dissolve grease from a frying pan. After the fat is dissolved, it is digested by enzymes from the pancreas and the lining of the intestine.

Absorption and Transport of Nutrients

Digested molecules of food, as well as water and minerals from the diet, are absorbed from the cavity of the upper small intestine. Most absorbed materials cross the mucosa into the blood and are carried off in the bloodstream to other parts of the body for storage or further chemical change. As already noted, this part of the process varies with different types of nutrients.

Carbohydrates. It is recommended that about 55 to 60 percent of total daily calories be from carbohydrates. Some of our most common foods contain mostly carbohydrates. Examples are bread, potatoes, legumes, rice, spaghetti, fruits, and vegetables. Many of these foods contain both starch and fiber.

The digestible carbohydrates are broken into simpler molecules by enzymes in the saliva, in juice produced by the pancreas, and in the lining of the small intestine. Starch is digested in two steps: First, an enzyme in the saliva and pancreatic juice breaks the starch into molecules called maltose; then an enzyme in the lining of the small intestine (maltase) splits the maltose into glucose molecules that can be absorbed into the blood. Glucose is carried through the bloodstream to the liver, where it is stored or used to provide energy for the work of the body.

Table sugar is another carbohydrate that must be digested to be useful. An enzyme in the lining of the small intestine digests table sugar into glucose and fructose, each of which can be absorbed from the intestinal cavity into the blood. Milk contains yet another type of sugar, lactose, which is changed into absorbable molecules by an enzyme called lactase, also found in the intestinal lining.

Protein. Foods such as meat, eggs, and beans consist of giant molecules of protein that must be digested by enzymes before they can be used to build and repair body tissues. An enzyme in the juice of the stomach starts the digestion of swallowed protein. Further digestion of the protein is completed in the small intestine. Here, several enzymes from the pancreatic juice and the lining of the intestine carry out the breakdown of huge protein molecules into small molecules called amino acids. These small molecules can be absorbed from the hollow of the small intestine into the blood and then be carried to all parts of the body to build the walls and other parts of cells.

Fats. Fat molecules are a rich source of energy for the body. The first step in digestion of a fat such as butter is to dissolve it into the watery content of the intestinal cavity. The bile acids produced by the liver act as natural detergents to dissolve fat in water and allow the enzymes to break the large fat molecules into smaller molecules, some of which are fatty acids and cholesterol. The bile acids combine with the fatty acids and cholesterol and help these molecules to move into the cells of the mucosa. In these cells the small molecules are formed back into large molecules, most of which pass into vessels (called lymphatics) near the intestine. These small vessels carry the reformed fat to the veins of the chest, and the blood carries the fat to storage depots in different parts of the body.

Vitamins. Another vital part of our food that is absorbed from the small intestine is the class of chemicals we call vitamins. The two different types of vitamins are classified by the fluid in which they can be dissolved: water-soluble vitamins (all the B vitamins and vitamin C) and fat-soluble vitamins (vitamins A, D, and K).

Water and salt. Most of the material absorbed from the cavity of the small intestine is water in which salt is dissolved. The salt and water come from the food and liquid we swallow and the juices secreted by the many digestive glands.

How is the digestive process controlled?

Hormone Regulators

A fascinating feature of the digestive system is that it contains its own regulators. The major hormones that control the functions of the digestive system are produced and released by cells in the mucosa of the stomach and small intestine. These hormones are released into the blood of the digestive tract, travel back to the heart and through the arteries, and return to the digestive system, where they stimulate digestive juices and cause organ movement.

The hormones that control digestion are gastrin, secretin, and cholecystokinin (CCK):

- *Gastrin* causes the stomach to produce an acid for dissolving and digesting some foods. It is also necessary for the normal growth of the lining of the stomach, small intestine, and colon.

- *Secretin* causes the pancreas to send out a digestive juice that is rich in bicarbonate. It stimulates the stomach to produce pepsin, an enzyme that digests protein, and it also stimulates the liver to produce bile.

- *CCK* causes the pancreas to grow and to produce the enzymes of pancreatic juice, and it causes the gallbladder to empty.

Additional hormones in the digestive system regulate appetite:

- *Ghrelin* is produced in the stomach and upper intestine in the absence of food in the digestive system and stimulates appetite.

- *Peptide YY* is produced in the GI tract in response to a meal in the system and inhibits appetite.

Both of these hormones work on the brain to help regulate the intake of food for energy.

Nerve Regulators

Two types of nerves help to control the action of the digestive system. Extrinsic (outside) nerves come to the digestive organs from the unconscious part of the brain or from the spinal cord. They release a chemical called acetylcholine and another called adrenaline. Acetylcholine causes the muscle of the digestive organs to squeeze with more force and increase the "push" of food and juice through the digestive tract. Acetylcholine also causes the stomach and pancreas to produce more digestive juice. Adrenaline relaxes the muscle of the stomach and intestine and decreases the flow of blood to these organs.

Even more important, though, are the intrinsic (inside) nerves, which make up a very dense network embedded in the walls of the esophagus, stomach, small intestine, and colon. The intrinsic nerves are triggered to act when the walls of the hollow organs are stretched by food. They release many different substances that speed up or delay the movement of food and the production of juices by the digestive organs.

Chapter 2

Common Gastrointestinal Symptoms

Chapter Contents

Section 2.1

Bleeding in the Digestive Tract

Reprinted from "Bleeding in the Digestive Tract," National Institute
of Diabetes and Digestive and Kidney Diseases, National Institutes of
Health, NIH Publication No. 05-1133, November 2004.

Bleeding in the digestive tract is a symptom of a disease rather than a disease itself. Bleeding can occur as the result of a number of different conditions, some of which are life threatening. Most causes of bleeding are related to conditions that can be cured or controlled, such as ulcers or hemorrhoids. The cause of bleeding may not be serious, but locating the source of bleeding is important.

The digestive or gastrointestinal (GI) tract includes the esophagus, stomach, small intestine, large intestine or colon, rectum, and anus (see Figure 2.1). Bleeding can come from one or more of these areas, that is, from a small area such as an ulcer on the lining of the stomach or from a large surface such as an inflammation of the colon. Bleeding can sometimes occur without the person noticing it. This type of bleeding is called occult or hidden. Fortunately, simple tests can detect occult blood in the stool.

What causes bleeding in the digestive tract?

Stomach acid can cause inflammation that may lead to bleeding at the lower end of the esophagus. This condition, usually associated with the symptom of heartburn, is called esophagitis or inflammation of the esophagus. Sometimes a muscle between the esophagus and stomach fails to close properly and allows the return of food and stomach juices into the esophagus, which can lead to esophagitis. In another, unrelated condition, enlarged veins (varices) at the lower end of the esophagus may rupture and bleed massively. Cirrhosis of the liver is the most common cause of esophageal varices. Esophageal bleeding can be caused by a tear in the lining of the esophagus (Mallory-Weiss syndrome). Mallory-Weiss syndrome usually results from vomiting but may also be caused by increased pressure in the abdomen from coughing, hiatal hernia, or childbirth. Esophageal cancer can cause bleeding.

The stomach is a frequent site of bleeding. Infections with *Helicobacter pylori* (*H. pylori*), alcohol, aspirin, aspirin-containing medicines, and various other medicines (NSAIDs, particularly those used for arthritis) can cause stomach ulcers or inflammation (gastritis). The stomach is often the site of ulcer disease. Acute or chronic ulcers may enlarge and erode through a blood vessel, causing bleeding. Also, patients suffering from burns, shock, head injuries, or cancer, or those who have undergone extensive surgery may develop stress ulcers. Bleeding can also occur from benign tumors or cancer of the stomach, although these disorders usually do not cause massive bleeding.

A common source of bleeding from the upper digestive tract is ulcers in the duodenum (the upper small intestine). Duodenal ulcers are most commonly caused by infection with *H. pylori* bacteria or drugs such as aspirin or NSAIDs.

In the lower digestive tract, the large intestine and rectum are frequent sites of bleeding. Hemorrhoids are the most common cause of visible blood in the digestive tract, especially blood that appears bright red. Hemorrhoids are enlarged veins in the anal area that can rupture and produce bright red blood, which can show up in the toilet or on toilet paper. If red blood is seen, however, it is essential to exclude

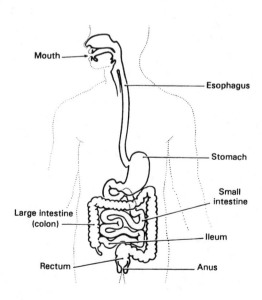

Figure 2.1. Gastrointestinal System

other causes of bleeding since the anal area may also be the site of cuts (fissures), inflammation, or cancer.

Benign growths or polyps of the colon are very common and are thought to be forerunners of cancer. These growths can cause either bright red blood or occult bleeding. Colorectal cancer is the third most frequent of all cancers in the United States and often causes occult bleeding at some time, but not necessarily visible bleeding.

Inflammation from various causes can produce extensive bleeding from the colon. Different intestinal infections can cause inflammation and bloody diarrhea. Ulcerative colitis can produce inflammation and extensive surface bleeding from tiny ulcerations. Crohn disease of the large intestine can also produce bleeding.

Diverticular disease caused by diverticula—pouches in the colon wall—can result in massive bleeding. Finally, as one gets older, abnormalities may develop in the blood vessels of the large intestine, which may result in recurrent bleeding.

Patients taking blood-thinning medications (warfarin) may have bleeding from the GI tract, especially if they take drugs like aspirin.

What are the common causes of bleeding in the digestive tract?

Esophagus

- inflammation (esophagitis)
- enlarged veins (varices)
- tear (Mallory-Weiss syndrome)
- cancer
- liver disease

Stomach

- ulcers
- inflammation (gastritis)
- cancer

Small Intestine

- duodenal ulcer
- inflammation (irritable bowel disease)
- cancer

Large Intestine and Rectum

- hemorrhoids
- infections
- inflammation (ulcerative colitis)
- colorectal polyps
- colorectal cancer
- diverticular disease

How is bleeding in the digestive tract recognized?

The signs of bleeding in the digestive tract depend upon the site and severity of bleeding. If blood is coming from the rectum or the lower colon, bright red blood will coat or mix with the stool. The stool may be mixed with darker blood if the bleeding is higher up in the colon or at the far end of the small intestine. When there is bleeding in the esophagus, stomach, or duodenum, the stool is usually black or tarry. Vomited material may be bright red or have a coffee-grounds appearance when one is bleeding from those sites. If bleeding is occult, the patient might not notice any changes in stool color.

If sudden massive bleeding occurs, a person may feel weak, dizzy, faint, short of breath, or have crampy abdominal pain or diarrhea. Shock may occur, with a rapid pulse, drop in blood pressure, and difficulty in producing urine. The patient may become very pale. If bleeding is slow and occurs over a long period of time, a gradual onset of fatigue, lethargy, shortness of breath, and pallor from the anemia will result. Anemia is a condition in which the blood's iron-rich substance, hemoglobin, is diminished.

How is bleeding in the digestive tract diagnosed?

The site of the bleeding must be located. A complete history and physical examination are essential. Symptoms such as changes in bowel habits, stool color (to black or red) and consistency, and the presence of pain or tenderness may tell the doctor which area of the GI tract is affected. Because the intake of iron, bismuth (Pepto-Bismol), or foods such as beets can give the stool the same appearance as bleeding from the digestive tract, a doctor must test the stool for blood before offering a diagnosis. A blood count will indicate whether the patient is anemic and also will give an idea of the extent of the bleeding and how chronic it may be.

Endoscopy: Endoscopy is a common diagnostic technique that allows direct viewing of the bleeding site. Because the endoscope can detect lesions and confirm the presence or absence of bleeding, doctors often choose this method to diagnose patients with acute bleeding. In many cases, the doctor can use the endoscope to treat the cause of bleeding as well.

The endoscope is a flexible instrument that can be inserted through the mouth or rectum. The instrument allows the doctor to see into the esophagus, stomach, duodenum (esophagoduodenoscopy), colon (colonoscopy), and rectum (sigmoidoscopy); to collect small samples of tissue (biopsies); to take photographs; and to stop the bleeding.

Small bowel endoscopy, or enteroscopy, is a procedure using a long endoscope. This endoscope may be used to localize unidentified sources of bleeding in the small intestine.

A new diagnostic instrument called a capsule endoscope is swallowed by the patient. The capsule contains a tiny camera that transmits images to a video monitor. It is used most often to find bleeding in portions of the small intestine that are hard to reach with a conventional endoscope.

Other Procedures: Several other methods are available to locate the source of bleeding. Barium x-rays, in general, are less accurate than endoscopy in locating bleeding sites. Some drawbacks of barium x-rays are that they may interfere with other diagnostic techniques if used for detecting acute bleeding, they expose the patient to x-rays, and they do not offer the capabilities of biopsy or treatment. Another type of x-ray is CT scan, particularly useful for inflammatory conditions and cancer.

Angiography is a technique that uses dye to highlight blood vessels. This procedure is most useful in situations when the patient is acutely bleeding such that dye leaks out of the blood vessel and identifies the site of bleeding. In selected situations, angiography allows injection of medicine into arteries that may stop the bleeding.

Radionuclide scanning is a noninvasive screening technique used for locating sites of acute bleeding, especially in the lower GI tract. This technique involves injection of small amounts of radioactive material. Then, a special camera produces pictures of organs, allowing the doctor to detect a bleeding site.

How is bleeding in the digestive tract treated?

Endoscopy is the primary diagnostic and therapeutic procedure for most causes of GI bleeding.

Active bleeding from the upper GI tract can often be controlled by injecting chemicals directly into a bleeding site with a needle introduced through the endoscope. A physician can also cauterize, or heat treat, a bleeding site and surrounding tissue with a heater probe or electrocoagulation device passed through the endoscope. Laser therapy is useful in certain specialized situations.

Once bleeding is controlled, medicines are often prescribed to prevent recurrence of bleeding. Medicines are useful primarily for *H. pylori*, esophagitis, ulcer, infections, and irritable bowel disease. Medical treatment of ulcers, including the elimination of *H. pylori*, to ensure healing and maintenance therapy to prevent ulcer recurrence can also lessen the chance of recurrent bleeding.

Removal of polyps with an endoscope can control bleeding from colon polyps. Removal of hemorrhoids by banding or various heat or electrical devices is effective in patients who suffer hemorrhoidal bleeding on a recurrent basis. Endoscopic injection or cautery can be used to treat bleeding sites throughout the lower intestinal tract.

Endoscopic techniques do not always control bleeding. Sometimes angiography may be used. However, surgery is often needed to control active, severe, or recurrent bleeding when endoscopy is not successful.

How do you recognize blood in the stool and vomit?

- bright red blood coating the stool
- dark blood mixed with the stool
- black or tarry stool
- bright red blood in vomit
- coffee-grounds appearance of vomit

What are the symptoms of acute bleeding?

- any of the bleeding symptoms above
- weakness
- shortness of breath
- dizziness
- crampy abdominal pain
- faintness
- diarrhea

What are the symptoms of chronic bleeding?

- any of the bleeding symptoms above
- weakness
- fatigue
- shortness of breath
- lethargy
- faintness

Section 2.2

Gas in the Digestive Tract

Reprinted from "Gas in the Digestive Tract," National Institute of Diabetes and Digestive and Kidney Diseases, National Institutes of Health, NIH Publication No. 04-883, March 2004.

Everyone has gas and eliminates it by burping or passing it through the rectum. However, many people think they have too much gas when they really have normal amounts. Most people produce about one to four pints a day and pass gas about fourteen times a day.

Gas is made primarily of odorless vapors—carbon dioxide, oxygen, nitrogen, hydrogen, and sometimes methane. The unpleasant odor of flatulence comes from bacteria in the large intestine that release small amounts of gases that contain sulfur.

Although having gas is common, it can be uncomfortable and embarrassing. Understanding causes, ways to reduce symptoms, and treatment will help most people find relief.

What causes gas?

Gas in the digestive tract (that is, the esophagus, stomach, small intestine, and large intestine) comes from two sources:

- swallowed air
- normal breakdown of certain undigested foods by harmless bacteria naturally present in the large intestine (colon)

18

Swallowed Air: Air swallowing (aerophagia) is a common cause of gas in the stomach. Everyone swallows small amounts of air when eating and drinking. However, eating or drinking rapidly, chewing gum, smoking, or wearing loose dentures can cause some people to take in more air.

Burping, or belching, is the way most swallowed air—which contains nitrogen, oxygen, and carbon dioxide—leaves the stomach. The remaining gas moves into the small intestine, where it is partially absorbed. A small amount travels into the large intestine for release through the rectum. (The stomach also releases carbon dioxide when stomach acid and bicarbonate mix, but most of this gas is absorbed into the bloodstream and does not enter the large intestine.)

Breakdown of Undigested Foods: The body does not digest and absorb some carbohydrates (the sugar, starches, and fiber found in many foods) in the small intestine because of a shortage or absence of certain enzymes.

This undigested food then passes from the small intestine into the large intestine, where normal, harmless bacteria break down the food, producing hydrogen, carbon dioxide, and, in about one-third of all people, methane. Eventually these gases exit through the rectum.

People who make methane do not necessarily pass more gas or have unique symptoms. A person who produces methane will have stools that consistently float in water. Research has not shown why some people produce methane and others do not.

Foods that produce gas in one person may not cause gas in another. Some common bacteria in the large intestine can destroy the hydrogen that other bacteria produce. The balance of the two types of bacteria may explain why some people have more gas than others.

Which foods cause gas?

Most foods that contain carbohydrates can cause gas. By contrast, fats and proteins cause little gas.

Sugars: The sugars that cause gas are raffinose, lactose, fructose, and sorbitol.

- *Raffinose:* Beans contain large amounts of this complex sugar. Smaller amounts are found in cabbage, Brussels sprouts, broccoli, asparagus, other vegetables, and whole grains.

- *Lactose:* Lactose is the natural sugar in milk. It is also found in milk products, such as cheese and ice cream, and processed foods, such as bread, cereal, and salad dressing. Many people, particularly those of African, Native American, or Asian background, normally have low levels of the enzyme lactase needed to digest lactose after childhood. Also, as people age, their enzyme levels decrease. As a result, over time people may experience increasing amounts of gas after eating food containing lactose.

- *Fructose:* Fructose is naturally present in onions, artichokes, pears, and wheat. It is also used as a sweetener in some soft drinks and fruit drinks.

- *Sorbitol:* Sorbitol is a sugar found naturally in fruits, including apples, pears, peaches, and prunes. It is also used as an artificial sweetener in many dietetic foods and sugar-free candies and gums.

Starches: Most starches, including potatoes, corn, noodles, and wheat, produce gas as they are broken down in the large intestine. Rice is the only starch that does not cause gas.

Fiber: Many foods contain soluble and insoluble fiber. Soluble fiber dissolves easily in water and takes on a soft, gel-like texture in the intestines. Found in oat bran, beans, peas, and most fruits, soluble fiber is not broken down until it reaches the large intestine, where digestion causes gas.

Insoluble fiber, on the other hand, passes essentially unchanged through the intestines and produces little gas. Wheat bran and some vegetables contain this kind of fiber.

What are some symptoms and problems of gas?

The most common symptoms of gas are flatulence, abdominal bloating, abdominal pain, and belching. However, not everyone experiences these symptoms. The determining factors probably are how much gas the body produces, how many fatty acids the body absorbs, and a person's sensitivity to gas in the large intestine.

Belching: An occasional belch during or after meals is normal and releases gas when the stomach is full of food. However, people who belch frequently may be swallowing too much air and releasing it before the air enters the stomach.

Sometimes a person with chronic belching may have an upper GI disorder, such as peptic ulcer disease, gastroesophageal reflux disease (GERD), or gastroparesis.

Occasionally, some people believe that swallowing air and releasing it will relieve the discomfort of these disorders, and these people may intentionally or unintentionally develop a habit of belching to relieve discomfort.

Gas-bloat syndrome may occur after fundoplication surgery to correct GERD. The surgery creates a one-way valve between the esophagus and stomach that allows food and gas to enter the stomach but often prevents normal belching and the ability to vomit. It occurs in about 10 percent of people who have this surgery but may improve with time.

Flatulence: Another common complaint is passage of too much gas through the rectum (flatulence). However, most people do not realize that passing gas fourteen to twenty-three times a day is normal. Too much gas may be the result of carbohydrate malabsorption.

Abdominal Bloating: Many people believe that too much gas causes abdominal bloating. However, people who complain of bloating from gas often have normal amounts and distribution of gas. They actually may be unusually aware of gas in the digestive tract.

Doctors believe that bloating is usually the result of an intestinal disorder, such as irritable bowel syndrome (IBS). The cause of IBS is unknown, but may involve abnormal movements and contractions of intestinal muscles and increased pain sensitivity in the intestine. These disorders may give a sensation of bloating because of increased sensitivity to gas.

Any disease that causes intestinal inflammation or obstruction, such as Crohn disease or colon cancer, may also cause abdominal bloating. In addition, people who have had many operations, adhesions (scar tissue), or internal hernias may experience bloating or pain. Finally, eating a lot of fatty food can delay stomach emptying and cause bloating and discomfort, but not necessarily too much gas.

Abdominal Pain and Discomfort: Some people have pain when gas is present in the intestine. When pain is on the left side of the colon, it can be confused with heart disease. When the pain is on the right side of the colon, it may mimic gallstones or appendicitis.

What diagnostic tests are used?

Because gas symptoms may be caused by a serious disorder, those causes should be ruled out. The doctor usually begins with a review of dietary habits and symptoms. The doctor may ask the patient to keep a diary of foods and beverages consumed for a specific time period.

If lactase deficiency is the suspected cause of gas, the doctor may suggest avoiding milk products for a period of time. A blood or breath test may be used to diagnose lactose intolerance.

In addition, to determine if someone produces too much gas in the colon or is unusually sensitive to the passage of normal gas volumes, the doctor may ask patients to count the number of times they pass gas during the day and include this information in a diary.

Careful review of diet and the amount of gas passed may help relate specific foods to symptoms and determine the severity of the problem.

Because the symptoms that people may have are so variable, the physician may order other types of diagnostic tests in addition to a physical exam, depending on the patient's symptoms and other factors.

How is gas treated?

Experience has shown that the most common ways to reduce the discomfort of gas are changing diet, taking medicines, and reducing the amount of air swallowed.

Diet: Doctors may tell people to eat fewer foods that cause gas. However, for some people this may mean cutting out healthy foods, such as fruits and vegetables, whole grains, and milk products.

Doctors may also suggest limiting high-fat foods to reduce bloating and discomfort. This helps the stomach empty faster, allowing gases to move into the small intestine.

Unfortunately, the amount of gas caused by certain foods varies from person to person. Effective dietary changes depend on learning through trial and error how much of the offending foods one can handle.

Nonprescription Medicines: Many nonprescription, over-the-counter medicines are available to help reduce symptoms, including antacids with simethicone. Digestive enzymes, such as lactase supplements, actually help digest carbohydrates and may allow people to eat foods that normally cause gas.

Antacids, such as Mylanta II, Maalox II, and Di-Gel, contain simethicone, a foaming agent that joins gas bubbles in the stomach so that gas is more easily belched away. However, these medicines have no effect on intestinal gas. Dosage varies depending on the form of medication and the patient's age.

The enzyme lactase, which aids with lactose digestion, is available in caplet and chewable tablet form without a prescription (Lactaid and Lactrase). Chewing lactase tablets just before eating helps digest foods that contain lactose. Also, lactose-reduced milk and other products are available at many grocery stores (Lactaid and Dairy Ease).

Beano, an over-the-counter digestive aid, contains the sugar-digesting enzyme that the body lacks to digest the sugar in beans and many vegetables. The enzyme comes in liquid and tablet form. Five drops are added per serving or one tablet is swallowed just before eating to break down the gas-producing sugars. Beano has no effect on gas caused by lactose or fiber.

Prescription Medicines: Doctors may prescribe medicines to help reduce symptoms, especially for people with a disorder such as IBS.

Reducing Swallowed Air: For those who have chronic belching, doctors may suggest ways to reduce the amount of air swallowed. Recommendations are to avoid chewing gum and to avoid eating hard candy. Eating at a slow pace and checking with a dentist to make sure dentures fit properly should also help.

Conclusion

Although gas may be uncomfortable and embarrassing, it is not life-threatening. Understanding causes, ways to reduce symptoms, and treatment will help most people find some relief.

Points to Remember

- Everyone has gas in the digestive tract.
- People often believe normal passage of gas to be excessive.
- Gas comes from two main sources: swallowed air and normal breakdown of certain foods by harmless bacteria naturally present in the large intestine.
- Many foods with carbohydrates can cause gas. Fats and proteins cause little gas.
- Foods that may cause gas include the following:
  - beans
  - vegetables, such as broccoli, cabbage, brussels sprouts, onions, artichokes, and asparagus

- fruits, such as pears, apples, and peaches

- whole grains, such as whole wheat and bran

- soft drinks and fruit drinks

- milk and milk products, such as cheese and ice cream, and packaged foods prepared with lactose, such as bread, cereal, and salad dressing

- foods containing sorbitol, such as dietetic foods and sugar-free candies and gums

- The most common symptoms of gas are belching, flatulence, bloating, and abdominal pain. However, some of these symptoms are often caused by an intestinal disorder, such as irritable bowel syndrome, rather than too much gas.

- The most common ways to reduce the discomfort of gas are changing diet, taking nonprescription medicines, and reducing the amount of air swallowed.

- Digestive enzymes, such as lactase supplements, actually help digest carbohydrates and may allow people to eat foods that normally cause gas.

Section 2.3

Abdominal Pain

© 2005 A.D.A.M., Inc. Reprinted with permission.

Alternative Names

Stomach pain; pain—abdomen; belly ache; abdominal cramps; acute abdomen

Definition

Abdominal pain is pain that you feel anywhere between your chest and groin. This is often referred to as the stomach region or belly.

Considerations

There are many organs in the abdomen. Pain in the abdomen can originate from any one of them, including:

- Organs related to digestion—the stomach, the end of the esophagus, the small and large intestines, the liver, the gall-bladder, and the pancreas.

- The aorta—a large blood vessel that runs straight down the inside of the abdomen.

- The appendix—an organ in the lower right abdomen that no longer serves much function.

- The kidneys—two bean-shaped organs that lie deep within the abdominal cavity.

However, the pain may originate from somewhere else—like your chest or pelvic region. You may also have a generalized infection affecting many parts of your body, like the flu or strep throat.

The intensity of the pain does not always reflect the seriousness of the condition causing the pain. Severe abdominal pain can be from mild conditions, such as gas or the cramping of viral gastroenteritis. On the other hand, relatively mild pain or no pain may be present with life-threatening conditions, such as cancer of the colon or early appendicitis.

Common Causes

Many different conditions can cause abdominal pain. The key is to know when you must seek medical care right away. In many cases you can simply wait, use home care remedies, and call your doctor at a later time only if the symptoms persist.

Possible causes include:

- Excessive gas;
- Chronic constipation;
- Lactose intolerance (milk intolerance);
- Viral gastroenteritis (stomach flu);
- Irritable bowel syndrome (sensitive stomach with intermittent episodes of diarrhea and constipation);
- Heartburn or indigestion;
- Gastroesophageal reflux;
- Ulcers;
- Cholecystitis (inflammation of the gallbladder) with or without gallstones;
- Appendicitis (inflammation of the appendix);
- Diverticular disease, including inflammation of small pouches that form in the large intestines (diverticulitis);
- Bowel obstruction—in addition to pain, this causes nausea, bloating, vomiting, and inability to pass gas or stool;
- Food allergy;
- Food poisoning (salmonella, shigella);
- Hernia;
- Kidney stones;
- Urinary tract infections;
- Pancreatitis (inflammation of the pancreas);
- Intussusception (telescoping intestines)—while uncommon, this is a serious possible cause of pain in an infant who may be drawing his or her knees to the chest and crying to indicate the pain;

- Dissecting abdominal aortic aneurysm—bleeding into the wall of the aorta;

- Parasite infections (*Giardia*);

- Sickle cell crisis;

- Crohn disease or ulcerative colitis (two different types of inflammatory bowel disease).

When an inflamed organ in the abdomen ruptures or leaks fluid, you not only have excruciating pain, your abdomen will be very stiff (board-like) and you will likely have a fever. This occurs when you have peritonitis due to an infection spreading in the abdominal cavity from the ruptured organ, like the appendix. This is a medical emergency.

In infants, prolonged unexplained crying (often called "colic") may be caused by abdominal pain that may end with the passage of gas or stool. Colic is often worse in the evening. Cuddling and rocking the child may bring some relief.

Abdominal pain that occurs during menstruation may be from menstrual cramps or it may indicate a problem in a reproductive organ. This includes conditions such as endometriosis (when tissue from the uterus is displaced to somewhere else like the pelvic wall or ovaries), uterine fibroids (thick bands of muscular and fibrous tissue in the uterus), ovarian cysts, ovarian cancer (rare), or pelvic inflammatory disease (PID)—infection of the reproductive organs, usually from a sexually transmitted disease.

Abdominal pain may actually be caused by an organ in the chest, like the lungs (for example, pneumonia) or the heart (like a heart attack). Or, it may stem from a muscle strain in the abdominal muscles.

Cancer of the colon, stomach, or pancreas are serious but uncommon causes of abdominal pain.

Other more unusual causes of abdominal pain include a type of emotional upset called somatization disorder, reflected as physical discomfort (including recurrent abdominal pain). Strep throat in children can cause abdominal pain.

Home Care

For mild pains:

- Sip water or other clear fluids.

- Avoid solid food for the first few hours. If there has been vomiting, wait six hours. Then, eat small amounts of mild foods.

- If the pain is high up in your abdomen and occurs after meals, antacids may provide some relief, especially if you feel heartburn or indigestion. Avoid citrus, high-fat foods, fried or greasy foods, tomato products, caffeine, alcohol, and carbonated beverages. You may also try H2 blockers (Tagamet, Pepcid, or Zantac) available over the counter. If any of these medicines worsen your pain, call your doctor right away.

- Avoid aspirin, ibuprofen, and narcotic pain medications unless your health care provider prescribes them. If you know that your pain is not related to your liver, you can try acetaminophen (Tylenol).

Call your health care provider if:

- Call 911 if you:
  - Have sudden, sharp abdominal pain;
  - Have chest, neck, or shoulder pain;
  - Are vomiting blood or have blood in your stool (especially if maroon or dark, tarry black);
  - Have a rigid, hard abdomen that is tender to touch;
  - Are unable to pass stool, especially if you are also vomiting.

- Call your doctor if you have:
  - Bloating that persists for more than two days;
  - Diarrhea for more than five days;
  - Abdominal discomfort that lasts one week or longer;
  - Fever (over 100°F for adults or 100.4°F for children) with your pain;
  - A burning sensation when you urinate or frequent urination;
  - Pain in your shoulder blades and nausea;
  - Pain that develops during pregnancy (or possible pregnancy);
  - Prolonged poor appetite;
  - Unexplained weight loss.

What to Expect at Your Health Care Provider's Office

From your medical history and physical examination, your doctor will try to determine the cause of your abdominal pain. Knowing the location of pain and its time pattern will help, as will the presence of other symptoms like fever, fatigue, general ill feeling, nausea, vomiting, or changes in stool.

During the physical examination, the doctor will test to see if the pain is localized to a single area (point tenderness) or whether it is diffuse. He or she will be checking to see if the pain is related to inflammation of the peritoneum (called peritonitis). If the health care provider finds evidence of peritonitis, the abdominal pain may be classified as an "acute abdomen," which may require surgery right away.

Your doctor may ask the following questions about your abdominal pain:

- Is the pain all over (diffuse or generalized) or in a specific location?

- What part of the abdomen is affected? Lower or upper? Right, left, or middle? Around the navel?

- Is the pain severe, sharp or cramping, persistent or constant, periodic and changing intensity over minutes?

- Does the pain awaken you at night?

- Have you had similar pain in past? How long has each episode lasted?

- How often do you have the pain?

- Does it occur within minutes following meals? Within two to three hours after meals?

- Is it getting increasingly more severe?

- Does it occur during menstruation (dysmenorrhea)?

- Does the pain go into your back, middle of the back, below the right shoulder blade, or your groin, buttocks, or legs?

- Does the pain get worse after lying on the back?

- Does the pain get worse after eating or drinking? After greasy foods, milk products, or alcohol?

- Does the pain get worse after stress? After straining efforts?

- Does the pain get better after eating or a bowel movement?

- Does the pain get better after milk or antacids?

- What medications are you taking?

- Have you had a recent injury?

- Are you pregnant?
- What other symptoms are occurring at the same time?

Diagnostic tests that may be performed include:

- Barium enema;
- Upper GI and small bowel series;
- Blood, urine, and stool tests;
- Endoscopy of upper GI (gastrointestinal) tract (EGD);
- Ultrasound of the abdomen;
- X-rays of the abdomen.

Prevention

For prevention of many types of abdominal pain:

- Eat small meals more frequently.
- Make sure that your meals are well balanced and high in fiber. Eat plenty of fruits and vegetables.
- Limit foods that produce gas.
- Drink plenty of water each day.
- Exercise regularly.

For prevention of symptoms from heartburn or gastroesophageal reflux disease:

- Quit smoking.
- Lose weight if you need to.
- Finish eating at least two hours before you go to bed.
- After eating, stay upright for at least thirty minutes.
- Elevate the head of your bed.

Section 2.4

Diarrhea

Reprinted from "Diarrhea," National Institute of Diabetes and Digestive and Kidney Diseases, National Institutes of Health, NIH Publication No. 04-2749, October 2003.

What is diarrhea?

Diarrhea—loose, watery stools occurring more than three times in one day—is a common problem that usually lasts a day or two and goes away on its own without any special treatment. However, prolonged diarrhea can be a sign of other problems. People with diarrhea may pass more than a quart of stool a day.

Diarrhea can cause dehydration, which means the body lacks enough fluid to function properly. Dehydration is particularly dangerous in children and the elderly, and it must be treated promptly to avoid serious health problems.

People of all ages can get diarrhea. The average adult has a bout of diarrhea about four times a year.

What causes diarrhea?

Diarrhea may be caused by a temporary problem, like an infection, or a chronic problem, like an intestinal disease. A few of the more common causes of diarrhea are

- *Bacterial infections.* Several types of bacteria, consumed through contaminated food or water, can cause diarrhea. Common culprits include *Campylobacter*, Salmonella, Shigella, and *Escherichia coli.*

- *Viral infections.* Many viruses cause diarrhea, including rotavirus, Norwalk virus, cytomegalovirus, herpes simplex virus, and viral hepatitis.

- *Food intolerances.* Some people are unable to digest some component of food, such as lactose, the sugar found in milk.

- *Parasites.* Parasites can enter the body through food or water and settle in the digestive system. Parasites that cause diarrhea

31

include *Giardia lamblia*, *Entamoeba histolytica*, and *Cryptosporidium*.

- *Reaction to medicines*, such as antibiotics, blood pressure medications, and antacids containing magnesium.

- *Intestinal diseases*, like inflammatory bowel disease or celiac disease.

- *Functional bowel disorders*, such as irritable bowel syndrome, in which the intestines do not work normally.

Some people develop diarrhea after stomach surgery or removal of the gallbladder. The reason may be a change in how quickly food moves through the digestive system after stomach surgery or an increase in bile in the colon that can occur after gallbladder surgery.

In many cases, the cause of diarrhea cannot be found. As long as diarrhea goes away on its own, an extensive search for the cause is not usually necessary.

People who visit foreign countries are at risk for traveler's diarrhea, which is caused by eating food or drinking water contaminated with bacteria, viruses, or, sometimes, parasites. Traveler's diarrhea is a particular problem for people visiting developing countries. Visitors to the United States, Canada, most European countries, Japan, Australia, and New Zealand do not face much risk for traveler's diarrhea.

What are the symptoms?

Diarrhea may be accompanied by cramping abdominal pain, bloating, nausea, or an urgent need to use the bathroom. Depending on the cause, a person may have a fever or bloody stools.

Diarrhea can be either acute (short-term) or chronic (long-term). The acute form, which lasts less than four weeks, is usually related to a bacterial, viral, or parasitic infection. Chronic diarrhea lasts more than four weeks and is usually related to functional disorders like irritable bowel syndrome or inflammatory bowel diseases like celiac disease.

Is diarrhea in children different from diarrhea in adults?

Children can have acute or chronic forms of diarrhea. Causes include bacteria, viruses, parasites, medications, functional disorders, and food sensitivities. Infection with the rotavirus is the most common cause of acute childhood diarrhea. Rotavirus diarrhea usually resolves in three to nine days.

Medications to treat diarrhea in adults can be dangerous to children and should be given only under a doctor's guidance.

Diarrhea can be dangerous in newborns and infants. In small children, severe diarrhea lasting just a day or two can lead to dehydration. Because a child can die from dehydration within a few days, the main treatment for diarrhea in children is rehydration.

Take your child to the doctor if any of the following symptoms appear:

- stools containing blood or pus, or black stools
- temperature above 101.4 degrees Fahrenheit
- no improvement after twenty-four hours
- signs of dehydration

What is dehydration?

General signs of dehydration include the following:

- thirst
- less frequent urination
- dry skin
- fatigue
- light-headedness
- dark-colored urine

Signs of dehydration in children include the following:

- dry mouth and tongue
- no tears when crying
- no wet diapers for three hours or more
- sunken abdomen, eyes, or cheeks
- high fever
- listlessness or irritability
- skin that does not flatten when pinched and released

If you suspect that you or your child is dehydrated, call the doctor immediately. Severe dehydration may require hospitalization.

When should a doctor be consulted?

Although usually not harmful, diarrhea can become dangerous or signal a more serious problem. You should see the doctor if any of the following is true:

- You have diarrhea for more than three days.
- You have severe pain in the abdomen or rectum.
- You have a fever of 102 degrees Fahrenheit or higher.
- You see blood in your stool or have black, tarry stools.
- You have signs of dehydration.

If your child has diarrhea, do not hesitate to call the doctor for advice. Diarrhea can be dangerous in children if too much fluid is lost and not replaced quickly.

What tests might the doctor do?

Diagnostic tests to find the cause of diarrhea include the following:

- *Medical history and physical examination.* The doctor will need to know about your eating habits and medication use and will examine you for signs of illness.
- *Stool culture.* Lab technicians analyze a sample of stool to check for bacteria, parasites, or other signs of disease or infection.
- *Blood tests.* Blood tests can be helpful in ruling out certain diseases.
- *Fasting tests.* To find out if a food intolerance or allergy is causing the diarrhea, the doctor may ask you to avoid lactose (found in milk products), carbohydrates, wheat, or other foods to see whether the diarrhea responds to a change in diet.
- *Sigmoidoscopy.* For this test, the doctor uses a special instrument to look at the inside of the rectum and lower part of the colon.
- *Colonoscopy.* This test is similar to sigmoidoscopy, but the doctor looks at the entire colon.

What is the treatment?

In most cases, replacing lost fluid to prevent dehydration is the only treatment necessary. Medicines that stop diarrhea may be helpful in some cases, but they are not recommended for people whose diarrhea is caused by a bacterial infection or parasite—stopping the diarrhea traps the organism in the intestines, prolonging the problem. Instead, doctors usually prescribe antibiotics. Viral causes are either treated with medication or left to run their course, depending on the severity and type of the virus.

Preventing Dehydration: Dehydration occurs when the body has lost too much fluid and electrolytes (the salts potassium and sodium). The fluid and electrolytes lost during diarrhea need to be replaced promptly—the body cannot function properly without them. Dehydration is particularly dangerous for children, who can die from it within a matter of days.

Although water is extremely important in preventing dehydration, it does not contain electrolytes. To maintain electrolyte levels, you could have broth or soups, which contain sodium, and fruit juices, soft fruits, or vegetables, which contain potassium.

For children, doctors often recommend a special rehydration solution that contains the nutrients they need. You can buy this solution in the grocery store without a prescription. Examples include Pedialyte, CeraLyte, and Infalyte.

Tips about Food: Until diarrhea subsides, try to avoid milk products and foods that are greasy, high-fiber, or very sweet. These foods tend to aggravate diarrhea.

As you improve, you can add soft, bland foods to your diet, including bananas, plain rice, boiled potatoes, toast, crackers, cooked carrots, and baked chicken without the skin or fat. For children, the pediatrician may recommend what is called the BRAT diet: bananas, rice, applesauce, and toast.

Preventing Traveler's Diarrhea

Traveler's diarrhea happens when you consume food or water contaminated with bacteria, viruses, or parasites. You can take the following precautions to prevent traveler's diarrhea when you go abroad:

- Do not drink any tap water, not even when brushing your teeth.
- Do not drink unpasteurized milk or dairy products.
- Do not use ice made from tap water.
- Avoid all raw fruits and vegetables (including lettuce and fruit salad) unless they can be peeled and you peel them yourself.

- Do not eat raw or rare meat and fish.

- Do not eat meat or shellfish that is not hot when served to you.

- Do not eat food from street vendors.

You can safely drink bottled water (if you are the one to break the seal), carbonated soft drinks, and hot drinks like coffee or tea.

Depending on where you are going and how long you are staying, your doctor may recommend that you take antibiotics before leaving to protect you from possible infection.

Points to Remember

- Diarrhea is a common problem that usually resolves on its own.

- Diarrhea is dangerous if a person becomes dehydrated.

- Causes include viral, bacterial, or parasitic infections; food intolerance; reactions to medicine; intestinal diseases; and functional bowel disorders.

- Treatment involves replacing lost fluids and electrolytes. Depending on the cause of the problem, a person might also need medication to stop the diarrhea or treat an infection. Children may need an oral rehydration solution to replace lost fluids and electrolytes.

- Call the doctor if a person with diarrhea has severe pain in the abdomen or rectum, a fever of 102 degrees Fahrenheit or higher, blood in the stool, signs of dehydration, or diarrhea for more than three days.

Section 2.5

Constipation

Reprinted from "Constipation," National Institute of Diabetes and Digestive and Kidney Diseases, National Institutes of Health, NIH Publication No. 03-2754, June 2003.

Constipation is passage of small amounts of hard, dry bowel movements, usually fewer than three times a week. People who are constipated may find it difficult and painful to have a bowel movement. Other symptoms of constipation include feeling bloated, uncomfortable, and sluggish.

Many people think they are constipated when, in fact, their bowel movements are regular. For example, some people believe they are constipated, or irregular, if they do not have a bowel movement every day. However, there is no right number of daily or weekly bowel movements. Normal may be three times a day or three times a week, depending on the person. Also, some people naturally have firmer stools than others.

At one time or another, almost everyone gets constipated. Poor diet and lack of exercise are usually the causes. In most cases, constipation is temporary and not serious. Understanding its causes, prevention, and treatment will help most people find relief.

Who gets constipated?

According to the 1996 National Health Interview Survey, about three million people in the United States have frequent constipation. Those reporting constipation most often are women and adults age sixty-five and over. Pregnant women may have constipation, and it is a common problem following childbirth or surgery.

Constipation is one of the most common gastrointestinal complaints in the United States, resulting in about two million doctor visits annually. However, most people treat themselves without seeking medical help, as is evident from the millions of dollars Americans spend on laxatives each year.

37

What causes constipation?

To understand constipation, it helps to know how the colon (large intestine) works. As food moves through the colon, it absorbs water while forming waste products, or stool. Muscle contractions in the colon push the stool toward the rectum. By the time stool reaches the rectum, it is solid because most of the water has been absorbed.

The hard and dry stools of constipation occur when the colon absorbs too much water or if the colon's muscle contractions are slow or sluggish, causing the stool to move through the colon too slowly. Common causes of constipation include the following:

• not enough fiber in the diet
• not enough liquids
• lack of exercise
• medications
• irritable bowel syndrome
• changes in life or routine such as pregnancy, older age, and travel
• abuse of laxatives
• ignoring the urge to have a bowel movement
• specific diseases such as stroke (by far the most common)
• problems with the colon and rectum
• problems with intestinal function (chronic idiopathic constipation)

Not Enough Fiber in the Diet: The most common cause of constipation is a diet low in fiber found in vegetables, fruits, and whole grains and high in fats found in cheese, eggs, and meats. People who eat plenty of high-fiber foods are less likely to become constipated.

Fiber—both soluble and insoluble—is the part of fruits, vegetables, and grains that the body cannot digest. Soluble fiber dissolves easily in water and takes on a soft, gel-like texture in the intestines. Insoluble fiber passes through the intestines almost unchanged. The bulk and soft texture of fiber help prevent hard, dry stools that are difficult to pass.

According to the National Center for Health Statistics,[1] Americans eat an average of five to fourteen grams of fiber daily, short of the twenty to thirty-five grams recommended by the American Dietetic

Association. Both children and adults eat too many refined and processed foods from which the natural fiber has been removed.

A low-fiber diet also plays a key role in constipation among older adults, who may lose interest in eating and choose convenience foods low in fiber. In addition, difficulties with chewing or swallowing may force older people to eat soft foods that are processed and low in fiber.

Not Enough Liquids: Liquids like water and juice add fluid to the colon and bulk to stools, making bowel movements softer and easier to pass. People who have problems with constipation should drink enough of these liquids every day, about eight 8-ounce glasses. Liquids that contain caffeine, like coffee and cola drinks, and alcohol have a dehydrating effect.

Lack of Exercise: Lack of exercise can lead to constipation, although doctors do not know precisely why. For example, constipation often occurs after an accident or during an illness when one must stay in bed and cannot exercise.

Medications: Some medications can cause constipation. They include the following:

• pain medications (especially narcotics)
• antacids that contain aluminum and calcium
• blood pressure medications (calcium channel blockers)
• antiparkinson drugs
• antispasmodics
• antidepressants
• iron supplements
• diuretics
• anticonvulsants

Irritable Bowel Syndrome (IBS): Some people with IBS, also known as spastic colon, have spasms in the colon that affect bowel movements. Constipation and diarrhea often alternate, and abdominal cramping, gassiness, and bloating are other common complaints. Although IBS can produce lifelong symptoms, it is not a life-threatening condition. It often worsens with stress, but there is no specific cause or anything unusual that the doctor can see in the colon.

Changes in Life or Routine: During pregnancy, women may be constipated because of hormonal changes or because the heavy uterus compresses the intestine. Aging may also affect bowel regularity because a slower metabolism results in less intestinal activity and muscle tone. In addition, people often become constipated when traveling because their normal diet and daily routines are disrupted.

Abuse of Laxatives: Myths about constipation have led to a serious abuse of laxatives. This is common among people who are preoccupied with having a daily bowel movement.

Laxatives usually are not necessary and can be habit-forming. The colon begins to rely on laxatives to bring on bowel movements. Over time, laxatives can damage nerve cells in the colon and interfere with the colon's natural ability to contract. For the same reason, regular use of enemas can also lead to a loss of normal bowel function.

Ignoring the Urge to Have a Bowel Movement: People who ignore the urge to have a bowel movement may eventually stop feeling the urge, which can lead to constipation. Some people delay having a bowel movement because they do not want to use toilets outside the home. Others ignore the urge because of emotional stress or because they are too busy. Children may postpone having a bowel movement because of stressful toilet training or because they do not want to interrupt their play.

Specific Diseases: Diseases that cause constipation include neurological disorders, metabolic and endocrine disorders, and systemic conditions that affect organ systems. These disorders can slow the movement of stool through the colon, rectum, or anus.

Several kinds of diseases can cause constipation:

Neurological Disorders

- multiple sclerosis
- Parkinson disease
- chronic idiopathic intestinal pseudo-obstruction
- stroke
- spinal cord injuries

Metabolic and Endocrine Conditions

- diabetes

- underactive or overactive thyroid gland
- uremia
- hypercalcemia

Systemic Disorders

- amyloidosis
- lupus
- scleroderma

Problems with the Colon and Rectum: Intestinal obstruction, scar tissue (adhesions), diverticulosis, tumors, colorectal stricture, Hirschsprung disease, or cancer can compress, squeeze, or narrow the intestine and rectum and cause constipation.

Problems with Intestinal Function (Chronic Idiopathic Constipation): Some people have chronic constipation that does not respond to standard treatment. This rare condition, known as idiopathic (of unknown origin) chronic constipation may be related to problems with intestinal function such as problems with hormonal control or with nerves and muscles in the colon, rectum, or anus. Functional constipation occurs in both children and adults and is most common in women.

Colonic inertia and delayed transit are two types of functional constipation caused by decreased muscle activity in the colon. These syndromes may affect the entire colon or may be confined to the lower or sigmoid colon.

Functional constipation that stems from abnormalities in the structure of the anus and rectum is known as anorectal dysfunction, or anismus. These abnormalities result in an inability to relax the rectal and anal muscles that allow stool to exit.

What diagnostic tests are used?

Most people with constipation do not need extensive testing and can be treated with changes in diet and exercise. For example, in young people with mild symptoms, a medical history and physical examination may be all the doctor needs to suggest successful treatment. The tests the doctor performs depend on the duration and severity of the constipation, the person's age, and whether blood in stools, recent changes in bowel movements, or weight loss have occurred.

Medical History: The doctor may ask a patient to describe his or her constipation, including duration of symptoms, frequency of bowel movements, consistency of stools, presence of blood in the stool, and toilet habits (how often and where one has bowel movements). A record of eating habits, medication, and level of physical activity or exercise will also help the doctor determine the cause of constipation.

The clinical definition of constipation is any two of the following symptoms for at least twelve weeks (not necessarily consecutive) in the previous twelve months:

- straining during bowel movements
- lumpy or hard stool
- sensation of incomplete evacuation
- sensation of anorectal blockage/obstruction
- fewer than three bowel movements per week

Physical Examination: A physical exam may include a rectal exam with a gloved, lubricated finger to evaluate the tone of the muscle that closes off the anus (anal sphincter) and to detect tenderness, obstruction, or blood. In some cases, blood and thyroid tests may be necessary to look for thyroid disease and serum calcium or to rule out inflammatory, neoplastic, metabolic, and other systemic disorders.

Extensive testing usually is reserved for people with severe symptoms, for those with sudden changes in number and consistency of bowel movements or blood in the stool, and for older adults. Additional tests that may be used to evaluate constipation include

- colorectal transit study
- anorectal function tests

Because of an increased risk of colorectal cancer in older adults, the doctor may use tests to rule out a diagnosis of cancer, including

- barium enema x-ray;
- sigmoidoscopy or colonoscopy.

Colorectal transit study. This test, reserved for those with chronic constipation, shows how well food moves through the colon. The patient swallows capsules containing small markers that are visible on an x-ray. The movement of the markers through the colon is monitored with abdominal x-rays taken several times three to seven days after the capsule is swallowed. The patient follows a high-fiber diet during the course of this test.

Anorectal function tests. These tests diagnose constipation caused by abnormal functioning of the anus or rectum (anorectal function). Anorectal manometry evaluates anal sphincter muscle function. For this test, a catheter or air-filled balloon inserted into the anus is slowly pulled back through the sphincter muscle to measure muscle tone and contractions.

Defecography is an x-ray of the anorectal area that evaluates completeness of stool elimination, identifies anorectal abnormalities, and evaluates rectal muscle contractions and relaxation. During the exam, the doctor fills the rectum with a soft paste that is the same consistency as stool. The patient sits on a toilet positioned inside an x-ray machine and then relaxes and squeezes the anus to expel the paste. The doctor studies the x-rays for anorectal problems that occurred as the paste was expelled.

Barium enema x-ray. This exam involves viewing the rectum, colon, and lower part of the small intestine to locate any problems. This part of the digestive tract is known as the bowel. This test may show intestinal obstruction and Hirschsprung disease, a lack of nerves within the colon.

The night before the test, bowel cleansing, also called bowel prep, is necessary to clear the lower digestive tract. The patient drinks a special liquid to flush out the bowel. A clean bowel is important, because even a small amount of stool in the colon can hide details and result in an incomplete exam.

Because the colon does not show up well on x-rays, the doctor fills it with barium, a chalky liquid that makes the area visible. Once the mixture coats the inside of the colon and rectum, x-rays are taken that reveal their shape and condition. The patient may feel some abdominal cramping when the barium fills the colon, but usually feels little discomfort after the procedure. Stools may be a whitish color for a few days after the exam.

Sigmoidoscopy or colonoscopy. An examination of the rectum and lower (sigmoid) colon is called a sigmoidoscopy. An examination of the rectum and entire colon is called a colonoscopy.

The patient usually has a liquid dinner the night before a sigmoidoscopy and takes an enema early the next morning. A light breakfast and a cleansing enema an hour before the test may also be necessary.

To perform a sigmoidoscopy, the doctor uses a long, flexible tube with a light on the end called a sigmoidoscope to view the rectum and lower colon. First, the doctor examines the rectum with a gloved, lubricated finger. Then, the sigmoidoscope is inserted through the anus into the rectum and lower colon. The procedure may cause a mild sensation of wanting to move the bowels and abdominal pressure. Sometimes the doctor fills the colon with air to get a better view. The air may cause mild cramping.

To perform a colonoscopy, the doctor uses a flexible tube with a light on the end called a colonoscope to view the entire colon. This tube is longer than a sigmoidoscope. The same bowel cleansing used for the barium x-ray is needed to clear the bowel of waste. The patient is lightly sedated before the exam. During the exam, the patient lies on his or her side and the doctor inserts the tube through the anus and rectum into the colon. If an abnormality is seen, the doctor can use the colonoscope to remove a small piece of tissue for examination (biopsy). The patient may feel gassy and bloated after the procedure.

How is constipation treated?

Although treatment depends on the cause, severity, and duration, in most cases dietary and lifestyle changes will help relieve symptoms of constipation and help prevent it.

Diet: A diet with enough fiber (20 to 35 grams each day) helps form soft, bulky stool. A doctor or dietitian can help plan an appropriate diet. High-fiber foods include beans, whole grains and bran cereals, fresh fruits, and vegetables such as asparagus, brussels sprouts, cabbage, and carrots. For people prone to constipation, limiting foods that have little or no fiber, such as ice cream, cheese, meat, and processed foods, is also important.

Lifestyle Changes: Other changes that can help treat and prevent constipation include drinking enough water and other liquids such as fruit and vegetable juices and clear soups, engaging in daily exercise, and reserving enough time to have a bowel movement. In addition, the urge to have a bowel movement should not be ignored.

Laxatives: Most people who are mildly constipated do not need laxatives. However, for those who have made diet and lifestyle changes and are still constipated, doctors may recommend laxatives or enemas for a limited time. These treatments can help retrain a chronically sluggish bowel. For children, short-term treatment with laxatives, along with retraining to establish regular bowel habits, also helps prevent constipation.

A doctor should determine when a patient needs a laxative and which form is best. Laxatives taken by mouth are available in liquid, tablet, gum, powder, and granule forms. They work in various ways:

- Bulk-forming laxatives generally are considered the safest but can interfere with absorption of some medicines. These laxatives, also known as fiber supplements, are taken with water. They absorb water in the intestine and make the stool softer. Brand names include Metamucil, Citrucel, Konsyl, and Serutan.

- Stimulants cause rhythmic muscle contractions in the intestines. Brand names include Correctol, Dulcolax, Purge, and Senokot. Studies suggest that phenolphthalein, an ingredient in some stimulant laxatives, might increase a person's risk for cancer. The Food and Drug Administration has proposed a ban on all over-the-counter products containing phenolphthalein. Most laxative makers have replaced or plan to replace phenolphthalein with a safer ingredient.

- Stool softeners provide moisture to the stool and prevent dehydration. These laxatives are often recommended after childbirth or surgery. Products include Colace and Surfak.

- Lubricants grease the stool, enabling it to move through the intestine more easily. Mineral oil is the most common example.

- Saline laxatives act like a sponge to draw water into the colon for easier passage of stool. Laxatives in this group include Milk of Magnesia and Haley's M-O.

People who are dependent on laxatives need to slowly stop using them. A doctor can assist in this process. In most people, this restores the colon's natural ability to contract.

Other Treatments: Treatment may be directed at a specific cause. For example, the doctor may recommend discontinuing medication or performing surgery to correct an anorectal problem such as rectal prolapse.

People with chronic constipation caused by anorectal dysfunction can use biofeedback to retrain the muscles that control release of bowel movements. Biofeedback involves using a sensor to monitor muscle activity that at the same time can be displayed on a computer screen, allowing for an accurate assessment of body functions. A health care professional uses this information to help the patient learn how to use these muscles.

Surgical removal of the colon may be an option for people with severe symptoms caused by colonic inertia. However, the benefits of this surgery must be weighed against possible complications, which include abdominal pain and diarrhea.

Can constipation be serious?

Sometimes constipation can lead to complications. These complications include hemorrhoids caused by straining to have a bowel movement or anal fissures (tears in the skin around the anus) caused when hard stool stretches the sphincter muscle. As a result, rectal bleeding may occur, appearing as bright red streaks on the surface of the stool. Treatment for hemorrhoids may include warm tub baths, ice packs, and application of a special cream to the affected area. Treatment for anal fissure may include stretching the sphincter muscle or surgical removal of tissue or skin in the affected area.

Sometimes straining causes a small amount of intestinal lining to push out from the anal opening. This condition, known as rectal prolapse, may lead to secretion of mucus from the anus. Usually eliminating the cause of the prolapse, such as straining or coughing, is the only treatment necessary. Severe or chronic prolapse requires surgery to strengthen and tighten the anal sphincter muscle or to repair the prolapsed lining.

Constipation may also cause hard stool to pack the intestine and rectum so tightly that the normal pushing action of the colon is not enough to expel the stool. This condition, called fecal impaction, occurs most often in children and older adults. An impaction can be softened with mineral oil taken by mouth and by an enema. After softening the impaction, the doctor may break up and remove part of the hardened stool by inserting one or two fingers into the anus.

Points to Remember

- Constipation affects almost everyone at one time or another.

- Many people think they are constipated when, in fact, their bowel movements are regular.

- The most common causes of constipation are poor diet and lack of exercise.

- Additional causes of constipation include medications, irritable bowel syndrome, abuse of laxatives, and specific diseases.

- A medical history and physical examination may be the only diagnostic tests needed before the doctor suggests treatment.

- In most cases, following these simple tips will help relieve symptoms and prevent recurrence of constipation:

  - Eat a well-balanced, high-fiber diet that includes beans, bran, whole grains, fresh fruits, and vegetables.

  - Drink plenty of liquids.

  - Exercise regularly.

  - Set aside time after breakfast or dinner for undisturbed visits to the toilet.

  - Do not ignore the urge to have a bowel movement.

  - Understand that normal bowel habits vary.

  - Whenever a significant or prolonged change in bowel habits occurs, check with a doctor.

- Most people with mild constipation do not need laxatives. However, doctors may recommend laxatives for a limited time for people with chronic constipation.

Notes

1. National Center for Health Statistics. Dietary Intake of Macronutrients, Micronutrients, and Other Dietary Constituents: United States, 1988–94. Vital and Health Statistics, Series 11, number 245. July 2002.

Section 2.6

Fecal Incontinence

Reprinted from "Fecal Incontinence," National Institute of Diabetes and Digestive and Kidney Diseases, NIH Publication No. 04-4866, March 2004.

Fecal incontinence is the inability to control your bowels. When you feel the urge to have a bowel movement, you may not be able to hold it until you can get to a toilet. Or stool may leak from the rectum unexpectedly.

More than 5.5 million Americans have fecal incontinence. It affects people of all ages—children as well as adults. Fecal incontinence is more common in women than in men and more common in older adults than in younger ones. It is not, however, a normal part of aging.

Loss of bowel control can be devastating. People who have fecal incontinence may feel ashamed, embarrassed, or humiliated. Some don't want to leave the house out of fear they might have an accident in public. Most try to hide the problem as long as possible, so they withdraw from friends and family. The social isolation is unfortunate but may be reduced because treatment can improve bowel control and make incontinence easier to manage.

Causes

Fecal incontinence can have several causes:

- constipation
- damage to the anal sphincter muscles
- damage to the nerves of the anal sphincter muscles or the rectum
- loss of storage capacity in the rectum
- diarrhea
- pelvic floor dysfunction

Constipation: Constipation is one of the most common causes of fecal incontinence. Constipation causes large, hard stools to become lodged in the rectum. Watery stool can then leak out around the hardened stool. Constipation also causes the muscles of the rectum to stretch, which weakens the muscles so they can't hold stool in the rectum long enough for a person to reach a bathroom.

Muscle Damage: Fecal incontinence can be caused by injury to one or both of the ring-like muscles at the end of the rectum called the anal internal and external sphincters. The sphincters keep stool inside. When damaged, the muscles aren't strong enough to do their job, and stool can leak out. In women, the damage often happens when giving birth. The risk of injury is greatest if the doctor uses forceps to help deliver the baby or does an episiotomy, which is a cut in the vaginal area to prevent it from tearing during birth. Hemorrhoid surgery can damage the sphincters as well.

Nerve Damage: Fecal incontinence can also be caused by damage to the nerves that control the anal sphincters or to the nerves that sense stool in the rectum. If the nerves that control the sphincters are injured, the muscle doesn't work properly and incontinence can occur. If the sensory nerves are damaged, they don't sense that stool

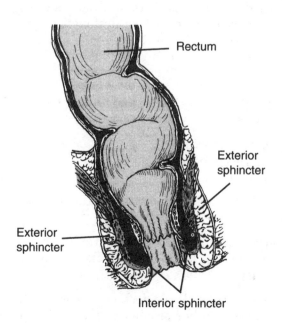

Figure 2.2. Anatomy of the rectum and anus.

is in the rectum. You then won't feel the need to use the bathroom until stool has leaked out. Nerve damage can be caused by childbirth, a long-term habit of straining to pass stool, stroke, and diseases that affect the nerves, such as diabetes and multiple sclerosis.

Loss of Storage Capacity: Normally, the rectum stretches to hold stool until you can get to a bathroom. But rectal surgery, radiation treatment, and inflammatory bowel disease can cause scarring that makes the walls of the rectum stiff and less elastic. The rectum then can't stretch as much and can't hold stool, and fecal incontinence results. Inflammatory bowel disease also can make rectal walls very irritated and thereby unable to contain stool.

Diarrhea: Diarrhea, or loose stool, is more difficult to control than solid stool that is formed. Even people who don't have fecal incontinence can have an accident when they have diarrhea.

Pelvic Floor Dysfunction: Abnormalities of the pelvic floor can lead to fecal incontinence. Examples of some abnormalities are decreased perception of rectal sensation, decreased anal canal pressures, decreased squeeze pressure of the anal canal, impaired anal sensation, a dropping down of the rectum (rectal prolapse), protrusion of the rectum through the vagina (rectocele), or generalized weakness and sagging of the pelvic floor. Often the cause of pelvic floor dysfunction is childbirth, and incontinence doesn't show up until the mid-forties or later.

Diagnosis

The doctor will ask health-related questions and do a physical exam and possibly other medical tests.

- Anal manometry checks the tightness of the anal sphincter and its ability to respond to signals, as well as the sensitivity and function of the rectum.

- Anorectal ultrasonography evaluates the structure of the anal sphincters.

- Proctography, also known as defecography, shows how much stool the rectum can hold, how well the rectum holds it, and how well the rectum can evacuate the stool.

- Proctosigmoidoscopy allows doctors to look inside the rectum for signs of disease or other problems that could cause fecal incontinence, such as inflammation, tumors, or scar tissue.

- Anal electromyography tests for nerve damage, which is often associated with obstetric injury.

Treatment

Treatment depends on the cause and severity of fecal incontinence; it may include dietary changes, medication, bowel training, or surgery. More than one treatment may be necessary for successful control since continence is a complicated chain of events.

Dietary Changes: Food affects the consistency of stool and how quickly it passes through the digestive system. If your stools are hard to control because they are watery, you may find that eating high-fiber foods adds bulk and makes stool easier to control. However people with well-formed stools may find that high fiber foods act as a laxative and contributes to the problem. Other foods that may make the problem worse are drinks containing caffeine, like coffee, tea, and chocolate, which relax the internal anal sphincter muscle.

You can adjust what and how you eat to help manage fecal incontinence.

- *Keep a food diary*. List what you eat, how much you eat, and when you have an incontinent episode. After a few days, you may begin to see a pattern involving certain foods and incontinence. After you identify foods that seem to cause problems, cut back on them and see whether incontinence improves. Foods that typically cause diarrhea, and so should probably be avoided, include the following:
  - caffeine
  - cured or smoked meat like sausage, ham, or turkey
  - spicy foods
  - alcohol
  - dairy products like milk, cheese, and ice cream
  - fruits like apples, peaches, or pears
  - fatty and greasy foods
  - sweeteners, like sorbitol, xylitol, mannitol, and fructose, which are found in diet drinks, sugarless gum and candy, chocolate, and fruit juices

- *Eat smaller meals more frequently*. In some people, large meals cause bowel contractions that lead to diarrhea. You can still eat the same amount of food in a day, but space it out by eating several small meals.

- *Eat and drink at different times.* Liquid helps move food through the digestive system. So if you want to slow things down, drink something half an hour before or after meals, but not with the meals.

- *Eat the right amounts of fiber.* For many people, fiber makes stool soft, formed, and easier to control. Fiber is found in fruits, vegetables, and grains. You'll need to eat twenty to thirty grams of fiber a day, but add it to your diet slowly so your body can adjust. Too much fiber all at once can cause bloating, gas, or even diarrhea. Also, too much insoluble, or undigestible, fiber can contribute to diarrhea. So if you find that eating more fiber makes your diarrhea worse, try cutting back to two servings each of fruits and vegetables and removing skins and seeds from your food.

- *Eat foods that make stool bulkier.* Foods that contain soluble, or digestible, fiber slow the emptying of the bowels. Examples are bananas, rice, tapioca, bread, potatoes, applesauce, cheese, smooth peanut butter, yogurt, pasta, and oatmeal.

- *Get plenty to drink.* You need to drink eight 8-ounce glasses of liquid a day to help prevent dehydration and to keep stool soft and formed. Water is a good choice, but avoid drinks with caffeine, alcohol, milk, or carbonation if you find that they trigger diarrhea.

Over time, diarrhea can rob you of vitamins and minerals. Ask your doctor if you need a vitamin supplement.

Medication: If diarrhea is causing the incontinence, medication may help. Sometimes doctors recommend using bulk laxatives to help people develop a more regular bowel pattern. Or the doctor may prescribe antidiarrheal medicines such as loperamide or diphenoxylate to slow down the bowel and help control the problem.

Bowel Training: Bowel training helps some people relearn how to control their bowels. In some cases, it involves strengthening muscles; in others, it means training the bowels to empty at a specific time of day.

- *Use biofeedback.* Biofeedback is a way to strengthen and coordinate the muscles and has helped some people. Special computer

equipment measures muscle contractions as you do exercises—
called Kegel exercises—to strengthen the rectum. These exercises work muscles in the pelvic floor, including those involved in controlling stool. Computer feedback about how the muscles are working shows whether you're doing the exercises correctly

Table 2.1. What Foods Have Fiber?

Breads, peas, and beans	Fiber
½ cup of black-eyed peas, cooked	4 grams
½ cup of kidney beans, cooked	5.7 grams
½ cup of lima beans, cooked	4.5 grams
1 slice of whole-wheat or multigrain bread	1.7 grams
Whole-grain cereal, cold	
½ cup of All-Bran	9.6 grams
¾ cup of Total	2.4 grams
¾ cup of Post Bran Flakes	5.3 grams
Whole-grain cereal, hot	
1 packet of whole-grain cereal, hot (oatmeal, Wheatena)	3 grams
Fruits	
1 medium apple	3.3 grams
1 medium peach	1.8 grams
½ cup of raspberries	4 grams
1 medium tangerine	1.9 grams
Vegetables	
1 cup of acorn squash, raw	2.1 grams
1 medium stalk of broccoli, raw	3.9 grams
5 brussels sprouts, raw	3.6 grams
1 cup of cabbage, raw	2 grams
1 medium carrot, raw	1.8 grams
1 cup of cauliflower, raw	2.5 grams
1 cup of spinach, cooked	4.3 grams
1 cup of zucchini, raw	1.4 grams

Source: USDA/ARS Nutrient Data Laboratory

and whether the muscles are getting stronger. Whether biofeed-back will work for you depends on the cause of your fecal incontinence, how severe the muscle damage is, and your ability to do the exercises.

- *Develop a regular pattern of bowel movements.* Some people—particularly those whose fecal incontinence is caused by constipation—achieve bowel control by training themselves to have bowel movements at specific times during the day, such as after every meal. The key to this approach is persistence—it may take a while to develop a regular pattern. Try not to get frustrated or give up if it doesn't work right away.

Surgery: Surgery may be an option for people whose fecal incontinence is caused by injury to the pelvic floor, anal canal, or anal sphincter. Various procedures can be done, from simple ones like repairing damaged areas, to complex ones like attaching an artificial anal sphincter or replacing anal muscle with muscle from the leg or forearm. People who have severe fecal incontinence that doesn't respond to other treatments may decide to have a colostomy, which involves removing a portion of the bowel. The remaining part is then either attached to the anus if it still works properly, or to a hole in the abdomen called a stoma, through which stool leaves the body and is collected in a pouch.

What to Do about Anal Discomfort

The skin around the anus is delicate and sensitive. Constipation and diarrhea or contact between skin and stool can cause pain or itching. Here's what you can do to relieve discomfort:

- Wash the area with water, but not soap, after a bowel movement. Soap can dry out the skin, making discomfort worse. If possible, wash in the shower with lukewarm water or use a sitz bath. Or try a no-rinse skin cleanser. Try not to use toilet paper to clean up—rubbing with dry toilet paper will only irritate the skin more. Premoistened, alcohol-free towelettes are a better choice.

- Let the area air dry after washing. If you don't have time, gently pat yourself dry with a lint-free cloth.

- Use a moisture barrier cream, which is a protective cream to help prevent skin irritation from direct contact with stool. However, talk to your health care professional before you try anal ointments and creams because some have ingredients that can be irritating. Also, you should clean the area well first to avoid trapping bacteria that could cause further problems. Your health care professional can recommend an appropriate cream or ointment.

- Try using nonmedicated talcum powder or corn starch to relieve anal discomfort.

- Wear cotton underwear and loose clothes that "breathe." Tight clothes that block air can worsen anal problems. Change soiled underwear as soon as possible.

- If you use pads or disposable undergarments, make sure they have an absorbent wicking layer on top. Products with a wicking layer protect the skin by pulling stool and moisture away from the skin and into the pad.

Emotional Considerations

Because fecal incontinence can cause distress in the form of embarrassment, fear, and loneliness, taking steps to deal with it is important. Treatment can help improve your life and help you feel better about yourself. If you haven't been to a doctor yet, make an appointment.

Everyday Practical Tips

- Take a backpack or tote bag containing cleanup supplies and a change of clothing with you everywhere.

- Locate public restrooms before you need them so you know where to go.

- Use the toilet before heading out.

- If you think an episode is likely, wear disposable undergarments or sanitary pads.

- If episodes are frequent, use oral fecal deodorants to add to your comfort level.

Fecal Incontinence in Children

If your child has fecal incontinence, you need to see a doctor to determine the cause and treatment. Fecal incontinence can occur in children because of a birth defect or disease, but in most cases it's because of chronic constipation.

Potty-trained children often get constipated simply because they refuse to go to the bathroom. The problem might stem from embarrassment over using a public toilet or unwillingness to stop playing and go to the bathroom. Yet if the child continues to hold in stool, the feces will accumulate and harden in the rectum. The child might have a stomachache and not eat much, despite being hungry. Furthermore, when he or she eventually does pass the stool, it can be painful, which can lead to fear of having a bowel movement.

A child who is constipated may soil his or her underpants. Soiling happens when liquid stool from farther up in the bowel seeps past the hard stool in the rectum and leaks out. Soiling is a sign of fecal incontinence. Try to remember that your child did not do this on purpose. He or she cannot control the liquid stool and may not even know it has passed.

The first step in treating the problem is passing the built-up stool. The doctor may prescribe one or more enemas or a drink that helps clean out the bowel, like magnesium citrate, mineral oil, or polyethylene glycol.

The next step is preventing future constipation. You will play a big role in this part of your child's treatment. You may need to teach your child bowel habits, which means training your child to have regular bowel movements. Experts recommend that parents of children with poor bowel habits encourage their child to sit on the toilet four times each day (after meals and at bedtime) for 5 minutes. Give rewards for bowel movements and remember that it is important not to punish your child for incontinent episodes.

Some changes in eating habits may be necessary too. Your child should eat more high-fiber foods to soften stool, avoid dairy products if they cause constipation, and drink plenty of fluids every day, including water and juices like prune, grape, or apricot, which help prevent constipation. If necessary, the doctor may prescribe laxatives.

It may take several months to break the pattern of withholding stool and constipation, and episodes may occur again in the future. The key is to pay close attention to your child's bowel habits. Some warning signs to watch for include the following:

- pain with bowel movements
- hard stool
- constipation
- refusal to go to the bathroom
- soiled underpants

- signs of holding back a bowel movement, like squatting, crossing the legs, or rocking back and forth

Why Children Get Constipated

- They were potty-trained too early.

- They refuse to have a bowel movement (because of painful ones in the past, embarrassment, stubbornness, or even a dislike of public bathrooms).

- They are in an unfamiliar place.

- They are reacting to family stress like a new sibling or their parents' divorce.

- They can't get to a bathroom when they need to go so they hold it. As the rectum fills with stool, the child may lose the urge to go and become constipated as the stool dries and hardens.

Chapter 3

Functional Abdominal Pain in Children

Children who complain of stomachaches for over three months are likely to have functional abdominal pains. The term "functional" refers to the fact that even after many tests, no clear explanation is found for the pain. There is no blockage, irritation, or infection to cause the discomfort. Yet the pain is very real.

Because of the pain, children might stop their usual activities and they often complain of nausea, excessive gas, diarrhea, or constipation. Fortunately, despite the chronic pain, the children grow well and keep their general good health.

How common is functional abdominal pain?

Functional pain is very common. About 10–15 percent of school-aged children will report episodes of recurrent pain. Another 15 percent will experience pain, but will not go to the doctor for this problem.

Why does it happen?

Your child's intestine has a complicated system of nerves and muscles that helps move food forward and carry out digestion. In some children, the nerves become very sensitive and pain is experienced even during normal intestinal activities. The pain can cause your child to cry, make his face pale or red, and he or she might break into a sweat.

An infection caused by a virus or bacteria, being under stress, or being tired may make the intestinal nerves more sensitive. Other family members may have a similar problem.

How is functional abdominal pain diagnosed?

A careful history of how the pain started, its location, and how it progressed often suggests the diagnosis for your child's problem. Blood, urine, and stool tests will be performed to rule out some conditions that can present with recurrent pain. A history of certain food intolerances, such as for dairy products or juices, can help explain crampy pain and excess gas. X-rays, CT scans, and endoscopy are recommended only for children where the history or exam raise questions about the diagnosis.

How is functional abdominal pain treated?

It is important to prevent the pain from becoming a reason for missing school, changing your child's social activities, or making it the center of everyone's attention at home.

You and your child should be reassured that there is no serious undiagnosed problem. Being positive about getting better will send the right signals to your child.

If diet can be modified, if the child can have a restful night, and if stress can be decreased, pains will improve. As much as possible, your child should continue with a normal life.

The use of medication in functional pain needs to be discussed with your physician. Muscle relaxers, antacids, or fiber supplements can be prescribed and are sometimes helpful in some children.

Chapter 4

Cyclic Vomiting Syndrome

In cyclic vomiting syndrome (CVS), people experience bouts or cycles of severe nausea and vomiting that last for hours or even days and alternate with longer periods of no symptoms. CVS occurs mostly in children, but the disorder can affect adults, too.

CVS has no known cause. Each episode is similar to the previous ones. The episodes tend to start at about the same time of day, last the same length of time, and present the same symptoms at the same level of intensity. Although CVS can begin at any age in children and adults, it usually starts between the ages of three and seven. In adults, episodes tend to occur less often than they do in children, but they last longer. Furthermore, the events or situations that trigger episodes in adults cannot always be pinpointed as easily as they can in children.

Episodes can be so severe that a person may have to stay in bed for days, unable to go to school or work. No one knows for sure how many people have CVS, but medical researchers believe that more people may have the disorder than is commonly thought (as many as one in fifty children in one study). Because other more common diseases and disorders also cause cycles of vomiting, many people with CVS are initially misdiagnosed until the other disorders can be ruled out. What is known is that CVS can be disruptive and frightening not just to people who have it, but to the entire family as well.

Reprinted from "Cyclic Vomiting Syndrome," National Institute of Diabetes and Digestive and Kidney Diseases, NIH Publication No. 04-4548, February 2004.

The Four Phases of CVS

CVS has four phases:

- prodrome
- episode
- recovery
- symptom-free interval

The **prodrome** phase signals that an episode of nausea and vomiting is about to begin. This phase, which is often marked by abdominal pain, can last from just a few minutes to several hours. Sometimes taking medicine early in the prodrome phase can stop an episode in progress. However, sometimes there is no warning: A person may simply wake up in the morning and begin vomiting.

The **episode** phase consists of nausea and vomiting; inability to eat, drink, or take medicines without vomiting; paleness; drowsiness; and exhaustion.

The **recovery** phase begins when the nausea and vomiting stop. Healthy color, appetite, and energy return.

The **symptom-free interval** phase is the period between episodes when no symptoms are present.

Triggers

Most people can identify a specific condition or event that triggered an episode. The most common trigger is an infection. Another, often found in children, is emotional stress or excitement, often from a birthday or vacation, for example. Colds, allergies, sinus problems, and the flu can also set off episodes in some people.

Other reported triggers include eating certain foods (such as chocolate or cheese), eating too much, or eating just before going to bed. Hot weather, physical exhaustion, menstruation, and motion sickness can also trigger episodes.

Symptoms

The main symptoms of CVS are severe vomiting, nausea, and retching (gagging). Episodes usually begin at night or first thing in the morning and may include vomiting or retching as often as six to twelve times an hour during the worst of the episode. Episodes usually last anywhere from one to five days, though they can last for up to ten days.

Other symptoms include pallor, exhaustion, and listlessness. Sometimes the nausea and vomiting are so severe that a person appears to be almost unconscious. Sensitivity to light, headache, fever, dizziness, diarrhea, and abdominal pain may also accompany an episode.

In addition, the vomiting may cause drooling and excessive thirst. Drinking water usually leads to more vomiting, though the water can dilute the acid in the vomit, making the episode a little less painful. Continuous vomiting can lead to dehydration, which means that the body has lost excessive water and salts.

Diagnosis

CVS is hard to diagnose because no clear tests—such as a blood test or x-ray—exist to identify it. A doctor must diagnose CVS by looking at symptoms and medical history and by excluding more common diseases or disorders that can also cause nausea and vomiting. Also, diagnosis takes time because doctors need to identify a pattern or cycle to the vomiting.

CVS and Migraine

The relationship between migraine and CVS is still unclear, but medical researchers believe that the two are related. First, migraine headaches, which cause severe pain in the head; abdominal migraine, which causes stomach pain; and CVS are all marked by severe symptoms that start quickly and end abruptly, followed by longer periods without pain or other symptoms.

Second, many of the situations that trigger CVS also trigger migraines. Those triggers include stress and excitement.

Third, research has shown that many children with CVS either have a family history of migraine or develop migraines as they grow older.

Because of the similarities between migraine and CVS, doctors treat some people with severe CVS with drugs that are also used for migraine headaches. The drugs are designed to prevent episodes, reduce their frequency, or lessen their severity.

Treatment

CVS cannot be cured. Treatment varies, but people with CVS are generally advised to get plenty of rest; sleep; and take medications that prevent a vomiting episode, stop or alleviate one that has already started, or relieve other symptoms.

Once a vomiting episode begins, treatment is supportive. It helps to stay in bed and sleep in a dark, quiet room. Severe nausea and vomiting may require hospitalization and intravenous fluids to prevent dehydration. Sedatives may help if the nausea continues.

Sometimes, during the prodrome phase, it is possible to stop an episode from happening altogether. For example, people who feel abdominal pain before an episode can ask their doctor about taking ibuprofen (Advil, Motrin) to try to stop it. Other medications that may be helpful are ranitidine (Zantac) or omeprazole (Prilosec), which help calm the stomach by lowering the amount of acid it makes.

During the recovery phase, drinking water and replacing lost electrolytes are very important. Electrolytes are salts that the body needs to function well and stay healthy. Symptoms during the recovery phase can vary: Some people find that their appetites return to normal immediately, while others need to begin by drinking clear liquids and then move slowly to solid food.

People whose episodes are frequent and long-lasting may be treated during the symptom-free intervals in an effort to prevent or ease future episodes. Medications that help people with migraine headaches—propranolol, cyproheptadine, and amitriptyline—are sometimes used during this phase, but they do not work for everyone. Taking the medicine daily for one to two months may be necessary to see if it helps.

In addition, the symptom-free phase is a good time to eliminate anything known to trigger an episode. For example, if episodes are brought on by stress or excitement, this period is the time to find ways to reduce stress and stay calm. If sinus problems or allergies cause episodes, those conditions should be treated.

Complications

The severe vomiting that defines CVS is a risk factor for several complications:

- **Dehydration.** Vomiting causes the body to lose water quickly.

- **Electrolyte imbalance.** Vomiting also causes the body to lose the important salts it needs to keep working properly.

- **Peptic esophagitis.** The esophagus (the tube that connects the mouth to the stomach) becomes injured from the stomach acid that comes up with the vomit.

- **Hematemesis.** The esophagus becomes irritated and bleeds, so blood mixes with the vomit.

- **Mallory-Weiss tear.** The lower end of the esophagus may tear open or the stomach may bruise from vomiting or retching.

- **Tooth decay.** The acid in the vomit can hurt the teeth by corroding the tooth enamel.

Points to Remember

- People with CVS have severe nausea and vomiting that come in cycles.

- CVS occurs mostly in children, but adults can have it, too.

- CVS has four phases: prodrome, episode, recovery, and symptom-free interval.

- Most people can identify a condition or event that triggers an episode of nausea and vomiting. Infections and emotional stress are two common triggers.

- The main symptoms of CVS are severe vomiting, nausea, and retching. Other symptoms include pallor and exhaustion.

- The only way a doctor can diagnose CVS is by looking at symptoms and medical history to rule out any other possible causes for the nausea and vomiting. Then the doctor must identify a pattern or cycle to the symptoms.

- CVS has no cure. Treatment varies by person, but people with CVS generally need to get plenty of rest and sleep. They may also be given drugs that may prevent an episode, stop one in progress, speed up recovery, or relieve symptoms.

- Complications include dehydration, loss of electrolytes, peptic esophagitis, hematemesis, Mallory-Weiss tear, and tooth decay.

Chapter 5

Smoking and Your Digestive System

Cigarette smoking causes a variety of life-threatening diseases, including lung cancer, emphysema, and heart disease. An estimated 430,000 deaths each year are directly caused by cigarette smoking. Smoking is responsible for changes in all parts of the body, including the digestive system. This fact can have serious consequences because it is the digestive system that converts foods into the nutrients the body needs to live.

Current estimates indicate that about one-third of all adults smoke, and while adult men seem to be smoking less, women and teenagers of both sexes seem to be smoking more. How does smoking affect the digestive system of all these people?

Harmful Effects

Smoking has been shown to have harmful effects on all parts of the digestive system, contributing to such common disorders as heartburn and peptic ulcers. It also increases the risk of Crohn disease and possibly gallstones. Smoking seems to affect the liver, too, by changing the way it handles drugs and alcohol. In fact, there seems to be enough evidence to stop smoking solely on the basis of digestive distress.

Reprinted from "Smoking and Your Digestive System," National Institute of Diabetes and Digestive and Kidney Diseases, NIH Publication No. 02-949, March 2002.

Heartburn

Heartburn is common among Americans. More than sixty million Americans have heartburn at least once a month, and about fifteen million have it daily.

Heartburn happens when acidic juices from the stomach splash into the esophagus. Normally, a muscular valve at the lower end of the esophagus, the lower esophageal sphincter (LES), keeps the acid solution in the stomach and out of the esophagus. Smoking decreases the strength of the esophageal valve, thereby allowing stomach acids to reflux, or flow backward into the esophagus.

Smoking also seems to promote the movement of bile salts from the intestine to the stomach, which makes the stomach acids more harmful. Finally, smoking may directly injure the esophagus, making it less able to resist further damage from refluxed fluids.

Peptic Ulcer

A peptic ulcer is an open sore in the lining of the stomach or duodenum, the first part of the small intestine. The exact cause of ulcers is not known. A relationship between smoking cigarettes and ulcers, especially duodenal ulcers, does exist. The 1989 Surgeon General's report stated that ulcers are more likely to occur, less likely to heal, and more likely to cause death in smokers than in nonsmokers.

Why is this so? Doctors are not really sure, but smoking does seem to be one of several factors that work together to promote the formation of ulcers.

For example, some research suggests that smoking might increase a person's risk of infection with the bacterium *Helicobacter pylori* (*H. pylori*). Most peptic ulcers are caused by this bacterium.

Stomach acid is also important in producing ulcers. Normally, most of this acid is buffered by the food we eat. Most of the unbuffered acid that enters the duodenum is quickly neutralized by sodium bicarbonate, a naturally occurring alkali produced by the pancreas. Some studies show that smoking reduces the bicarbonate produced by the pancreas, interfering with the neutralization of acid in the duodenum. Other studies suggest that chronic cigarette smoking may increase the amount of acid secreted by the stomach.

Whatever causes the link between smoking and ulcers, two points have been repeatedly demonstrated: People who smoke are more likely to develop an ulcer, especially a duodenal ulcer, and ulcers in smokers are less likely to heal quickly in response to otherwise effective treatment. This research tracing the relationship between smoking and ulcers strongly suggests that a person with an ulcer should stop smoking.

Liver Disease

The liver is an important organ that has many tasks. Among other things, the liver is responsible for processing drugs, alcohol, and other toxins to remove them from the body. There is evidence that smoking alters the ability of the liver to handle such substances. In some cases, this may influence the dose of medication necessary to treat an illness. Some research also suggests that smoking can aggravate the course of liver disease caused by excessive alcohol intake.

Crohn Disease

Crohn disease causes inflammation deep in the lining of the intestine. The disease, which causes pain and diarrhea, usually affects the small intestine, but it can occur anywhere in the digestive tract. Research shows that current and former smokers have a higher risk of developing Crohn disease than nonsmokers do. Among people with the disease, smoking is associated with a higher rate of relapse, repeat surgery, and immunosuppressive treatment. In all areas, the risk for women, whether current or former smokers, is slightly higher than for men. Why smoking increases the risk of Crohn disease is unknown, but some theories suggest that smoking might lower the intestine's defenses, decrease blood flow to the intestines, or cause immune system changes that result in inflammation.

Gallstones

Several studies suggest that smoking may increase the risk of developing gallstones and that the risk may be higher for women. However, research results on this topic are not consistent, and more study is needed.

Can the Damage Be Reversed?

Some of the effects of smoking on the digestive system appear to be of short duration. For example, the effect of smoking on bicarbonate production by the pancreas does not appear to last. Within a half-hour after smoking, the production of bicarbonate returns to normal.

The effects of smoking on how the liver handles drugs also disappear when a person stops smoking. However, people who no longer smoke still remain at risk for Crohn disease. Clearly, this question needs more study.

Chapter 6

Effects of Common Medicines on the Gastrointestinal Tract

Many medications affect the gastrointestinal tract, either directly or indirectly. While patients often ask about the effects of prescription medications, many over-the-counter drugs also have significant potential gastrointestinal side effects. This chapter provides an overview of some common medications that influence the gastrointestinal tract.

Acetaminophen (Tylenol®, Generics)

Acetaminophen is one of the most widely used over-the-counter (OTC) pain relievers and fever reducers. It is also an ingredient in a many OTC and prescription combination medications, including most cold and flu preparations.

Properly used, acetaminophen is quite safe for the gastrointestinal tract. Unlike aspirin and NSAIDs (see following), it rarely causes stomach upset, and it does not cause peptic ulcers. However, in overdose, it is among the most lethal OTC medications.

When taken in overdose, the body converts acetaminophen into a form that is highly toxic to the liver, and will rapidly destroy it. If not quickly treated, an acetaminophen overdose will cause fatal liver failure within days. An antidote is available, but it must be given soon after the overdose to be effective. Once liver failure develops, an emergency liver transplant may be the only hope for survival.

"Effects of Common Medicines on the Gastrointestinal Tract," by David A. Cooke, M.D., © 2005 Omnigraphics, Inc.

The best way to avoid acetaminophen toxicity is to follow the dosing instructions on the package. Read medication ingredients carefully to make sure you are not taking more than one medication at the same time that contain acetaminophen.

For most adults, up to a maximum of 4,000 mg (twelve regular tablets or eight extra-strength tablets) can be safely taken over a twenty-four hour period. However, if you regularly drink three or more alcoholic drinks per day, or if you have liver disease, a lower maximum daily dose of 2,500 mg is recommended.

Keep in mind that dosing instructions are present for a reason. The assumption that "if two is good, four is better" is definitely not true with acetaminophen!

Antibiotics

Antibiotics are used to treat a wide variety of infections. They work by selectively killing harmful bacteria without harming your body's cells. However, they also kill the beneficial bacteria that live in your intestine and are important to normal bowel function. This often results in diarrhea following antibiotic use. While some antibiotics are more likely to cause diarrhea than others, virtually any antibiotic can cause this problem.

Less frequently, antibiotic use can lead to a serious condition called *C. difficile* colitis. *Clostridium difficile* is a bacterial species that is present in small numbers in many peoples' intestines; in these quantities, it is not harmful. However, *C. difficile* is resistant to many antibiotics, so it may survive when other intestinal bacteria are killed. With its competition gone, it can grow in large numbers. Toxins produced by *C. difficile* cause a severe diarrhea and intestinal inflammation, which can be fatal. *C. difficile* should be suspected when diarrhea is very severe and persistent, and especially among people who have been recently hospitalized.

Antihistamines

Antihistamines are often used over-the-counter or by prescription for various allergic complaints. Some commonly used antihistamines include diphenhydramine (Benadryl®, generics), chlorpheniramine (Chlor-Trimeton®, generics), and clemastine (Tavist®, generics).

Antihistamines may cause dry mouth, and less frequently, constipation. These potential side effects should be kept in mind when using these medications.

A newer generation of "nonsedating" antihistamines have become available, including loratadine (Claritin®, generics), fexofenadine

(Allegra®), and cetirizine (Zyrtec®). They have the potential to cause the same side effects as other antihistamines, but this is considerably less frequent.

Aspirin

Aspirin has been a popular pain reliever and fever reducer for over one hundred years. More recently, it has also been used to lower the risk of heart attacks. While aspirin remains a very useful and valuable medication, it is important to be aware of its potential negative effects on the gastrointestinal tract.

Aspirin blocks enzymes involved in maintaining the protective lining of the stomach. This can lead to irritation of the stomach, known as gastritis, which may cause stomach upset and abdominal pain. In more severe cases, aspirin can cause ulcers in the stomach or small intestine, which often bleed. Because aspirin also interferes with the clotting of blood, bleeding from an ulcer can be life-threatening.

Various formulations such as buffered or enteric-coated aspirin are available, and are often advertised as being less upsetting to the stomach. While they will cause less indigestion for some people, the risk of stomach ulceration is the same.

The risk of ulcers from aspirin increases with the dose, but even "baby aspirin" doses can cause ulcers in some people. Risk of aspirin-induced ulcers is increased in the sick, the elderly, those who have had ulcers in the past, and those infected with *H. pylori* bacteria. It is also increased in patients taking corticosteroids. Physicians will sometimes recommend that acid-reducing medications or misoprostol (Cytotec®, generics) be taken with aspirin to reduce risk of ulcers in especially vulnerable patients.

If you experience abdominal pain, vomiting, or black stools while using aspirin, you should stop using it immediately and consult your physician. However, severe bleeding often occurs with no warning signs, so the absence of symptoms does not rule out ulcers.

Laxatives

A number of medications are available to stimulate bowel movements when constipation is a problem. There are several different classes, which have different modes of action.

Most laxatives are intended for short-term or occasional use only. If regular use is necessary, you should consult a physician about which drugs are recommended. Some types of laxatives, particularly stimulant laxatives, can cause permanent damage to the intestinal nerves if used chronically. This can result in more severe constipation and an inability to have a bowel movement without a laxative.

Nonsteroidal Anti-inflammatory Drugs (NSAIDs)

This group includes some of the most commonly used medications for pain, fever, and arthritis. Three of these drugs are currently available over-the-counter: ibuprofen (Motrin®, Advil®, generics), naproxen (Aleve®, Naprosyn®, generics), and ketoprofen (Orudis®, generics). There are more than a dozen additional drugs of this class available by prescription, including diclofenac (Cataflam®, Voltaren®, generics), nabumetone (Relafen®, generics), piroxicam (Feldene®, generics), oxaprozin (Daypro®, generics), and meloxicam (Mobic®).

While these drugs are quite useful, it is important to realize they are closely related to aspirin, and work in a very similar manner. As a result, they have the same potential to cause peptic ulcers and gastrointestinal bleeding. Thousands of Americans are hospitalized or die from this every year.

As with aspirin, you should stop using NSAIDs immediately and consult your doctor if you have abdominal pain, vomiting, or black stools. However, NSAIDs can also cause severe gastrointestinal bleeding without any preceding symptoms or warning signs.

More recently, a group of medications known as selective cyclooxygenase-2 inhibitors (COX-2 inhibitors) was introduced. These include celecoxib (Celebrex®), rofecoxib (Vioxx®), and valdecoxib (Bextra®). They work very similarly to NSAIDs, but were believed to have a much lower risk of causing gastrointestinal bleeding.

Unfortunately, it became clear with wider use of the COX-2 inhibitors that ulcers and bleeding can occur with these drugs as well. While the risk of these complications appears to be lower than with traditional NSAIDs, how much lower this risk is has become a matter of scientific debate. More recently, the overall safety of these drugs has been called into question due to studies suggesting that they increase the risk of heart attacks. At the time of this writing, Vioxx® and Bextra® have been withdrawn from the market due to these safety concerns, and only Celebrex® remains available. The advisability and future of these drugs remain in question.

Opiates

Opiates, also known as narcotics, are prescription medications for moderate to severe pain. Common examples include codeine (Tylenol #3®, generics), fentanyl (Duragesic®, generics), hydrocodone (Vicodin®, Lorcet®, generics), oxycodone (OxyContin®, generics), methadone (Methadose®, generics), morphine (Oramorph, MS-Contin®, generics), and propoxyphene (Darvocet®, generics).

All medications of this class cause constipation, which can be quite severe. If long-term use is anticipated, a laxative is often prescribed with it. Nausea and vomiting are also common side effects of these medications, although this may vary considerably from one drug to another.

Part Two

Diagnostic and Surgical Procedures Used for Gastrointestinal Disorders

Chapter 7

Endoscopic Procedures and Related Concerns

Chapter Contents

Section 7.1

Colonoscopy

What is a colonoscopy?

Colonoscopy enables your doctor to examine the lining of your colon (large intestine) for abnormalities by inserting a flexible tube as thick as your finger into your anus and slowly advancing it into the rectum and colon. If your doctor has recommended a colonoscopy, this section will give you a basic understanding of the procedure—how it's performed, how it can help, and what side effects you might experience. It can't answer all of your questions since much depends on the individual patient and the doctor. Please ask your doctor about anything you don't understand.

What preparation is required?

Your doctor will tell you what dietary restrictions to follow and what cleansing routine to use. In general, the preparation consists of consuming either a large volume of a special cleansing solution or clear liquids and special oral laxatives. The colon must be completely clean for the procedure to be accurate and complete, so be sure to follow your doctor's instructions carefully.

Can I take my current medications?

Most medications can be continued as usual, but some medications can interfere with the preparation or the examination. Inform your doctor about medications you're taking, particularly aspirin products, arthritis medications, anticoagulants (blood thinners), insulin, or iron products. Also, be sure to mention allergies you have to medications.

Alert your doctor if you require antibiotics prior to dental procedures, because you might need antibiotics before a colonoscopy as well.

What happens during colonoscopy?

Colonoscopy is well tolerated and rarely causes much pain. You might feel pressure, bloating, or cramping during the procedure. Your doctor might give you a sedative to help you relax and better tolerate any discomfort.

You will lie on your side or back while your doctor slowly advances a colonoscope through your large intestine to examine the lining. Your doctor will examine the lining again as he or she slowly withdraws the colonoscope. The procedure itself usually takes fifteen to sixty minutes, although you should plan on two to three hours for waiting, preparation, and recovery.

In some cases, the doctor cannot pass the colonoscope through the entire colon to where it meets the small intestine. Although another examination might be needed, your doctor might decide that the limited examination is sufficient.

What if the colonoscopy shows something abnormal?

If your doctor thinks an area needs further evaluation, he or she might pass an instrument through the colonoscope to obtain a biopsy (a sample of the colon lining) to be analyzed. Biopsies are used to identify many conditions, and your doctor might order one even if he or she doesn't suspect cancer. If colonoscopy is being performed to identify sites of bleeding, your doctor might control the bleeding through the colonoscope by injecting medications or by electrocoagulation (sealing off bleeding vessels with heat treatment). Your doctor might also find polyps during colonoscopy, and he or she will most likely remove them during the examination. These procedures don't usually cause any pain.

What are polyps and why are they removed?

Polyps are abnormal growths in the colon lining that are usually benign (noncancerous). They vary in size from a tiny dot to several inches. Your doctor can't always tell a benign polyp from a malignant (cancerous) polyp by its outer appearance, so he or she might send removed polyps for analysis. Because cancer begins in polyps, removing them is an important means of preventing colorectal cancer.

How are polyps removed?

Your doctor might destroy tiny polyps by fulguration (burning) or by removing them with wire loops called snares or with biopsy instruments.

Your doctor might use a technique called "snare polypectomy" to remove larger polyps. That technique involves passing a wire loop through the colonoscope and removing the polyp from the intestinal wall using an electrical current. You should feel no pain during the polypectomy.

What happens after a colonoscopy?

Your physician will explain the results of the examination to you, although you'll probably have to wait for the results of any biopsies performed.

If you have been given sedatives during the procedure, someone must drive you home and stay with you. Even if you feel alert after the procedure, your judgment and reflexes could be impaired for the rest of the day. You might have some cramping or bloating because of the air introduced into the colon during the examination. This should disappear quickly when you pass gas.

You should be able to eat after the examination, but your doctor might restrict your diet and activities, especially after polypectomy.

What are the possible complications of colonoscopy?

Colonoscopy and polypectomy are generally safe when performed by doctors who have been specially trained and are experienced in these procedures.

One possible complication is a perforation, or tear, through the bowel wall that could require surgery. Bleeding might occur at the site of biopsy or polypectomy, but it's usually minor. Bleeding can stop on its own or be controlled through the colonoscope; it rarely requires follow-up treatment. Some patients might have a reaction to the sedatives or complications from heart or lung disease.

Although complications after colonoscopy are uncommon, it's important to recognize early signs of possible complications. Contact your doctor if you notice severe abdominal pain, fever and chills, or rectal bleeding of more than one-half cup. Note that bleeding can occur several days after the procedure.

Section 7.2

Virtual Colonoscopy

Reprinted from "Virtual Colonoscopy," National Institute of Diabetes and Digestive and Kidney Diseases, NIH Publication No. 03-5095, May 2003.

Virtual colonoscopy (VC) uses x-rays and computers to produce two- and three-dimensional images of the colon (large intestine) from the lowest part, the rectum, all the way to the lower end of the small intestine and display them on a screen. The procedure is used to diagnose colon and bowel disease, including polyps, diverticulosis, and cancer. VC can be performed with computed tomography (CT), sometimes called a CAT scan, or with magnetic resonance imaging (MRI).

VC Procedure

While preparations for VC vary, you will usually be asked to take laxatives or other oral agents at home the day before the procedure to clear stool from your colon. You may also be asked to use a suppository to cleanse your rectum of any remaining fecal matter.

VC takes place in the radiology department of a hospital or medical center. The examination takes about ten minutes and does not require sedatives. During the procedure,

- The doctor will ask you to lie on your back on a table.

- A thin tube will be inserted into your rectum, and air will be pumped through the tube to inflate the colon for better viewing.

- The table moves through the scanner to produce a series of two-dimensional cross-sections along the length of the colon. A computer program puts these images together to create a three-dimensional picture that can be viewed on the video screen.

- You will be asked to hold your breath during the scan to avoid distortion on the images.

- The scanning procedure will then be repeated with you lying on your stomach.

After the examination, the information from the scanner will need to be processed to create the computer picture or image of your colon. A radiologist will evaluate the results to identify any abnormalities.

You may resume normal activity after the procedure, although your doctor may ask you to wait while the test results are analyzed. If abnormalities are found and you need conventional colonoscopy, it may be performed the same day.

Conventional Colonoscopy

In a conventional colonoscopy, the doctor inserts a colonoscope—a long, flexible, lighted tube—into the patient's rectum and slowly guides it up through the colon. Pain medication and a mild sedative help the patient stay relaxed and comfortable during the thirty- to sixty-minute procedure. A tiny camera in the scope transmits an image of the lining of the colon, so the doctor can examine it on a video monitor. If an abnormality is detected, the doctor can remove it or take tissue samples using tiny instruments passed through the scope.

Advantages of VC

VC is more comfortable than conventional colonoscopy for some people because it does not use a colonoscope. As a result, no sedation is needed, and you can return to your usual activities or go home after the procedure without the aid of another person. VC provides clearer, more detailed images than a conventional x-ray using a barium enema, sometimes called a lower gastrointestinal (GI) series. It also takes less time than either a conventional colonoscopy or a lower GI series.

Disadvantages of VC

The doctor cannot take tissue samples or remove polyps during VC, so a conventional colonoscopy must be performed if abnormalities are found. Also, VC does not show as much detail as a conventional colonoscopy, so polyps smaller than ten millimeters in diameter may not show up on the images.

Section 7.3

Upper Endoscopy

What is upper endoscopy?

Upper endoscopy lets your doctor examine the lining of the upper part of your gastrointestinal tract, which includes the esophagus, stomach, and duodenum (first portion of the small intestine). Your doctor will use a thin, flexible tube called an endoscope, which has its own lens and light source, and will view the images on a video monitor. You might hear your doctor or other medical staff refer to upper endoscopy as upper GI endoscopy, esophagogastroduodenoscopy (EGD) or panendoscopy. If your doctor has recommended upper endoscopy, this section will give you a basic understanding of the procedure—how it's performed, how it can help, and what side effects you might experience. It can't answer all of your questions, since a lot depends on the individual patient and the doctor. Please ask your doctor about anything you don't understand.

Why is upper endoscopy done?

Upper endoscopy helps your doctor evaluate symptoms of persistent upper abdominal pain, nausea, vomiting, or difficulty swallowing. It's an excellent test for finding the cause of bleeding from the upper gastrointestinal tract. It's also more accurate than x-ray films for detecting inflammation, ulcers, and tumors of the esophagus, stomach, and duodenum.

Your doctor might use upper endoscopy to obtain a biopsy (small tissue samples). A biopsy helps your doctor distinguish between benign and malignant (cancerous) tissues. Remember, biopsies are taken for many reasons, and your doctor might order one even if he or she does not suspect cancer. For example, your doctor might use a biopsy to test for *Helicobacter pylori*, bacterium that causes ulcers.

Your doctor might also use upper endoscopy to perform a cytology test, where he or she will introduce a small brush to collect cells for analysis.

Upper endoscopy is also used to treat conditions of the upper gastrointestinal tract. Your doctor can pass instruments through the endoscope to directly treat many abnormalities with little or no discomfort. For example, your doctor might stretch a narrowed area, remove polyps (usually benign growths), or treat bleeding.

How should I prepare for the procedure?

An empty stomach allows for the best and safest examination, so you should have nothing to eat or drink, including water, for approximately six hours before the examination. Your doctor will tell you when to start fasting.

Tell your doctor in advance about any medications you take; you might need to adjust your usual dose for the examination. Discuss any allergies to medications as well as medical conditions, such as heart or lung disease.

Also, alert your doctor if you require antibiotics prior to undergoing dental procedures, because you might need antibiotics prior to upper endoscopy as well.

What can I expect during upper endoscopy?

Your doctor might start by spraying your throat with a local anesthetic or by giving you a sedative to help you relax. You'll then lie on your side, and your doctor will pass the endoscope through your mouth and into the esophagus, stomach, and duodenum. The endoscope doesn't interfere with your breathing, Most patients consider the test only slightly uncomfortable, and many patients fall asleep during the procedure.

What happens after upper endoscopy?

You will be monitored until most of the effects of the medication have worn off. Your throat might be a little sore, and you might feel bloated because of the air introduced into your stomach during the test. You will be able to eat after you leave unless your doctor instructs you otherwise.

Your doctor generally can tell you your test results on the day of the procedure; however, the results of some tests might take several days.

If you received sedatives, you won't be allowed to drive after the procedure even though you might not feel tired. You should arrange for someone to accompany you home because the sedatives might affect your judgment and reflexes for the rest of the day.

What are the possible complications of upper endoscopy?

Although complications can occur, they are rare when doctors who are specially trained and experienced in this procedure perform the test. Bleeding can occur at a biopsy site or where a polyp was removed, but it's usually minimal and rarely requires follow-up. Other potential risks include a reaction to the sedative used, complications from heart or lung diseases, and perforation (a tear in the gastrointestinal tract lining). It's important to recognize early signs of possible complications. If you have a fever after the test, trouble swallowing, or increasing throat, chest, or abdominal pain, tell your doctor immediately.

Section 7.4

Capsule Endoscopy

Reprinted from "Incredible Journey Through the Digestive System,"
FDA *Consumer Magazine*, March–April 2005.

Lights! Camera! Swallow!

Through the marvels of miniaturization, people with symptoms that indicate a possible problem in the gastrointestinal tract can now swallow a tiny camera that takes snapshots inside the body for a physician to evaluate.

The miniature camera, along with a light, transmitter, and batteries, is housed in a capsule the size of a large vitamin pill. The capsule, called the PillCam, is used in a procedure known as capsule endoscopy, a noninvasive and painless way of looking into the esophagus and small intestine. The procedure requires no sedation and no recovery time, as in a conventional endoscopy where the physician pushes a lighted instrument (endoscope) down the patient's throat to view interior regions. The disposable PillCam passes naturally and painlessly out of the body in eight to seventy-two hours.

In November 2004, the Food and Drug Administration cleared the PillCam ESO for use in adults to help detect abnormalities in the esophagus. In 2001, the agency cleared the PillCam SB for detecting problems in the small bowel, or small intestine, in adults and children at least ten years old. Both types of PillCam are made by Given Imaging Ltd., an Israel-based company with North American headquarters in Norcross, Georgia.

Physicians use the PillCam ESO to look for conditions such as gastroesophageal reflux disease (GERD). GERD occurs when a muscle valve in the esophagus malfunctions, allowing stomach acid to flow up into the esophagus and cause heartburn. Left untreated, GERD may lead to a pre-cancerous condition called Barrett's esophagus.

Blair Lewis, M.D., a gastroenterologist at Mount Sinai School of Medicine in New York City, notes that the PillCam ESO views only the esophagus—not the stomach or the beginning of the small intestine where peptic ulcers may form. "It does not replace conventional endoscopy," Lewis says, because endoscopy allows the physician to view these areas and to take a tissue sample (biopsy). If a capsule endoscopy suggests a serious problem, the patient will still need conventional endoscopy to confirm a diagnosis, he says.

Lewis uses the PillCam ESO for patients "who are reticent to have an upper endoscopy but are still concerned that they may develop problems such as Barrett's esophagus." Capsule endoscopy, as with traditional endoscopy, can help guide treatment, he says.

The PillCam SB, which views the small intestine, can help determine the cause of persistent abdominal pain, unexplained rectal bleeding, or diarrhea. Physicians use it to detect polyps, cancer, and other causes of bleeding and anemia, such as Crohn disease, a chronic inflammation of the digestive tract that can cause abdominal cramps, diarrhea, and anemia.

"[The PillCam] can see lesions that indicate sources of gastrointestinal bleeding," says Jamie Barkin, M.D., professor of medicine at the University of Miami and chief of gastroenterology at Mount Sinai Medical Center in Miami Beach, Florida. "Crohn disease is not apparent on x-rays," he says, "so it can find Crohn at an earlier stage and tell us the extent of Crohn.

"The advantage of capsule endoscopy is that it sees areas that were never seen before—areas that were overlooked by conventional endoscopy and small bowel x-ray," adds Barkin. Only about 20 percent of the small intestine can be seen with conventional endoscopy, he says.

The PillCam SB allows doctors to see the entire twenty-foot-long small intestine; however, it does not photograph the large intestine—the site of colon cancer. "It doesn't replace the colonoscopy," says Jeffrey Cooper, D.V.M., an FDA medical officer who evaluated the PillCam. "The battery has an eight-hour life expectancy, which generally is long enough to photograph the small intestine but not the entire gastrointestinal tract," he says.

The Procedure

A person must fast for ten hours prior to undergoing capsule endoscopy for the small intestine, but can eat four hours after swallowing the capsule. Lewis says he schedules patients early in the morning, so they can eat lunch and dinner. Wire leads with sensors on the end are affixed to the patient's abdomen and connected to a data-recording device worn on a belt around the waist.

The PillCam SB takes about eight hours to move through the small intestine, taking two pictures per second with its single camera. During this time, the person can leave the doctor's office and go about a regular routine while wearing the sensors and recorder. Later, the person returns to hand over the sensors and data recorder. The physician downloads about 57,000 color images into a computer, which compresses them to form a video. The physician then views the video on a monitor to determine the next step in treatment.

A two-hour fast is required before taking the PillCam ESO, which views the esophagus. Wire leads with sensors are placed on the patient's chest and connected to a recording device. The person swallows the capsule with water while lying flat on the back. Every two minutes over a six-minute period, the person is raised by thirty-degree angles until sitting upright, then remains upright for an additional fifteen minutes to make sure the capsule has traveled through the entire esophagus.

The gradual rise to a sitting position slows down the movement of the PillCam ESO, giving it additional time to take pictures. In contrast to the PillCam SB, which moves slowly through the snake-like turns of the small intestine over several hours, the PillCam ESO "moves through the esophagus in minutes," says Cooper. Given Imaging added a second miniature camera to the ESO capsule, putting one camera at either end, to take about 2,600 total color images of the esophagus.

Few Side Effects

The FDA clearance of the PillCam devices was based on their safety, ability to detect abnormalities in the small intestine and esophagus, and lack of side effects.

No cramping or discomfort has been reported with the PillCam, says Lewis, who has conducted clinical studies involving the device. People have "no clue it's there," he says, adding that he's gotten calls from some patients who insisted that it did not pass in their stool and requested an x-ray to confirm it was no longer there.

The size of the capsule—a little more than an inch long and a little less than one-half inch wide—may be daunting for some individuals. "Children and people who have trouble swallowing pills may have a hard time swallowing the capsule," says Cooper.

"Once inside, if a patient has a small blockage, the device could get hung up, sometimes requiring surgery to remove it," he says. The device is not for use in a person with a known intestinal blockage or a significantly narrowed small intestine.

Lewis notes that, in studies worldwide involving a total of 150 patients, the esophageal capsule never became lodged in the body. In larger studies, the capsule for the small intestine became lodged in the gastrointestinal tract in less than 1 percent of those studied.

Most insurance carriers will reimburse patients for the capsule endoscopy for the small intestine, says Lewis. However, the newer esophageal capsule endoscopy is not yet widely accepted by carriers, who consider it on a case-by-case basis.

Section 7.5

Endoscopic Ultrasound

You've been referred to have an endoscopic ultrasonography, or EUS, which will help your doctor evaluate or treat your condition. This section will give you a basic understanding of the procedure—how it is performed, how it can help, and what side effects you might experience. It can't answer all of your questions, since a lot depends on the individual patient and the doctor. Please ask your doctor about anything you don't understand. Endoscopists are highly trained specialists who welcome your questions regarding their credentials, training, and experience

What is EUS?

EUS allows your doctor to examine the lining and the walls of your upper and lower gastrointestinal tract. The upper tract is the esophagus, stomach, and duodenum; the lower tract includes your colon and rectum. EUS is also used to study internal organs that lie next to the gastrointestinal tract, such as the gall bladder and pancreas.

Your endoscopist will use a thin, flexible tube called an endoscope. Your doctor will pass the endoscope through your mouth or anus to the area to be examined. Your doctor then will turn on the ultrasound component to produce sound waves that create visual images of the digestive tract.

Why is EUS done?

EUS provides your doctor more detailed pictures of your digestive tract anatomy. Your doctor can use EUS to diagnose the cause of conditions such as abdominal pain or abnormal weight loss. Or, if your doctor has ruled out certain conditions, EUS can confirm your diagnosis and give you a clean bill of health.

EUS is also used to evaluate an abnormality, such as a growth, that was detected at a prior endoscopy or by x-ray. EUS provides a detailed picture of the growth, which can help your doctor determine its nature and decide upon the best treatment.

In addition, EUS can be used to diagnose diseases of the pancreas, bile duct, and gallbladder when other tests are inconclusive.

Why is EUS used for patients with cancer?

EUS helps your doctor determine the extent of certain cancers of the digestive and respiratory systems. EUS allows your doctor to accurately assess the cancer's depth and whether it has spread to adjacent lymph glands or nearby vital structures such as major blood vessels. In some patients, EUS can be used to obtain tissue samples to help your doctor determine the proper treatment.

How should I prepare for EUS?

For EUS of the upper gastrointestinal tract, you should have nothing to eat or drink, not even water, usually six hours before the examination. Your doctor will tell you when to start this fasting.

For EUS of the rectum or colon, your doctor will instruct you to either consume a large volume of a special cleansing solution or to follow a clear liquid diet combined with laxatives or enemas prior to the examination. The procedure might have to be rescheduled if you don't follow your doctor's instructions carefully.

What about my current medications or allergies?

Tell your doctor in advance of the procedure about all medications that you're taking and about any allergies you have to medication. He or she will tell you whether or not you can continue to take your medication as usual before the EUS examination. In general, you can safely take aspirin and nonsteroidal anti-inflammatories (Motrin, Advil, Aleve, etc.) before an EUS examination, but it's always best to discuss their use with your doctor. Check with your doctor about which medications you should take the morning of the EUS examination, and take essential medication with only a small cup of water.

If you have an allergy to latex you should inform your doctor prior to your test. Patients with latex allergies often require special equipment and may not be able to have an EUS examination.

Do I need to take antibiotics?

Antibiotics aren't generally required before or after EUS examinations, but tell your doctor if you take antibiotics before dental procedures. If your doctor feels you need antibiotics, antibiotics might be ordered during the EUS examination or after the procedure to help prevent an infection. Your doctor might prescribe antibiotics if you're having specialized EUS procedures, such as to drain a fluid collection or a cyst using EUS guidance. Again, tell your doctor about any allergies to medications.

Should I arrange for help after the examination?

If you receive sedatives, you won't be allowed to drive after the procedure, even if you don't feel tired. You should arrange for a ride home. You should also plan to have someone stay with you at home after the examination, because the sedatives could affect your judgment and reflexes for the rest of the day.

What can I expect during EUS?

Practices vary among doctors, but for an EUS examination of the upper gastrointestinal tract, your endoscopist might spray your throat with a local anesthetic before the test begins. Most often you will receive sedatives intravenously to help you relax. You will most likely begin by lying on your left side. After you receive sedatives, your endoscopist will pass the ultrasound endoscope through your mouth, esophagus, and stomach into the duodenum. The instrument does not interfere with your ability to breathe. The actual examination generally takes between fifteen and forty-five minutes. Most patients consider it only slightly uncomfortable, and many fall asleep during it.

An EUS examination of the lower gastrointestinal tract can often be performed safely and comfortably without medications, but you will probably receive a sedative if the examination will be prolonged or if the doctor will examine a significant distance into the colon. You will start by lying on your left side with your back toward the doctor. Most EUS examinations of the lower gastrointestinal tract last from ten to thirty minutes.

What happens after EUS?

If you received sedatives, you will be monitored in the recovery area until most of the sedative medication's effects have worn off. If you had an upper EUS, your throat might be sore. You might feel bloated because of the air and water that were introduced during the examination. You'll be able to eat after you leave the procedure area, unless you're instructed otherwise.

Your doctor generally can inform you of the results of the procedure that day, but the results of some tests will take longer.

What are the possible complications of EUS?

Although complications can occur, they are rare when doctors with specialized training and experience perform the EUS examination. Bleeding might occur at a biopsy site, but it's usually minimal and rarely requires follow-up. You might have a sore throat for a day or more. Nonprescription anesthetic-type throat lozenges and painkillers help relieve the sore throat. Other potential, but uncommon, risks of EUS include a reaction to the sedatives used; backwash of stomach contents into your lungs; infection; and complications from heart or lung diseases. One major, but very uncommon, complication of EUS is perforation. This is a tear through the lining of the intestine that might require surgery to repair.

The possibility of complications increases slightly if a deep needle aspiration is performed during the EUS examination. These risks must be balanced against the potential benefits of the procedure and the risks of alternative approaches to the condition.

Additional Questions?

If you have any questions about your need for EUS, alternative approaches to your problem, the cost of the procedure, methods of billing, or insurance coverage, do not hesitate to speak to your doctor or doctor's office staff about it.

Section 7.6

Flexible Sigmoidoscopy

What is flexible sigmoidoscopy?

Flexible sigmoidoscopy lets your doctor examine the lining of the rectum and a portion of the colon (large intestine) by inserting a flexible tube about the thickness of your finger into the anus and slowly advancing it into the rectum and lower part of the colon. If your doctor has recommended a flexible sigmoidoscopy, this section will give you a basic understanding of the procedure—how it is performed, how it can help, and what side effects you might experience. It can't answer all of your questions, since a lot depends of the individual patient and the doctor. Please ask your doctor about anything you don't understand.

What preparation is required?

Your doctor will tell you what cleansing routine to use. In general, preparation consists of one or two enemas prior to the procedure but could include laxatives or dietary modifications as well. However, in some circumstances your doctor might advise you to forgo any special preparation. Because the rectum and lower colon must be completely empty for the procedure to be accurate, it's important to follow your doctor's instructions carefully.

Should I continue my current medications?

Most medications can be continued as usual. Inform your doctor about medications that you're taking—particularly aspirin products or anticoagulants (blood thinners)—as well as any allergies you have to medications. Also, tell your doctor if you require antibiotics prior to dental procedures, because you might need antibiotics prior to sigmoidoscopy as well.

What can I expect during flexible sigmoidoscopy?

Flexible sigmoidoscopy is usually well tolerated. You might experience a feeling of pressure, bloating, or cramping during the procedure. You will lie on your side while your doctor advances the sigmoidoscope through the rectum and colon. As your doctor withdraws the instrument, your doctor will carefully examine the lining of the intestine.

What if the flexible sigmoidoscopy finds something abnormal?

If your doctor sees an area that needs further evaluation, your doctor might take a biopsy (sample of the colon lining) to be analyzed. Biopsies are used to identify many conditions, and your doctor might order one even if he or she doesn't suspect cancer.

If your doctor finds polyps, he or she might take a biopsy of them as well. Polyps, which are growths from the lining of the colon, vary in size and types. Polyps known as "hyperplastic" might not require removal, but benign polyps known as "adenomas" are potentially precancerous. Your doctor might ask you to have a colonoscopy (a complete examination of the colon) to remove any large polyps or any small adenomas.

What happens after a flexible sigmoidoscopy?

Your doctor will explain the results to you when the procedure is done. You might feel bloating or some mild cramping because of the air that was passed into the colon during the examination. This will disappear quickly when you pass gas. You should be able to eat and resume your normal activities after leaving your doctor's office or the hospital, assuming you did not receive any sedative medication.

What are possible complications of flexible sigmoidoscopy?

Flexible sigmoidoscopy and biopsy are safe when performed by doctors who are specially trained and experienced in these endoscopic procedures. Complications are rare, but it's important for you to recognize early signs of possible complications. Contact your doctor if you notice severe abdominal pain, fevers and chills, or rectal bleeding of more than one-half cup. Note that rectal bleeding can occur several days after the biopsy.

Section 7.7

Endoscopic Retrograde Cholangiopancreatography (ERCP)

Reprinted from "ERCP (Endoscopic Retrograde Cholangiopancreatography)," National Institute of Diabetes and Digestive and Kidney Diseases, NIH Publication No. 05-4336, November 2004.

Endoscopic retrograde cholangiopancreatography (ERCP) enables the physician to diagnose problems in the liver, gallbladder, bile ducts, and pancreas. The liver is a large organ that, among other things, makes a liquid called bile that helps with digestion. The gallbladder is a small, pear-shaped organ that stores bile until it is needed for digestion. The bile ducts are tubes that carry bile from the liver to the gallbladder and small intestine. These ducts are sometimes called the biliary tree. The pancreas is a large gland that produces chemicals that help with digestion and hormones such as insulin.

ERCP is used primarily to diagnose and treat conditions of the bile ducts, including gallstones, inflammatory strictures (scars), leaks (from trauma and surgery), and cancer. ERCP combines the use of x-rays and an endoscope, which is a long, flexible, lighted tube. Through the endoscope, the physician can see the inside of the stomach and duodenum, and inject dyes into the ducts in the biliary tree and pancreas so they can be seen on x-rays.

For the procedure, you will lie on your left side on an examining table in an x-ray room. You will be given medication to help numb the back of your throat and a sedative to help you relax during the exam. You will swallow the endoscope, and the physician will then guide the scope through your esophagus, stomach, and duodenum until it reaches the spot where the ducts of the biliary tree and pancreas open into the duodenum. At this time, you will be turned to lie flat on your stomach, and the physician will pass a small plastic tube through the scope. Through the tube, the physician will inject a dye into the ducts to make them show up clearly on x-rays. X-rays are taken as soon as the dye is injected.

If the exam shows a gallstone or narrowing of the ducts, the physician can insert instruments into the scope to remove or relieve the obstruction. Also, tissue samples (biopsy) can be taken for further testing.

Possible complications of ERCP include pancreatitis (inflammation of the pancreas), infection, bleeding, and perforation of the duodenum. Except for pancreatitis, such problems are uncommon. You may have tenderness or a lump where the sedative was injected, but that should go away in a few days.

ERCP takes thirty minutes to two hours. You may have some discomfort when the physician blows air into the duodenum and injects the dye into the ducts. However, the pain medicine and sedative should keep you from feeling too much discomfort. After the procedure, you will need to stay at the hospital for one to two hours until the sedative wears off. The physician will make sure you do not have signs of complications before you leave. If any kind of treatment is done during ERCP, such as removing a gallstone, you may need to stay in the hospital overnight.

Preparation

Your stomach and duodenum must be empty for the procedure to be accurate and safe. You will not be able to eat or drink anything after midnight the night before the procedure, or for six to eight hours beforehand, depending on the time of your procedure. Also, the physician will need to know whether you have any allergies, especially to iodine, which is in the dye. You must also arrange for someone to take you home—you will not be allowed to drive because of the sedatives. The physician may give you other special instructions.

Section 7.8

Therapeutic ERCP

What is a therapeutic ERCP?

Endoscopic retrograde cholangiopancreatography, or ERCP, is a study of the ducts that drain the liver and pancreas. Ducts are drainage routes into the bowel. The ones that drain the liver and gallbladder are called bile or biliary ducts. The one that drains the pancreas is called the pancreatic duct. The bile and pancreatic ducts join together just before they drain into the upper bowel, about three inches from the stomach. The drainage opening is called the papilla. The papilla is surrounded by a circular muscle, called the sphincter of Oddi.

Diagnostic ERCP is when x-ray contrast dye is injected into the bile duct, the pancreatic duct, or both. This contrast dye is squirted through a small tube called a catheter that fits through the ERCP endoscope. X-rays are taken during ERCP to get pictures of these ducts. That is called diagnostic ERCP. However, most ERCPs are actually done for treatment and not just picture taking. When an ERCP is done to allow treatment, it is called therapeutic ERCP.

What treatments can be done through an ERCP scope?

Sphincterotomy: Sphincterotomy is cutting the muscle that surrounds the opening of the ducts, or the papilla. This cut is made to enlarge the opening. The cut is made while your doctor looks through the ERCP scope at the papilla, or duct opening. A small wire on a specialized catheter uses electric current to cut the tissue. A sphincterotomy does not cause discomfort because you do not have nerve endings there. The actual cut is quite small, usually less than half an inch. This small cut allows various treatments in the ducts. Most commonly

the cut is directed toward the bile duct, called a biliary sphincterotomy. Occasionally, the cut is directed toward the pancreatic duct,
depending on the type of treatment you need.

Stone Removal: The most common treatment through an ERCP
scope is removal of bile duct stones. These stones may have formed
in the gallbladder and traveled into the bile duct or may form in the
duct itself years after your gallbladder has been removed. After a
sphincterotomy is performed to enlarge the opening of the bile duct,
stones can be pulled from the duct into the bowel. A variety of balloons and baskets attached to specialized catheters can be passed
through the ERCP scope into the ducts, allowing stone removal. Very
large stones may require crushing in the duct with a specialized basket so the fragments can be pulled out through the sphincterotomy.

Stent Placement: Stents are placed into the bile or pancreatic
ducts to bypass strictures, or narrowed parts of the duct. These narrowed areas of the bile or pancreatic duct are due to scar tissue or
tumors that cause blockage of normal duct drainage. There are two
types of stents that are commonly used. The first is made of plastic
and looks like a small straw. A plastic stent can be pushed through
the ERCP scope into a blocked duct to allow normal drainage. The
second type of stent is made of metal wires that looks like the cross
wires of a fence. The metal stent is flexible and springs open to a larger
diameter than plastic stents. Both plastic and metal stents tend to
clog up after several months and you may require another ERCP to
place a new stent. Metal stents are permanent while plastic stents
are easily removed at a repeat procedure. Your doctor will choose the
best type of stent for your problem.

Balloon Dilation: There are ERCP catheters fitted with dilating
balloons that can be placed across a narrowed area or stricture. The
balloon is then inflated to stretch out the narrowing. Dilation with
balloons is often performed when the cause of the narrowing is benign (not a cancer). After balloon dilation, a temporary stent may be
placed for a few months to help maintain the dilation.

Tissue Sampling: One procedure that is commonly performed
through the ERCP scope is to take samples of tissue from the papilla
or from the bile or pancreatic ducts. There are several different sampling techniques although the most common is to brush the area with
subsequent examination of the cells obtained. Tissue samples can help

decide if a stricture, or narrowing, is due to a cancer. If the sample is positive for cancer it is very accurate. Unfortunately, a tissue sampling that does not show cancer may not be accurate.

What can you expect before, during, and after a therapeutic ERCP?

You should not eat for at least six hours before the procedure. You should tell your doctor about medications that you take regularly and whether you have any allergies to medications or contrast material.

You will have an intravenous needle placed in your arm so you can receive medicine during the procedure. You will be given sedatives that will make you comfortable during the ERCP. Some patients require antibiotics before the procedure. The procedure is performed on an x-ray table. After the ERCP is complete you will go to a recovery area until the sedation effects reside. Some patients are admitted to the hospital for a day but many go home from the recovery unit. You should not drive a car for the rest of the day although most patients can return to full activity the next day.

What are possible complications of therapeutic ERCP?

The overall ERCP complication rate requiring hospitalization is 6–10 percent. Depending on your age, your other medical problems, what therapy is performed, and the indication for your procedure, your complication rate may be higher or lower than the average. Your doctor will discuss your likelihood of complications before you undergo the test. The most common complication is pancreatitis, or inflammation of the pancreas. Other complications include bleeding, infection, an adverse reaction to the sedative medication, or bowel perforation. Most complications are managed without surgery but may require you to stay in the hospital for treatment.

Chapter 8

Upper and Lower GI Series

Chapter Contents

Section 8.1

Upper GI and Small Bowel Series

Alternative Names

GI series; barium swallow x-ray; upper GI series

Definition

An upper GI and small bowel series is a set of x-rays taken to examine the esophagus, stomach, and small intestine. X-rays are taken after the patient has swallowed a barium suspension (contrast medium).

X-rays are a form of electromagnetic radiation like light, but of higher energy, so they can penetrate the body to form an image on film. Structures that are dense (such as bone) will appear white, air will be black, and other structures will be shades of gray Barium is very dense and will appear white on the x-ray film.

How the Test Is Performed

This test may be done in an office or in a hospital radiology department. You will be sitting or standing up while your heart, lungs, and abdomen are examined with a fluoroscope (a type of x-ray that projects images onto a monitor like a TV screen).

You may be given an injection of a medication that will temporarily slow bowel movement, so structures can be more easily imaged. You will then be given a drink like a milk shake that has a barium mixture in it. You must drink sixteen to twenty ounces for the examination.

The passage of the barium through the esophagus, stomach, and small intestine is monitored on the fluoroscope. Pictures are taken with you in a variety of positions. The test usually takes around three hours. However, in some cases, it may take up to six hours to complete.

A GI series may include this test or a barium enema.

How to Prepare for the Test

You may be given a restricted diet for two or three days before the test. You will likely be told not to smoke or eat for a period of time before the test. Generally, oral medications may be taken.

Be sure to check with your health care provider regarding any dietary or medication restrictions before the test. Never discontinue or decrease medications without consulting your health care provider.

Remove all jewelry before the test.

Infants and Children

The physical and psychological preparation you can provide for this or any test or procedure depends on your child's age, interests, previous experience, and level of trust.

How the Test Will Feel

The x-ray causes no discomfort. The barium milk shake has a chalky texture.

Why the Test Is Performed

The purpose of the test is to detect anatomic or functional abnormalities of the esophagus, stomach, and small intestine.

Normal Values

The esophagus, stomach, and small intestine are normal in size and contour.

What Abnormal Results Mean

In the esophagus, abnormal results may mean:

- Esophageal cancer;
- Esophageal stricture (benign);
- Hiatal hernia (a portion of the stomach protrudes through the esophageal opening);
- Diverticula (a pouch-like sac that protrudes from the walls of an organ);
- Ulcers (open sores);
- Achalasia (esophagus fails to relax).

In the stomach, abnormal results may mean:

- Gastric cancer;
- Gastric ulcer; benign;
- Polyps (a tumor that is usually noncancerous that grows on the mucous membrane);
- Gastritis (inflammation of the stomach);
- Pyloric stenosis (a narrowing of the opening from the stomach).

In the small intestines the test may reveal:

- Tumors;
- Malabsorption syndrome (inadequate absorption of nutrients in the intestinal tract);
- Inflammation of the small intestines.

Additional conditions under which the test may be performed:

- Alcoholic neuropathy;
- Annular pancreas;
- CMV gastroenteritis/colitis;
- Cystic fibrosis;
- Duodenal ulcer;
- Gastroesophageal reflux disease;
- Gastroparesis;
- Intestinal obstruction;
- Lower esophageal ring (Schatzki);
- Ovarian cancer;
- Primary or idiopathic intestinal pseudo-obstruction.

What the Risks Are

There is low radiation exposure, which carries a measurable but small risk of cancer. X-rays are monitored and regulated to provide the minimum amount of radiation exposure needed to produce the image. Most experts feel that the risk is low compared with the benefits.

Pregnant women and children are more sensitive to the risks of x-rays.

Barium may cause constipation. Consult your health care provider if the barium has not passed through your system by two or three days after the exam.

Special Considerations

The upper GI series should be performed after other x-ray procedures, because the barium that is retained may obscure details in other imaging tests.

Section 8.2

Lower GI Series (Barium Enema)

"Barium Enema," © 2005, A.D.A.M., Inc. Reprinted with Permission.

Definition

A barium enema is given in order to perform an x-ray examination of the large intestines. Pictures are taken after rectal instillation of barium sulfate (a radiopaque contrast medium).

How the Test Is Performed

This test may be done in an office or a hospital radiology department. You lie on the x-ray table and a preliminary x-ray is taken. You are asked to lie on your side while a well-lubricated enema tube is inserted gently into your rectum.

Barium, a radiopaque (shows up on x-ray) contrast medium, is then allowed to flow into your colon. A small balloon at the tip of the enema tube may be inflated to help keep the barium inside. The flow of the barium is monitored by the health care provider on an x-ray fluoroscope screen (like a TV monitor). Air may be puffed into the colon to distend (expand) it and provide better images.

You are asked to move into different positions and the table is slightly tipped to get different views. At certain times when the x-ray pictures are taken, you must hold your breath and be still for a few seconds so the images won't be blurry.

The enema tube is removed after the pictures are taken and you are given a bedpan or helped to the toilet. You then expel as much of the barium as possible. One or two x-rays may be taken after the barium is expelled.

If a double or air-contrast examination is being done, the enema tube will be reinserted gently and a small amount of air will be gently introduced into the colon, and more x-ray pictures taken. This gives a more detailed picture. The enema tube is then removed, and you again empty the colon.

How to Prepare for the Test

Thorough cleaning of the large intestine is necessary for accurate pictures. Test preparations include a clear liquid diet, drinking a bottle of magnesium citrate (a laxative), and warm water enemas to clear out any stool particles.

For Infants and Children

The preparation you can provide for this test depends on your child's age and experience.

How the Test Will Feel

There is a feeling of fullness during the procedure, moderate to severe cramping, the urge to defecate, and a general discomfort. The x-rays themselves are painless.

Why the Test Is Performed

The test is used to detect colon cancer. The barium enema may also be used to diagnose and evaluate the extent of inflammatory bowel diseases.

Normal Values

Barium should fill the colon uniformly and show normal bowel contour, patency (should be freely open), and position.

What Abnormal Results Mean

Abnormal findings may include cancer, diverticulitis (small pouches formed on the colon wall that can become inflamed), polyps (a tumor, usually noncancerous, that grows on the mucous membrane), inflammation of the inner lining of the intestine (ulcerative colitis), and irritable colon. An acute appendicitis or twisted loop of the bowel may also be seen.

Additional conditions under which the test may be performed:

- annular pancreas;
- CMV gastroenteritis/colitis;
- colorectal polyps;
- Crohn disease (regional enteritis);
- Hirschsprung disease;
- intestinal obstruction;
- intussusception (children);
- pyloric stenosis.

What the Risks Are

There is low radiation exposure. X-rays are monitored and regulated to provide the minimum amount of radiation exposure needed to produce the image. Most experts feel that the risk is low compared with the benefits. Pregnant women and children are more sensitive to the risks of the x-ray.

A more serious risk is a perforated colon, which is very rare.

Special Considerations

CT scans and ultrasounds are now the tests of choice for the initial evaluation of abdominal masses.

Chapter 9

Diagnostic Liver Tests

Chapter Contents

Section 9.1

Liver Function Tests

Liver function tests (LFTs) measure liver injury, rather than liver function. They are a group of blood tests that measure substances in the blood that reflect whether the liver has been injured and the extent of the injuries. Sometimes these tests are also called a liver panel. The tests usually include the following: alanine transaminase (ALT), aspartate transaminase (AST), alkaline phosphatase (ALP), albumin, total protein, and total and direct bilirubin.

The liver is a complex organ, located in the upper right corner of the abdomen, which has many vital roles. The liver stores fuel for the body that has been produced from sugars, and it is involved in the processing of fats and proteins. Bile produced by the liver is involved in the digestion and absorption of fat in the intestines. The liver also makes proteins that are essential for blood clotting, and it helps remove poisons and toxins from the body.

When a blood sample is collected from a child to measure LFTs, the skin is cleaned with alcohol first, then a needle is inserted into a vein and blood is drawn into specific tubes. These blood samples are then sent to a laboratory and processed by machines. The tests are done simultaneously, which takes about twenty minutes. Emergency test results are reported within an hour. For routine tests processed at the site of collection, results are usually available within three to six hours. If samples are shipped to a central processing facility, they are usually available the next day.

The Liver Function Tests

Alanine Transaminase (ALT)

Alanine transaminase is an enzyme that is important in the processing of proteins. This enzyme is found in large amounts in the liver, and small amounts of this enzyme are also found in the heart, muscle, and kidney. When the liver is injured or inflamed, the levels of ALT in blood usually rise; therefore, this test is done to check for signs of liver disease. The ALT is elevated, for example, in some viral infections of childhood that may affect the liver, such as mononucleosis.

Aspartate Transaminase (AST)

Aspartate transaminase is an enzyme that plays a role in many aspects of body metabolism. This enzyme is found in many body tissues including the heart, muscle, kidney, brain, and lung. It is also present in the liver. If there is cell injury or death in any of these tissues, AST is released into the bloodstream; therefore, elevated AST levels can be seen in a variety of conditions, including liver disease. For example, the AST may be elevated in viral hepatitis, mononucleosis, or following a heart attack.

Alkaline Phosphatase (ALP)

Alkaline phosphatase is an enzyme found in the liver and bone. Blood levels of the enzyme are elevated in some types of liver disease. Children—especially teens—normally have higher blood levels of ALP than adults. This is related to rapid growth of their bones. Compared to the transaminases, alkaline phosphatase tends to be higher in diseases associated with injury to the bile-secreting part of the liver's activity.

Albumin and Total Protein

Albumin and total protein levels in the blood reflect the protein-building function of the liver. Found throughout the body, proteins perform many functions: hold cells together, carry information from place to place, control chemical reactions, fight infections, transport oxygen—and much more. Albumin is a protein made by the liver found in large amounts in the blood. In fact, it's similar to the protein in egg whites. In some types of liver disease, the ability of the organ to make proteins is affected. In these cases the blood levels of total protein and albumin are low. Low total protein and albumin levels are also seen in kids who are malnourished.

Because most proteins, including albumin, have fairly long half lives, the liver's incapacity to produce proteins must last weeks to months to be reflected in lowered blood levels of total protein or albumin.

Total and Direct Bilirubin

Total and direct bilirubin levels in blood are also measured as part of the liver function tests. Bilirubin is the chemical substance that gives bile, a fluid produced by the liver, its yellow-green color. Jaundice, the yellow discoloration of the skin seen in some types of liver disease, occurs because high levels of bilirubin accumulating in the blood lead to some of the substance becoming deposited in the skin. Bilirubin is produced from hemoglobin, which is released when red blood cells break down. The liver takes bilirubin and attaches conjugated sugar molecules to it so it can leave the body through the urine. This type of bilirubin is called conjugated direct (because it can be measured directly in a water solution) bilirubin. In liver disease, bilirubin levels in blood can become high. Measurements of total and direct bilirubin can be helpful in diagnosing specific liver problems.

Section 9.2

Hepatitis Virus Test or Panel

Alternative Names

Hepatitis A antibody test; hepatitis B antibody test; hepatitis C antibody test; hepatitis D antibody test

Definition

Hepatitis virus blood tests detect the presence of antibodies to viruses that cause the disease hepatitis (inflammation of the liver). The tests are specific to hepatitis A, hepatitis B, or hepatitis C viruses. A "panel" of tests can be used to screen blood samples for more than one kind of hepatitis virus at the same time.

How the Test Is Performed

Blood is drawn from a vein on the inside of the elbow or the back of the hand. The puncture site is cleaned with antiseptic, and an elastic band is placed around the upper arm to apply pressure and restrict blood flow through the vein. This causes veins below the band to fill with blood.

A needle is inserted into the vein, and the blood is collected in an air-tight vial or a syringe. During the procedure, the band is removed to restore circulation. Once the blood has been collected, the needle is removed and the puncture site is covered to stop any bleeding.

For an infant or young child, the area is cleansed with antiseptic and punctured with a sharp needle or a lancet. The blood may be collected in a pipette (small glass tube), on a slide, onto a test strip, or into a small container. Cotton or a bandage may be applied to the puncture site if there is any continued bleeding.

How the Test Will Feel

When the needle is inserted to draw blood, some people feel moderate pain, while others feel only a prick or stinging sensation. Afterward, there may be some throbbing.

Why the Test Is Performed

These tests are performed to detect infection by hepatitis-causing viruses. Hepatitis is an inflammation of the liver. Three common viruses can cause hepatitis—the viruses are called hepatitis A, hepatitis B, and hepatitis C.

Hepatitis A virus (HAV) is usually spread when something contaminated with infected stool is placed in the mouth. It has an incubation period of two to six weeks.

Hepatitis B virus (HBV) is most frequently transmitted by blood contact, but can also be transmitted through other body fluids. HBV can cause a severe and unrelenting form of hepatitis ending in liver failure and death. The incidence of HBV is higher among blood transfusion recipients, male homosexuals, dialysis patients, organ transplant patients, and IV drug users. It has a long incubation period (five weeks to six months).

The hepatitis B virus is made up of an inner core surrounded by an outer capsule. The outer capsule contains a protein called HBsAg (Hep B surface antigen). The inner core contains HBcAg (Hep B core antigen). A third protein called HBeAg is also found within the core. In addition to detecting hepatitis B virus itself, tests can detect antibodies a patient has made to these antigens. The antibodies are called HBsAb, HBcAb, and HBeAb.

Hepatitis C virus (HCV) is transmitted in a manner similar to hepatitis B. The incubation period is two to twelve weeks after exposure. The symptoms and course of the illness are similar to HBV.

Hepatitis D causes disease only when hepatitis B is also present. It is not routinely checked on a hepatitis antibody panel.

Normal Values

No presence of antibodies (a negative test) is normal.

What Abnormal Results Mean

Serology tests have been developed to detect the presence of antibodies to each of the hepatitis viruses in serum. IgM antibodies appear three to four weeks after exposure and usually return to normal in about eight weeks. IgG antibodies appear about two weeks after the IgM antibodies start to increase; such antibodies may persist forever.

If the IgM antibody is elevated in the absence of IgG antibody, acute hepatitis is suspected. If IgG antibody is increased, but not IgM antibody, a convalescent or chronic state is likely.

Positive tests may indicate:

- hepatitis A;
- hepatitis B;
- hepatitis C;
- chronic hepatitis B or hepatitis B carrier state;
- hepatitis D, when found in conjunction with hepatitis B.

Additional conditions under which the test may be performed:

- chronic persistent hepatitis;
- delta agent (hepatitis D);
- nephrotic syndrome.

What the Risks Are

The risks associated with having blood drawn are:

- excessive bleeding;
- fainting or feeling light-headed;
- hematoma (blood accumulating under the skin);
- infection (a slight risk any time the skin is broken);
- multiple punctures to locate veins.

Special Considerations

Veins and arteries vary in size from one patient to another and from one side of the body to the other. Obtaining a blood sample from some people may be more difficult than from others.

Section 9.3

Liver Biopsy

Reprinted from "Liver Biopsy," National Institute of Diabetes and Digestive and Kidney Diseases, NIH Publication No. 05-4731, November 2004.

In a liver biopsy, the physician examines a small piece of tissue from your liver for signs of damage or disease. A special needle is used to remove the tissue from the liver. The physician decides to do a liver biopsy after tests suggest that the liver does not work properly. For example, a blood test might show that your blood contains higher than normal levels of liver enzymes or too much iron or copper. An x-ray could suggest that the liver is swollen. Looking at liver tissue itself is the best way to determine whether the liver is healthy or what is causing it to be damaged.

Preparation

Before scheduling your biopsy, the physician will take blood samples to make sure your blood clots properly. Be sure to mention any medications you take, especially those that affect blood clotting, like blood thinners. One week before the procedure, you will have to stop taking aspirin, ibuprofen, and anticoagulants.

You must not eat or drink anything for eight hours before the biopsy, and you should plan to arrive at the hospital about an hour before the scheduled time of the procedure. Your physician will tell you whether to take your regular medications during the fasting period and may give you other special instructions.

Procedure

Liver biopsy is considered minor surgery, so it is done at the hospital. For the biopsy, you will lie on a hospital bed on your back with your right hand above your head. After marking the outline of your liver and injecting a local anesthetic to numb the area, the physician will make a small incision in your right side near your rib cage, then insert the biopsy needle and retrieve a sample of liver tissue. In some cases, the physician may use an ultrasound image of the liver to help guide the needle to a specific spot.

You will need to hold very still so that the physician does not nick the lung or gallbladder, which are close to the liver. The physician will ask you to hold your breath for five to ten seconds while he or she puts the needle in your liver. You may feel pressure and a dull pain. The entire procedure takes about twenty minutes.

Two other methods of liver biopsy are also available. For a laparoscopic biopsy, the physician inserts a special tube called a laparoscope through an incision in the abdomen. The laparoscope sends images of the liver to a monitor. The physician watches the monitor and uses instruments in the laparoscope to remove tissue samples from one or more parts of the liver. Physicians use this type of biopsy when they need tissue samples from specific parts of the liver.

Transvenous biopsy involves inserting a tube called a catheter into a vein in the neck and guiding it to the liver. The physician puts a biopsy needle into the catheter and then into the liver. Physicians use this procedure when patients have blood-clotting problems or fluid in the abdomen.

Chapter 10

Other Diagnostic Tests of the Gastrointestinal Tract

Chapter Contents

Section 10.1

Esophageal Manometry Testing

"Esophageal Manometry Testing," © 2005 The Cleveland Clinic Foundation, 9500 Euclid Avenue, Cleveland, OH 44195, www.clevelandclinic.org. Additional information is available from the Cleveland Clinic Health Information Center, 216-444-3771, toll-free 800-223-2273 extension 43771, or at http://www.clevelandclinic.org/health.

What Is Esophageal Manometry?

Esophageal manometry is a test used to measure the function of the lower esophageal sphincter (the valve that prevents reflux of gastric acid into the esophagus). This test will tell your doctor if your esophagus is able to move food to your stomach normally.

The manometry test is commonly given to people who have:

- Difficulty swallowing;
- Pain when swallowing;
- Heartburn;
- Chest pain;
- Chronic cough or hoarseness.

The Swallowing and Digestive Processes

To know why you might be experiencing a problem with your digestive system, it helps to understand the swallowing and digestive processes.

When you swallow, food moves down your esophagus and into your stomach with the assistance of a wavelike motion called peristalsis. Disruptions in this wavelike motion may cause chest pain or problems with swallowing.

In addition, the muscular valve connecting the esophagus with the stomach, called the esophageal sphincter, prevents food and acid from backing up out of the stomach into the esophagus. If this valve does not work properly, food and stomach acids can enter the esophagus and cause a condition called esophageal reflux (GERD).

Manometry will indicate not only how well the esophagus is able to move food down the esophagus but also how well the esophageal sphincter is working to prevent reflux.

Before the Test

Special Conditions

- Tell the physician if you have a lung or heart condition, have any other diseases, or have allergies to any medications.

Medications

Please follow the following instructions (unless told otherwise by your doctor):

- One day (twenty-four hours) before the test, stop taking:
  - Calcium channel blockers such as Calan, Isoptin (verapamil), Adalat, Pro-cardia (nifedipine), or Cardizem (diltiazem).
  - Nitrate and nitroglycerin products such as Isordil (isosorbide), Nitro-Bid, Nitrodisc, Nitro-Dur, Nitrogard, Transderm-Nitro, or Tridil.
- Twelve hours before the test, do not take sedatives such as Valium (diazepam) or Xanax (alprazolam).
- Do not stop taking any other medication without first talking with your doctor.

Day of Test

Eating and Drinking

- Do not eat or drink anything four to six hours before the test.
- Do not wear perfume or cologne.

During the Test

- You are not sedated, however, a topical anesthetic (pain-relieving medication) will be applied to your nose to make the passage of the tube more comfortable.
- A small (about ¼ inch in diameter), flexible tube is passed through your nose, down your esophagus, and into your stomach. The tube

121

does not interfere with your breathing. You are seated while the tube is inserted.

- You may feel some discomfort as the tube is being placed, but it takes only about a minute to place the tube. Most patients quickly adjust to the tube's presence. Vomiting and coughing are possible when the tube is being placed, but are rare.

- After the tube is inserted, you are asked to lie on your left side. The end of the tube exiting your nose is connected to a machine that records the pressure exerted on the tube. The tube is then slowly withdrawn. Sensors at various locations on the tubing sense the strength of the lower esophageal sphincter. During the test, you will be asked to swallow a small amount of water to evaluate how well the sphincter is working. As the tube is pulled into the esophagus, the sensors measure the strength and coordination of the contractions in the esophagus as you swallow.

- The test lasts twenty to thirty minutes. When the test is over, the tube is removed. The gastroenterologist will interpret the recordings that were made during the test.

After the Test

- Your physician will notify you when the test results are available or will discuss the results with you at your next scheduled appointment.

- You may resume your normal diet and activities and any medications that were withheld for this test.

- You may feel a temporary soreness in your throat. Lozenges or gargling with salt water may help.

- If you think you may be experiencing any unusual symptoms or side effects, call your doctor.

Section 10.2

Gastric Analysis (Stomach Acid Test)

Reprinted from "Gastric Analysis," National Institutes of Health, Warren Grant Magnuson Clinical Center, 1999. Reviewed by David A. Cooke, M.D., August 2005.

This test measures how much acid your stomach makes. For this test, the contents of your stomach will be collected through a nasogastric (stomach) tube.

Preparation

- Do not eat or drink after midnight on the day of the test, until the test is over.

- You may be taking medications that will affect the test results. Your doctor will decide which medications you should stop taking before the test.

- For your comfort during the test, empty your bladder before the test.

- Tell your doctor if you have a deviated septum or have had a broken nose.

Procedure

- The test will be done in your room or in the endoscopy suite.

- A small nasogastric tube will be inserted into your nose. You will swallow this tube into your stomach with sips of water. You may feel pressure at the back of your nose for about five minutes.

- You will be asked to lie on your back or on your left side.

- A nurse will collect the contents of your stomach in a container.

- You may be given medications during the test by injection. You may also have an intravenous (IV) line inserted. Blood samples may also be taken.

- The procedure usually starts early in the morning and lasts two hours or longer, depending on the type of test your doctor ordered.

After the Procedure

After the test, the nasogastric tube will be removed.

If you have questions about the procedure, please ask. Your nurse and doctor are ready to assist you at all times.

Section 10.3

Helicobacter Pylori *Test*

"Helicobacter Pylori: The Test Sample, the Test," © 2005 American Association for Clinical Chemistry. Reprinted with permission. For additional information about clinical testing, visit www.labtestsonline.org.

What is being tested?

These tests are looking for evidence of an infection by a bacterium, known as *Helicobacter pylori*. This bacterium is now known to be a major cause of peptic ulcer disease. *H. pylori* is also associated with the development of gastric cancer.

How is the sample collected for testing?

What is collected depends on the test your doctor orders. It may be as simple as submitting a stool sample to look for the *H. pylori* antigen or a blood sample from your vein to detect antibody to the bacteria.

A more invasive test will require a procedure called an endoscopy, which means putting a tube down the throat into the stomach to take a small piece of tissue (a biopsy) from the stomach lining. A biopsy can be used to detect other reasons for stomach pain, as well as be tested in the laboratory for *H. pylori*. *H. pylori* produces urease, a special enzyme that allows it to survive in the acidic environment of the stomach. The lab can detect the presence of this bacterium by looking for this enzyme in the tissue sample. The tissue may also be examined under a microscope by a pathologist, who will look for these bacteria or any other signs of disease that may explain your symptoms.

Sometimes a breath test can be used instead of a biopsy. You will be asked to drink a special liquid containing a harmless radioactive material. If *H. pylori* is present in your GI tract, the material will be broken down into radio-labeled carbon dioxide gas. By testing the expelled air collected from your breath sample, the laboratory can determine if this organism is in your body.

How is it used?

A positive test for *H. pylori* indicates that your gastrointestinal pain may be caused by this bacterium. Taking antibiotics will kill the bacteria and may stop the pain and the ulceration.

When is it ordered?

If you are experiencing gastrointestinal pain and symptoms of an ulcer, your doctor may order one of the *H. pylori* tests to determine if there is evidence of this disease. These tests may also be ordered after you finish taking the prescribed antibiotics, to prove that the *H. pylori* bacteria are gone from your body. A follow-up test is not performed on every patient.

What does the test result mean?

A positive *H. pylori* test, antibody, antigen, or breath test signifies that you have been infected with this organism. In recent years, scientific data support that this bacteria causes stomach ulcers and appropriate treatment can destroy the bacteria and stop the disease.

Is there anything else I should know?

People have gastrointestinal pain for many reasons—*H. pylori* is only one.

Section 10.4

Celiac Disease Tests

What is being tested?

Celiac disease tests are a group of assays developed to help diagnose celiac disease and a few other gluten-sensitive conditions. These tests detect autoantibodies that the body creates as part of an immune response to dietary proteins (gluten and gliadin) found in wheat, rye, and barley. These autoantibodies cause intestinal inflammation and damage in the lining of the intestinal wall. This causes symptoms associated with malnutrition and malabsorption, such as: diarrhea, weakness, weight loss, abdominal pain, abdominal distention, fatigue, oral ulceration, bleeding tendency, bone and joint pain, and anemia. Adults may also experience depression and a general feeling of illness while children are frequently irritable and may have delayed growth and development.

In the past the only way to diagnose celiac disease was with a biopsy of the small intestine. While this microscopic evaluation is still considered the gold standard and is still used to confirm a diagnosis of celiac disease, the availability of less invasive blood tests used to screen for celiac disease have reduced the number of biopsies needed. Autoantibody blood tests that are available include:

- **Anti-tissue Transglutaminase Antibody (tTG), IgA:** Tissue transglutaminase is an enzyme responsible for cross-linking certain proteins. It has been identified as the antigen that the body responds to when it creates anti-EMA antibodies. Gliadin in grains triggers the development of tTG autoantibodies. Although "tissue" is in the name of this autoantibody, it nevertheless involves testing blood and not tissue.

- **Anti-Endomysial Antibodies (EMA), IgA:** Endomysium is the thin connective tissue layer that covers individual muscle fibers. Anti-endomysial antibodies are developed in reaction to the ongoing damage to the intestinal lining. Almost 100 percent of patients with active celiac disease and 70 percent of patients with dermatitis herpetiformis (another gluten-sensitive enteropathy that causes an itchy burning blistering rash on the skin) will have anti-EMA, IgA antibodies. Anti-tTG and anti-EMA antibodies measure the same tissue damage.

- **Anti-Gliadin Antibodies (AGA), IgG and IgA:** Gliadin is part of the gluten protein found in wheat (similar proteins are found in rye, barley, and oats). AGA is an autoantibody against the gliadin portion. It is created by those who are sensitive to it when they are exposed to gluten over a period of time.

- **Anti-Reticulin Antibodies (ARA), IgA:** Anti-ARA is not ordered as frequently as it once was as it is not as specific or sensitive as the other autoantibodies. It is found in about 60 percent of celiac disease patients and about 25 percent of patients with dermatitis herpetiformis. When used, ARA is ordered along with other celiac disease tests to help diagnose celiac disease.

Each of the celiac blood tests available measures the amount of a particular autoantibody in the blood and is available in both an IgG and an IgA version. IgG and IgA are two of the five classes of antibody proteins that the immune system creates in response to a perceived threat.

While both IgG and IgA types of each autoantibody will be present in the blood, they are not equally specific for celiac disease. In general, the IgA forms of the tests tend to be more specific, and in some cases are used almost exclusively. IgG versions may be ordered either to complement the IgA testing or ordered because someone has an overall deficiency in IgA. This happens about 2 percent of the time with celiac disease and can lead to some false negative test results.

How is the sample collected for testing?

A blood sample is obtained by inserting a needle into a vein in the arm.

How is it used?

Celiac disease tests are used to screen for and help diagnose celiac disease and a few other gluten-sensitive conditions (such as dermatitis herpetiformis). They are usually ordered on those patients with symptoms suggesting celiac disease, but may also be ordered to help rule out celiac disease as a cause for conditions such as anemia and abdominal pain. Since those with celiac disease may also experience conditions such as lactose intolerance, celiac tests may be done in conjunction with other intolerance and allergy testing.

Sometimes celiac testing is ordered to screen for asymptomatic celiac disease in those who have close relatives with celiac disease (about 10 percent of those who have close relatives with celiac disease will develop it themselves) or in those who have other autoimmune diseases (those with autoimmune diseases often have more than one disease).

A doctor may order one or more celiac disease tests, along with tests to evaluate the status and extent of a patient's malnutrition and malabsorption. There are four autoantibodies that are related to celiac disease that can be measured. The doctor will often order an anti-tissue transglutaminase antibody (tTG), IgA first to screen for celiac disease. If this test is positive, it is likely that the patient has celiac disease. The doctor may perform an intestinal biopsy to confirm that there is damage to the intestine. If the anti-tTG is negative but the physician still suspects celiac disease, he may order other tests that include:

- **Anti-Gliadin Antibodies (AGA), IgG and IgA:** These tests are often useful when testing young symptomatic children but they are found in fewer cases of celiac disease than anti-tTG and they can also be positive in other diseases. AGA IgG and IgA are often ordered together so that their results can be compared. If one is positive, both should be—unless the patient has an IgA deficiency. They can be used to monitor dietary compliance.

- **Anti-Endomysial Antibodies (EMA), IgA:** This test is being replaced by the anti-tTG test as they both measure the autoantibodies causing the tissue damage associated with celiac disease. Anti-EMA is, however, still being ordered at this time by many physicians and may be used to monitor dietary compliance.

- **Anti-Reticulin Antibodies (ARA), IgA:** Anti-ARA is not ordered as frequently as it once was as it is not as specific or sensitive as the other autoantibodies. It is found in about 60 percent of celiac disease patients and about 25 percent of patients with dermatitis herpetiformis.

tTG can also be used for monitoring dietary compliance.

These autoantibody tests are often ordered along with other tests to help determine the severity of the disease and the extent of a patient's malnutrition, malabsorption, and organ involvement. Other tests might include a:

- CBC (complete blood count) to look for anemia;
- ESR (erythrocyte sedimentation rate) to evaluate inflammation;
- CRP (C-Reactive protein) to evaluate inflammation;
- CMP (complete metabolic panel) to determine electrolyte, protein, and calcium levels, and to verify the status of the kidney and liver;
- Vitamin D, E, and B_{12} to measure vitamin deficiencies;
- Stool fat, to help evaluate malabsorption.

When is it ordered?

Celiac disease tests are ordered when someone has symptoms suggesting celiac disease, malnutrition, or malabsorption—such as diarrhea, abdominal pain, weakness, fatigue, weight loss, and joint pain. They may be ordered as part of an investigation of anemia, osteoporosis, infertility, or seizures (certain types are linked to celiac disease). In children, celiac disease tests may be ordered when a child exhibits delayed development, short stature, or a failure to thrive.

Asymptomatic people may be tested if they have a close relative with celiac disease, but celiac disease testing is not recommended at this time as a screen for the general population.

Autoantibody levels may also be ordered when a patient with celiac disease has been on a gluten-free diet for a period of time. This is done to verify that antibody levels have decreased and to verify that the diet has been effective in relieving symptoms and reversing the intestinal lining damage (this is sometimes still confirmed with a second biopsy). When a patient's symptoms have not subsided, celiac disease tests may be ordered to check for dietary compliance, and to help the doctor and patient look for either hidden gluten in the patient's diet or for other reasons for his or her unrelieved symptoms.

What does the test result mean?

In general, if your anti-tTG test is positive, then it is likely that you have celiac disease. If the anti-tTG test is negative, then it is most likely that you do not have celiac disease. However, your anti-tTG levels may be very low or undetectable if you have been avoiding wheat, rye, and barley for a period of time or if you are one of the small percentage of patients with celiac disease who are also deficient in IgA. This may lead to a false negative result and may prompt your doctor to do additional testing.

If several of the other autoantibodies are present in high concentrations but tTG is negative, then you may have celiac disease. If only one autoantibody is high, or if one or more are present, but only at low concentrations, then your symptoms may be due to celiac disease or due to another cause. If any of the blood test results are positive (or indeterminate) your doctor will usually do an intestinal biopsy to confirm or rule out celiac disease.

If you have been diagnosed with celiac disease and have removed gluten from your diet, then your autoantibody levels should fall. If they do not, and your symptoms do not diminish, then there may either be hidden forms of gluten in your diet that have not been eliminated (gluten is often found in unexpected places, from salad dressings to cough syrup) or you may have one of the rare forms of celiac disease that does not respond to dietary changes. In most cases, when celiac disease tests are used to monitor progress, rising levels of autoantibodies indicate some form of noncompliance with a gluten-free diet.

If you have changed your diet, eliminating gluten days or weeks prior to visiting your doctor, then your celiac disease may not be detectable. In this case your doctor may do a gluten challenge—have you put gluten back into your diet for several weeks or months to see if the symptoms return, then do a biopsy to check for villous atrophy (damage to the villi in your intestine).

Is there anything else I should know?

Although celiac disease is relatively common—about one in three hundred people in the United States are thought to be affected—most people who have the disease are not aware of it. This is partly due to the fact that the symptoms are variable—they may be mild or even absent, even when intestinal damage is present on biopsied tissue. Since these symptoms may also be due to a variety of other conditions, a diagnosis of celiac disease may be missed or delayed—sometimes for years.

Section 10.5

Diagnostic Laparoscopy

Definition

Diagnostic laparoscopy is a procedure that allows a health care provider to look directly at the contents of a patient's abdomen or pelvis, including the fallopian tubes, ovaries, uterus, small bowel, large bowel, appendix, liver, and gallbladder.

The purpose of this examination is to actually see if a problem exists that has not been found with noninvasive tests. Inflammation of the gallbladder (cholecystitis), appendix (appendicitis), pelvic organs (pelvic inflammatory disease), or tumors of the ovaries may be diagnosed laparoscopically.

Additionally, the provider may wish to exclude abdominal trauma following an accident by using laparoscopy rather than a large abdominal incision.

Major procedures to treat cancer, such as surgery to remove an organ, may begin with laparoscopy to exclude the presence of additional tumors (metastatic disease), which would change the course of treatment.

How the Test Is Performed

The procedure is usually done in the hospital or outpatient surgical center under general anesthesia (while the patient is unconscious and pain-free). However, this procedure may also be done using local anesthesia, which merely numbs the area affected by the surgery and allows the patient to stay awake.

A small incision is made below the navel, a needle is inserted into the incision, and carbon dioxide gas is injected to elevate the abdominal wall, creating a larger space to work in. This allows for easier viewing and manipulation of the organs. A tube called a trocar is inserted through the incision, which allows passage of a tiny video camera into the abdomen.

The laparoscope is then inserted so that the organs of the pelvis and abdomen can be examined. Additional small incisions may be made for instruments that allow the surgeon to move organs for a clearer view.

In the case of gynecologic laparoscopy, dye may be injected through the cervical canal to make the fallopian tubes easier to view.

Following the examination, the laparoscope is removed, the incisions are closed, and bandages are applied.

How to Prepare for the Test

Do not consume any food or fluid for eight hours before the test. You must sign a consent form.

Infants and Children

The preparation you can provide for this test depends on your child's age, previous experiences, and level of trust.

How the Test Will Feel

If you are under general anesthesia, you will feel no pain during the procedure, although the incisions may throb and be slightly painful afterward. A pain reliever may be given by your physician.

With local anesthesia, you may feel a prick and a burning sensation when the local anesthetic is given. Pain may occur at the incision site. The laparoscope may cause pressure, but there should be no pain during the procedure. Afterward, the incision site may throb for several hours and may be slightly painful. A pain reliever may be given by your physician.

Additionally, you may experience shoulder pain for a few days, because the carbon dioxide can irritate the diaphragm, which shares some of the same nerves as the shoulder. You may also experience an increased urge to urinate, since the gas can put pressure on the bladder.

Why the Test Is Performed

The examination helps identify the cause of pain in the abdomen and pelvic area. It may detect the following conditions:

* Endometriosis (tissues normally found in the uterus growing in other areas)

- Ectopic pregnancy (in which the fertilized egg develops outside of the uterus)
- Pelvic inflammatory disease (an inflammation in the pelvic cavity)
- Cancer
- Cholecystitis
- Appendicitis

Normal Values

There is no blood in the abdomen, no hernias, no intestinal obstruction, and no cancer in any visible organs. The uterus, fallopian tubes, and ovaries are of normal size, shape, and color. The liver is normal.

What Abnormal Results Mean

The procedure may detect the following:

- Ovarian cysts
- Abnormal union of body surfaces (such as adhesions following prior surgery)
- Endometriosis
- Uterine fibroids
- Tumors
- Pelvic inflammatory disease
- Appendicitis
- Cholecystitis
- Metastatic cancer
- Signs of trauma

What the Risks Are

There is a risk of puncturing an organ, which could cause leakage of intestinal contents, or bleeding into the abdominal cavity. These complications may result in the conversion of laparoscopy to open surgery (laparotomy).

There is also some risk of infection. However, antibiotics are usually given as a precaution.

Section 10.6

Fecal Occult Blood Tests

"Stool Guaiac Test," and "Flushable Reagent Stool Blood Test,"
both © 2005 A.D.A.M., Inc. Reprinted with permission.

Stool Guaiac Test

Alternative Names

Guaiac smear test; fecal occult blood test—guaiac smear; stool occult blood test— guaiac smear

Definition

The stool guaiac test is a test that detects the presence of hidden (occult) blood in the stool (bowel movement). The stool guaiac is the most common form of fecal occult blood test (FOBT) in use today.

Brand names include Hemoccult, Hemoccult SENSA, Coloscreen, Coloscreen-ES, Seracult, and Seracult Plus®.

How the Test Is Performed

A stool sample from three consecutive bowel movements is collected, smeared on a card, and mailed to a laboratory for processing. In order to ensure the accuracy of the guaiac test, it is important to follow, whenever available, the manufacturer's instruction on how to collect the stool.

Adults and Children: There are many ways to collect the samples. You can catch the stool on plastic wrap that is loosely placed over the toilet bowl and held in place by the toilet seat. Then put the sample in a clean container. One test kit supplies a special toilet tissue that you use to collect the sample, then put the sample in a clean container. Do not sample stool specimen from within the toilet bowl water, as this can cause measurement errors.

Infants and Young Children: For children wearing diapers, you can line the diaper with plastic wrap. If the plastic wrap is positioned so that it isolates the stool from any urine output, mixing of urine and stool can be prevented for a better sample.

Laboratory procedures may vary. In one type of test, a small sample of stool is placed on a paper card. A drop or two of testing solution is applied to the opposite side of the card. A color change indicates the presence of blood in the stool.

How to Prepare for the Test

Do not consume red meat, any blood-containing food, cantaloupe, uncooked broccoli, turnip, radish, or horseradish for three days prior to the test.

You may need to discontinue drugs that can interfere with the test such as vitamin C and aspirin if possible. Check with your health care provider regarding medication changes that may be necessary. Never discontinue or decrease any medication without consulting your health care provider.

How the Test Will Feel

Because this test involves normal bowel functions, there is no discomfort.

Why the Test Is Performed

This test is a screening test to detect blood in the gastrointestinal tract.

Normal Values

A negative test result is normal.

What Abnormal Results Mean

Abnormal results may indicate:

- Colon polyps;
- Colon cancer or other gastrointestinal (GI) tumors;
- Esophagitis;
- Gastritis;
- GI trauma or bleeding from recent GI surgery;
- Hemorrhoids;

- Inflammatory bowel disease;
- Peptic ulcer;
- Angiodysplasia of the GI tract;
- GI infections;
- Esophageal varices and portal hypertensive gastropathy.

Additional non-GI related causes of positive guaiac test may include:

- Nose bleed;
- Coughing up blood.

Abnormal tests require follow-up with your physician.

What the Risks Are

There can be false-positive and false-negative results. Using proper stool collection technique, avoiding certain drugs, and observing dietary restrictions can minimize these measurement errors.

Flushable Reagent Stool Blood Test

Alternative Names

Stool occult blood test—flushable home test; fecal occult blood test—flushable home test

Definition

This is a test performed at home with disposable pads that detects the presence of hidden (occult) blood in the stool. The pads are available at drugstores without a prescription.
Brand names include EZ-Detect™ and ColoCARE.

How the Test Is Performed

There is no direct handling of stool with this test. You simply note any changes on a card and then mail the results card to your physician.
Urinate if you need to, then flush the toilet before you defecate. After the bowel movement, place the chemically treated tissue pad in the toilet. Watch for a change of color on the test area of the pad (results usually appear within two minutes). Repeat for two more

consecutive bowel movements. Note the results on the card provided. Then flush the pad away.

The different tests have different methods to check for water quality. Check the package for instructions.

How to Prepare for the Test

Some drugs may interfere with this test.

Check with your health care provider regarding medication changes that may be necessary. Never discontinue or decrease any medication without consulting your health care provider.

Check package instructions for dietary restrictions.

How the Test Will Feel

This test involves only normal bowel functions, and there is no discomfort.

Why the Test Is Performed

This test is mainly performed for colorectal cancer screening. It may also be recommended in the evaluation of anemia.

Normal Values

A negative result is normal.

What Abnormal Results Mean

Abnormal results of the flushable test may indicate the same issues as the guaiac smear test:

- Colon polyps
- Colon cancer or other GI (gastrointestinal) tumors
- Esophagitis
- Gastritis
- GI trauma or bleeding from recent GI surgery
- Hemorrhoids
- Inflammatory bowel disease
- Peptic ulcer
- Angiodysplasia of the GI tract

- GI infections
- Esophageal varices and portal hypertensive gastropathy

Additional non-GI related causes of positive guaiac test may include:

- Nose bleed;
- Coughing up blood.

Abnormal test results require follow-up with your physician.

What the Risks Are

There can be false-positive or false-negative results. These are similar as for the traditional guaiac smear tests.

Chapter 11

Common Gastrointestinal Surgical Procedures

Chapter Contents

139

Section 11.1

Frequently Asked Questions about Ostomy Surgery

As always, in order to obtain answers to your individually specific questions, be sure to consult with your doctor or ostomy nurse for help.

Who should I tell? What should I say about my surgery?

You should tell those who need to know, such as healthcare providers, your spouse or significant others, and people who are involved in your recuperative care.

You need not feel you have to explain your surgery to everyone who asks. Those who are just curious need to know only that you had abdominal surgery, or that you had part or all of your colon or bladder removed.

If you are considering marriage, thorough discussions with your future spouse about life with an ostomy and its effect on sex, children, and family acceptance will help alleviate misconceptions and fear on the part of the spouse.

If you have children, answer their questions simply and truthfully. A simple explanation will be enough for them. You may want to confide in your employer or a good friend at work because keeping it a complete secret may cause practical difficulties.

Will I be able to continue my daily activities once I recover from surgery?

As your strength returns, you can go back to your regular activities. Most people can return to their previous line of work; however, communicate with your healthcare team about your daily routines, so they can assist you in returning to maximum health as early as possible.

An ostomy should not limit your participation in sports. Many physicians do not allow contact sports because of possible injury to the stoma from a severe blow or because the pouching system may slip, but these problems can be overcome with special ostomy supplies. Weight lifting may result in a hernia at the stoma. Check with your doctor about such sports. There are many people who are distance runners, skiers, swimmers, and participants in many other types of athletics.

What about showering and bathing? Should I bathe with or without my pouch?

You may bathe with or without your pouching system in place. If you wish to take a shower or bath with your pouch off, you can do so. Normal exposure to air or contact with soap and water will not harm the stoma, and water does not enter the opening. Choose a time for bathing when the bowel is less active. You can also leave your pouch on while bathing.

What can I eat? Will I need to change my diet?

There may be some modifications in your diet according to the type of ostomy surgery.

People with colostomy and ileostomy surgery should return to their normal diet after a period of adjustment. Introduce foods back into your diet a little at a time and monitor the effect of each food on the ostomy function. Chew your food well and drink plenty of fluids. Some less digestible or high roughage foods are more likely to create potential for blockage problems (i.e., corn, coconut, mushrooms, nuts, raw fruits and vegetables).

There are no eating restrictions as a result of urostomy surgery. Urostomates should drink plenty of liquids each day following the healthcare team's recommendations.

Will I be able to wear the same clothes as before?

Whatever you wore before surgery, you can wear afterward with very few exceptions. Many pouching systems are made today that are unnoticeable even when wearing the most stylish, form fitting clothing for men and women.

Depending on your stoma location you might find belts uncomfortable or restrictive. Some people choose to wear higher or looser waistbands on trousers and skirts.

Cotton knit or stretch underpants or panty hose may give the support and security you need. Some men find that jockey type shorts help support the pouch.

Women may want to choose a swimsuit that has a lining to provide a smoother profile. Stretch panties (with Lycra) can also be worn under a swimsuit to add support and smooth out any bulges or outlines. Men may prefer to wear a tank shirt and trunks if the stoma is above the belt line.

What about sex and intimacy? Will I be able to get pregnant after surgery?

Sexual relationships and intimacy are important and fulfilling aspects of your life that should continue after ostomy surgery. Your attitude is a key factor in re-establishing sexual expression and intimacy. A period of adjustment after surgery is to be expected. Sexual function in women is usually not impaired, while sexual potency of men may sometimes be affected, usually only temporarily. Discuss any problems with your physician or ostomy nurse.

Your ability to conceive does not change, and pregnancy and delivery should be normal after ostomy surgery. However, if you are thinking about becoming pregnant, you should first check with your doctor about any other health problems.

Is travel possible?

All methods of travel are open to you. Many people with ostomies travel extensively, from camping trips to cruises to plane excursions around the world. Take along enough supplies to last the entire trip plus some extra, double what you think you may need. Checked luggage sometimes gets lost, so carry an extra pouching system and other supplies on the plane with you. When traveling by car, keep your supplies in the coolest part, and avoid the trunk or back window ledge. Seat belts will not harm the stoma when adjusted comfortably.

When traveling abroad, take an adequate amount of supplies, referral lists for physicians and medical centers, and some medication to control any diarrhea and stop the fluid and electrolyte loss. When going through customs or luggage inspection, a note from your doctor stating that you need to carry ostomy supplies and medications by hand may be helpful.

What about medications? Can I take vitamins?

Absorption may vary with individuals and types of medication. Certain drug problems may arise depending on the type of ostomy you have and the medications you are taking. Make sure all your healthcare providers know the type of ostomy you have and the location of the stoma. This information will help your pharmacist and other health-care providers monitor your situation (i.e., time-released and enteric coated medications may pass through the system of ileostomates too quickly to be effective).

Will I always be wearing the same size and type of pouch?

The type of pouching system that was used in the hospital may need to be changed as the healing process takes place. Your stoma may shrink and may require a change in the size opening of your pouch. Your lifestyle may necessitate a change of the pouching system after a recuperative period. Make an appointment with your ostomy nurse to evaluate your management system.

Got any tips on emptying the pouch?

Check the pouch occasionally to see if it needs emptying before it gets too full and causes a leakage problem. Always empty prior to go-ing out of the house and away from a convenient toilet. Most people find the easiest way to empty the pouch is to sit on the toilet with the pouch between the legs. Hold the bottom of the pouch up and remove the clamp. Slowly unroll the tail of the pouch into the toilet. Clean the outside and inside of the pouch tail with toilet paper. Replace the clamp.

How often should I change the pouch?

The adhesiveness and durability of pouching systems vary. Any-where from three to seven days is to be expected. Itching or burning are signs that the wafer should be changed. Changing too frequently or wearing one too long may be damaging to the skin.

What should I do if hospitalized again?

Take your ostomy supplies with you since the hospital may not have your brand in supply. If you are in doubt about any procedure, ask to talk to your doctor.

Ask to have the following information listed on your chart:

1. Type of ostomy or continent diversion

2. Whether or not your rectum is intact

3. Detailed description of your management routine and a list of the ostomy products used

4. **For urinary stomas:** Instructions not to take a urine specimen from the urostomy pouch, but to use a catheter inserted into the stoma

Where can I purchase supplies?

Supplies may be ordered from a mail order company or from a medical supply or pharmacy in your town. Check the Yellow Pages under "Ostomy Supplies," "Surgical Supplies," or "Hospital Supplies."

Does insurance cover the cost of ostomy supplies?

Medicare Part B covers ostomy equipment. Medicare allows only a predetermined maximum quantity each month.

Medicaid is the federal/state insurance of last resort for low-income persons. Check with the state Medicaid office for specifics.

Most individual health insurance plans typically will pay you 80 percent of the "reasonable and customary" costs after the deductible is met.

When should I seek medical assistance?

You should call the doctor or ostomy nurse when you have:

- severe cramps lasting more than two or three hours;
- a deep cut in the stoma;
- excessive bleeding from the stoma opening (or a moderate amount in the pouch at several emptyings);
- continuous bleeding at the junction between the stoma and skin;
- severe skin irritation or deep ulcers;
- unusual change in stoma size and appearance;
- severe watery discharge lasting more than five or six hours;
- continuous nausea and vomiting;
- or if the ostomy does not have any output for four to six hours and is accompanied by cramping and nausea..

Section 11.2

Colostomy

© 2005 A.D.A.M., Inc. Reprinted with permission.

Alternative Names

Intestinal opening

Definition

Colostomy is a surgical procedure that creates an opening (stoma) on the abdomen for the drainage of stool from the large intestine (colon). The procedure is usually done after bowel resections or injuries and it may be temporary or permanent.

Description

The procedure is done while the patient is under general anesthesia (unconscious and pain-free). An incision is made in the abdomen and the bowel resection or repair is performed as needed.

For the colostomy, the proximal (nearer to the small intestine) end of the healthy bowel tissue is then passed through the abdominal wall, and the edges are stitched to the skin of the abdominal wall. An adhesive drainage bag (stoma appliance) is placed around the opening. The abdominal incision is closed.

Indications

There are a number of reasons to perform a colostomy:

- When the lower large intestine, rectum, or anus is unable to function normally

- When the lower large intestine, rectum, or anus needs rest from normal functions

- When infection or contamination from stool within the resected colon would prevent healing

Whether a colostomy is temporary or permanent depends on the disease process or injury being treated. In most cases, colostomies are temporary and can be closed with another operation at a later date. If a large portion of the bowel is removed, or if the distal (far) end of the colon is too diseased to be reconnected to the proximal intestine, the colostomy may be permanent.

Risks

Risks for any anesthesia are:

- Reactions to medications;
- Problems breathing.

Risks for any surgery are:

- Bleeding;
- Infection.

Additional risks are:

- Narrowing or obstruction of the colostomy opening (stoma);
- Development of a hernia at the incision site;
- Skin irritation.

Expectations after Surgery

The colostomy functions to drain stool (feces) from the colon into the colostomy bag. Most colostomy stool is softer and more liquid than normally passed stool. The degree of liquidity of the stool depends on the location of the intestinal segment used to form the colostomy.

Convalescence

Hospital stay is usually seven to ten days. After two to four days, the patient will be able to resume eating. Complete healing may take one to two months. Learning to clean the abdomen and change the colostomy bag will be necessary. Most people can eventually change the bag at regular and convenient times.

Section 11.3

Ileostomy

An ileostomy is a surgically created opening in the abdominal wall through which digested food passes. The end of the ileum (the lowest part of the small intestine) is brought through the abdominal wall to form a stoma. An ileostomy may be performed when a disease or injured colon cannot be treated successfully with medicine.

Reasons for Surgery

Ulcerative colitis, Crohn disease, familial polyposis

Care of Ileostomy

A pouching system is worn. Pouches are odor free and different manufacturers have disposable or reusable varieties to fit your lifestyle. Ostomy supplies are available at drugstores, at ostomy supply houses, and through the mail.

Living with an Ileostomy

Work: With the possible exception of jobs requiring very heavy lifting, an ileostomy should not interfere with work. People with ileostomies are successful business people, teachers, carpenters, welders, and so on.

Sex and Social Life: Physically, the creation of an ileostomy usually does not affect sexual function. If there is a problem, it is almost always related to the removal of the rectum. The ileostomy itself should not interfere with normal sexual activity or pregnancy. It does not prevent one from dating, marriage, or having children.

Clothing: Usually one is able to wear the same clothing as before surgery, including swimwear.

147

Sports and Activities: With a securely attached pouch one can swim, camp out, play baseball, and participate in practically all types of sports. Caution is advised in heavy body contact sports. Travel is not restricted in any way. Bathing and showering may be done with or without the pouch in place.

Diet: Usually there are no dietary restrictions and foods can be enjoyed as before.

Section 11.4

Ileoanal Reservoir (Pouch) Surgery

"Overview of Ileoanal Reservoir (Pouch) Surgery" by Linda B. Hurd, RN, MSN, © 2004. Reprinted with permission of the author.

The ileoanal reservoir procedure is a surgical treatment option for chronic ulcerative colitis, colon cancer, and familial polyposis patients who need to have their large intestine (colon) removed. An ileoanal reservoir (or pouch) is an internal pouch formed of small intestine. This pouch provides a storage place for stool in the absence of the large intestine. Anal sphincter muscles assist in holding in the stool. Several times a day, stool is passed through the anus.

Ileoanal reservoir surgery is a widely accepted surgical treatment for ulcerative colitis or familial polyposis because it eliminates the disease, gives the patient control of bowel movements, and does not require a permanent ileostomy. Each patient considering this surgery is carefully evaluated to determine if this procedure is appropriate for them. This procedure is performed in one, two, or three stages, but is most often done in two stages, usually two to three months apart.

Stage 1

The first surgery removes the entire large bowel and the lining of the rectum, but leaves the rectal muscle intact. A reservoir or "pouch" is made out of small intestine and then is connected to the anus. Next, a temporary ileostomy is made. An ileostomy is a surgically created opening between the small bowel and the skin of the abdomen through which stool and gas are passed. This temporary ileostomy diverts the stool, protecting the reservoir (pouch) while it heals.

What to Expect after the First Surgery

In the initial weeks after surgery, waste material coming through the ileostomy is liquid but then begins to thicken. A good diet with increased fluid intake is needed to keep well hydrated and nourished. Patients wear an ileostomy appliance over the ileostomy that collects the waste as it passes through the ostomy (or opening) on the abdomen. Learning to care for the ileostomy is a little tricky but with practice becomes very manageable. Patients also may occasionally pass small amounts of mucus or blood through the rectum.

Approximately four to six weeks after the first surgery, an x-ray study of the pouch is performed. If the study shows that the pouch is healed, then the second surgery can be scheduled.

Stage 2

The second surgery (usually done two to three months after the first) "takes down" or removes the ileostomy and reconnects the bowel. The pouch now becomes functional so that waste passes into the pouch, where it is stored. When an "urge" is felt, the stool can be passed through the anus, out of the body.

In most cases, the second surgery can be done at the ileostomy site without reopening the first incision. The skin at the former ileostomy site is usually left to close on its own.

What to Expect after the Second Surgery

Once a patient starts passing stool through the anus, stools are frequent and liquid. There may be accompanying urgency and leakage of stool. All of these aspects improve over time as the anal sphincter muscles strengthen and the pouch adapts to its new function. Stools become thicker as the small intestine absorbs more water. In addition, medications to decrease bowel activity and bulk-forming agents to thicken the stool may be prescribed.

Patients can help during this adaptation process by avoiding foods that may cause gas, diarrhea, and anal irritation. Careful skin care around the anus will protect the skin from the irritation of frequent stools. Continuing anal sphincter muscle exercises (Kegel exercises) during this time are also beneficial.

After six months, most people can expect about five to six semi-formed bowel movements during the day and one at night. The pouch takes up to one year to fully adapt. In most patients, functioning of the pouch continues to improve over time.

General Considerations

When considering and undergoing this surgery, all patients and their loved ones have concerns and questions. Sometimes they feel isolated and frightened. It is helpful for all involved to receive general information about this surgery and understand what to expect during the course of these procedures. In addition, patients and family members may be interested in contacting an ileoanal support group, which provides a place to learn more about this surgery and to meet others with similar concerns and experiences. Be sure to talk with your gastroenterologist, surgeon, or ET nurse about these issues and keep in close contact with them during the surgeries and throughout the rehabilitation process. Patient satisfaction with this surgery is high and with both ulcerative colitis and familial polyposis patients, their disease is cured!

Section 11.5

Percutaneous Endoscopic Gastrostomy (PEG)

What is a PEG?

PEG stands for percutaneous endoscopic gastrostomy, a procedure through which a flexible feeding tube is placed through the abdominal wall and into the stomach. It allows nutrition, fluids, or medications to be put directly into the stomach, bypassing the mouth and esophagus. This section will give you a basic understanding of the procedure—how it's performed, how it can help, and what side effects you might experience. It can't answer all of your questions, since a lot depends on the individual patient and the doctor's professional judgment. Please ask your doctor about anything you don't understand.

How is the PEG performed?

Your doctor will use a lighted flexible tube called an endoscope to guide the creation of a small opening through the skin of the abdomen and directly into the stomach. This procedure allows the doctor to place and secure a feeding tube into the stomach. Patients generally receive a mild sedative and local anesthesia, and an antibiotic is given by vein prior to the procedure. Patients can usually go home the day of the procedure or the next day.

Who can benefit from a PEG?

Patients who have difficulty swallowing, problems with their appetite, or an inability to take enough nutrition through the mouth can benefit from this procedure.

How should I care for the PEG tube?

A dressing will be placed on the PEG site following the procedure. This dressing is usually removed after one or two days. After that you should clean the site once a day with diluted soap and water and keep the site dry between cleansings. No special dressing or covering is needed.

How are feedings given? Can I still eat and drink?

Liquid nutritional supplements are given through the PEG tube using a large syringe, a gravity drip using a tube connected to a hanging plastic bag, or a mechanical pump. Your doctor or other health care provider will give you complete instructions and a demonstration. A PEG does not prevent a patient from eating or drinking, but your doctor and you might decide to limit eating or drinking depending on any associated medical conditions.

Are there complications from PEG placement?

Complications can occur with the PEG placement. Possible complications include pain at the PEG site, leakage of stomach contents around the tube site, and dislodgment or malfunction of the tube. Possible complications include infection of the PEG site, aspiration (inhalation of gastric contents into the lungs), bleeding and perforation (an unwanted hole in the bowel wall). Your doctor can describe for you symptoms that could indicate a possible complication.

How long do these tubes last? How are they removed?

PEG tubes can last for months or years. However, because they can break down or become clogged over extended periods of time, they might need to be replaced. Your doctor can easily remove or replace a tube without sedatives or anesthesia, although your doctor might opt to use sedation and endoscopy in some cases. Your doctor will pull out the tube using firm traction and will either insert a new tube or let the opening close if no replacement is needed. PEG sites close quickly once the tube is removed, so accidental dislodgment requires immediate attention.

Section 11.6

Gastric Bypass

© 2005 A.D.A.M., Inc. Reprinted with permission.

Alternative Names

Bariatric surgery—gastric bypass; Roux-en-Y gastric bypass

Definition

Gastric bypass surgery is one type of procedure that can be used to cause significant weight loss if you are very obese. The surgery reduces your body's intake of calories.

Calorie reduction is accomplished in two ways:

1. After the surgery, your stomach is smaller. You feel full faster and learn to reduce the amount that you eat at any given time.

2. Part of your stomach and small intestines are literally bypassed (skipped over) so that fewer calories are absorbed. Unfortunately, sometimes nutrients are lost as well.

The surgery is only right for you if you meet certain strict criteria described later in this section.

Description

Prior to any weight loss operation, your doctor will give you a complete medical examination and evaluate your overall health.

A psychological evaluation will be given to you. This will determine whether you are ready to adhere to a healthier lifestyle. If you are not ready to make lifestyle changes (and have not tried hard to do so already), you will not be considered eligible for the procedure. Without changing your lifestyle, the surgery will not be a success.

You will also receive extensive nutritional counseling before (and after) your surgery.

The surgery is performed under anesthesia. There are two basic steps:

Step 1: The first step in the surgical procedure makes your stomach smaller. The surgeon divides the stomach into a small upper section and a larger bottom section using staples that are similar to stitches. The top section of the stomach (called the pouch) will hold your food.

Step 2: After the stomach has been divided, the surgeon connects a section of the small intestine to the pouch. When you eat, the food will now travel from the pouch through this new connection ("Roux limb"), bypassing the lower portion of the stomach. The surgeon will then reconnect the base of the Roux limb with the remaining portion of the small intestines from the bottom of the stomach, forming a y-shape.

This "y-connection" allows food to mix with pancreatic fluid and bile, aiding the absorption of important vitamins and minerals. You still may experience poor absorption of certain nutrients.

The risk of malabsorption is of greater concern in gastric surgeries that skip over a larger portion of the small intestines. These are performed much less commonly than the Roux-en-Y gastric bypass as described.

Laparoscopy

Gastric bypass can be performed using a laparoscope. This less-invasive technique allows the surgeon to make smaller incisions, which lowers the risk of large scars and hernias after the procedure.

First, small incisions are made in your abdomen. The surgeon passes slender surgical instruments through these narrow openings. The surgeon also passes a camera (laparoscope) through one of these small openings and watches through a lens and video monitor to do the surgery.

Types of Weight Loss Surgeries

Weight loss surgery can be divided into three types:

- **Restrictive procedures** reduce the size of your stomach.

- **Malabsorptive procedures** alter the flow from your stomach to your intestine, causing poor absorption of calories, vitamins, and minerals in the intestine.

- **Combination procedures** involve characteristics of both restrictive and malabsorptive procedures.

Gastric bypass surgeries are combination procedures that use both restriction and malabsorption to achieve weight loss.

Because it is a combination approach, it tends to be more successful for weight loss than purely restrictive surgeries. However, your body may not absorb vitamins and minerals properly.

Restrictive-only procedures are not as successful. It is easy to "cheat" and eat too much food, over-stretching the newly created stomach pouch.

Indications

Gastric bypass surgery may be an option if you are significantly obese and have tried unsuccessfully to lose weight on diet and exercise programs and are unlikely to lose weight successfully with non-surgical methods.

Gastric bypass surgery is not a "quick fix" for obesity. The surgery can take several hours and has risks and possible complications. For example, vomiting following the surgery is not uncommon because of eating more than the new, small stomach can accommodate.

Your commitment to diet and exercise must be very strong because even after the surgery, you must adhere to these lifestyle changes. Otherwise, complications from the surgery are likely to develop.

The procedure may be considered for obese individuals who have:

- A body mass index (BMI) of 40 or more. BMI is a calculation based on height and weight that is used to determine whether you are of normal weight or are overweight. Someone with a BMI of 40 or more is at least one hundred pounds over their recommended weight. A normal BMI is between 18.5 and 25.

- A BMI of 35 or more along with a life-threatening illness that can be made better with weight loss, such as sleep apnea, type 2 diabetes, and heart disease.

Laparoscopy

Not everyone is a candidate for the laparoscopic (minimally invasive) approach. If you weigh more than 350 pounds or if you have had abdominal surgery in the past, you are probably *not* a good candidate for laparoscopy. Your surgeon will determine the best and safest approach for you.

Risks

The risks of gastric bypass surgery include:

- Bleeding;
- Infections;
- Follow-up surgeries to correct complications, or to remove excess skin;
- Gallstones due to significant weight loss in a short amount of time;
- Gastritis (inflammation of the lining of the stomach);
- Vomiting from eating more than the stomach pouch can hold;
- Iron or vitamin B_{12} deficiencies (if they occur) can lead to anemia;
- Calcium deficiency (if it occurs) can contribute to the development of early osteoporosis or other bone disorders.

Follow-up surgeries may be less likely if gastric bypass is performed with a laparoscope.

Another common complication from gastric bypass is "dumping syndrome." The symptoms often include:

- Nausea and vomiting;
- Diarrhea;
- Bloated feeling;
- Dizziness;
- Sweating.

You can lessen these symptoms by following your dietitian's guidelines very carefully, especially during the first two months after surgery.

Expectations after Surgery

The weight loss results of gastric bypass surgery are generally good. Most patients lose an average of ten pounds per month and reach a stable weight between eighteen and twenty-four months after surgery. Often, the greatest rate of weight loss occurs in the very beginning (that is, just following the surgery when you are still on a liquid diet).

After the surgery, you will need to follow up with your doctor fairly often during the first year. During those visits, your physician will be evaluating your physical and mental health status, including any change in weight and your nutritional needs. You will likely see a dietitian during those visits as well.

The surgery is not a solution in and of itself. While it can train you to eat smaller quantities and feel full more quickly, you still have to do much of the work. To achieve weight loss and avoid complications from the procedure, you must exercise and eat properly—according to important, healthy guidelines that your doctor and nutritionist will teach you.

Convalescence

You will usually need to stay in the hospital for four to five days after gastric bypass surgery. Your doctor will approve your discharge to home once you can do the following:

- Move without too much discomfort
- Eat liquid or pureed food without vomiting
- No longer require pain medication given by injection

You will remain on liquid or pureed food for several weeks after the surgery. Even after that time, you will feel full very quickly, sometimes only being able to take a few bites of solid food. This is because the new stomach pouch initially only holds a tablespoonful of food. The pouch eventually expands. However, it will hold no more than about one cup of thoroughly chewed food (a normal stomach can hold up to one quart).

Upon follow up, your doctor will determine if you need replacement of iron, calcium, vitamin B_{12}, or other nutrients. Supplements, such as a multivitamin with minerals, will be prescribed to provide any nutrients that you may not be getting from your diet. This lack of nutrients can occur because you are eating less and because the food moves through your digestive system more quickly.

Once your diet begins to consist of more solid food, remember to chew each bite very slowly and thoroughly.

You will be instructed on eating small meals frequently throughout the day, rather than large meals that your stomach cannot accommodate.

Your new stomach probably won't be able to handle both solid food and fluids at the same time. So, you should separate fluid and food intake by at least thirty minutes and only sip what you are drinking.

You won't be able to tolerate large amounts of fat, alcohol, or sugar. You should reduce your fat intake, especially fast food meals, deep-fried foods, and high-fat foods, as well as high-sugar foods like cakes, cookies, and candy.

Exercise and the support of others (for example, joining a support group with people who have undergone weight loss surgery) are extremely important to help you lose weight and maintain that loss following gastric bypass. You can generally resume exercise six weeks after the operation. Even sooner than that, you will be able to take short walks at a comfortable pace, with the approval and guidance of your doctor. Exercise improves your metabolism, while both exercise and attending a group support can boost your self-esteem and help you stay motivated.

Part Three

Disorders of the Upper Gastrointestinal Tract

Chapter 12

Dyspepsia

What is dyspepsia?

Dyspepsia is a pain or an uncomfortable feeling in the upper middle part of your stomach. The pain might come and go, but it's usually there most of the time.

People of any age can get dyspepsia. Both men and women get it. About one of every four persons gets dyspepsia at some time.

What are the signs of dyspepsia?

Here are some of the signs of dyspepsia:

- A gnawing or burning stomach pain
- Bloating (a feeling of fullness in your stomach)
- Heartburn (stomach contents coming back up into your throat)
- Upset stomach (nausea)
- Vomiting
- Burping

If you have these signs, or any kind of stomach pain or discomfort, talk to your family doctor.

Reproduced with permission from "Dyspepsia: What It Is and What to Do about It," February 2003, http://familydoctor.org/474.xml, updated March 2005. © 2005 American Academy of Family Physicians. All rights reserved.

What causes dyspepsia?

Often, dyspepsia is caused by a stomach ulcer or acid reflux disease. If you have acid reflux disease, stomach acid backs up into your esophagus (the tube leading from your mouth to your stomach). This causes pain in your chest. Your doctor may do some tests to find out if you have an ulcer or acid reflux disease.

If you have dyspepsia, your doctor will ask if you take certain medicines. Some medicines, like anti-inflammatory medicines, can cause dyspepsia.

Rarely, dyspepsia is caused by stomach cancer, so you should take this problem seriously. Sometimes no cause of dyspepsia can be found.

Is dyspepsia a serious condition?

Most often, medicine can take care of this condition.

Sometimes dyspepsia can be the sign of a serious problem—for example, a deep stomach ulcer.

If you have dyspepsia, talk to your family doctor. This is especially important if any one of the following is true for you:

- You're over fifty years of age
- You recently lost weight without trying to
- You have trouble swallowing
- You have severe vomiting
- You have black, tarry bowel movements
- You can feel a mass in your stomach area

How is dyspepsia treated?

If you have a stomach ulcer, it can be cured. You may need to take an acid-blocking medicine. If you have an infection in your stomach, you may also need to take an antibiotic.

If your doctor thinks that a medicine you're taking causes your dyspepsia, you might take another medicine.

A medicine that cuts down on the amount of acid in your stomach might help your pain. This medicine can also help if you have acid reflux disease.

Your doctor might want you to have an endoscopy if:

- You still have stomach pain after you take a dyspepsia medicine for eight weeks.

- The pain goes away for a while but comes back again.

In an endoscopy, a small tube with a camera inside it is put into your mouth and down into your stomach. Then your doctor can look inside your stomach to try to find a cause for your pain.

Do the medicines for dyspepsia have side effects?

The medicines for dyspepsia most often have only minor side effects that go away on their own. Some medicines can make your tongue or stools black. Some cause headaches, nausea, or diarrhea.

If you have side effects that make it hard for you to take medicine for dyspepsia, talk to your family doctor. Your doctor may have you take a different medicine or may suggest something you can do to make the side effects less bothersome.

Remember to take medicines just the way your doctor tells you. If you need to take an antibiotic, take all of the pills, even when you start feeling better.

Can I do anything else to avoid dyspepsia?

You can do quite a bit to help yourself feel better:

- If you smoke, stop smoking.
- If some foods bother your stomach, try to avoid eating them.
- Try to reduce the stress in your life.
- If you have acid reflux, don't eat right before bedtime. Raising the head of your bed with blocks under two legs may also help.
- Unless your doctor tells you otherwise, don't take a lot of anti-inflammatory medicines like ibuprofen, aspirin, naproxen (brand name: Aleve), and ketoprofen (brand name: Orudis). Acetaminophen (brand name: Tylenol) is a better choice for pain, because it doesn't hurt your stomach.

Source

Evaluation and Management of Dyspepsia (*American Family Physician*, October 15, 1999, http://www.aafp.org/afp/991015ap/1773.html).

Chapter 13

Barrett Esophagus

Barrett esophagus is a condition in which the esophagus, the muscular tube that carries food and saliva from the mouth to the stomach, changes so that some of its lining is replaced by a type of tissue similar to that normally found in the intestine. This process is called intestinal metaplasia.

While Barrett esophagus may cause no symptoms itself, a small number of people with this condition develop a relatively rare but often deadly type of cancer of the esophagus called esophageal adenocarcinoma. Barrett esophagus is estimated to affect about seven hundred thousand adults in the United States. It is associated with the very common condition gastroesophageal reflux disease or GERD.

Normal Function of the Esophagus

The esophagus seems to have only one important function in the body—to carry food, liquids, and saliva from the mouth to the stomach. The stomach then acts as a container to start digestion and pump food and liquids into the intestines in a controlled process. Food can then be properly digested over time, and nutrients can be absorbed by the intestines.

The esophagus transports food to the stomach by coordinated contractions of its muscular lining. This process is automatic and people

Reprinted from "Barrett's Esophagus," National Institute of Diabetes and Digestive and Kidney Diseases, NIH Publication No. 05-4546, December 2004.

are usually not aware of it. Many people have felt their esophagus when they swallow something too large, try to eat too quickly, or drink very hot or very cold liquids. They then feel the movement of the food or drink down the esophagus into the stomach, which may be an uncomfortable sensation.

The muscular layers of the esophagus are normally pinched together at both the upper and lower ends by muscles called sphincters. When a person swallows, the sphincters relax automatically to allow food or drink to pass from the mouth into the stomach. The muscles then close rapidly to prevent the swallowed food or drink from leaking out of the stomach back into the esophagus or into the mouth. These sphincters make it possible to swallow while lying down or even upside-down. When people belch to release swallowed air or gas from carbonated beverages, the sphincters relax and small amounts of food or drink may come back up briefly; this condition is called reflux. The esophagus quickly squeezes the material back into the stomach. This amount of reflux and the reaction to it by the esophagus are considered normal.

While these functions of the esophagus are obviously an important part of everyday life, people who must have their esophagus removed, for example because of cancer, can live a relatively healthy life without it.

Gastroesophageal Reflux Disease (GERD)

Having occasional liquid or gas reflux is considered normal. When it happens frequently, particularly when not trying to belch, and causes other symptoms, it is considered a medical problem or disease. However, it is not necessarily a serious one that requires seeing a physician.

The stomach produces acid and enzymes to digest food. When this mixture refluxes into the esophagus more frequently than normal, or for a longer period of time than normal, it may produce symptoms. These symptoms, often called acid reflux, are usually described by people as heartburn, indigestion, or "gas." The symptoms typically consist of a burning sensation below and behind the lower part of the breastbone or sternum.

Almost everyone has experienced these symptoms at least once, typically after overeating. GERD symptoms can also result from being overweight, eating certain types of foods, or being pregnant. In most people, GERD symptoms last only a short time and require no treatment at all. More persistent symptoms are often quickly relieved by over-the-counter acid-reducing agents such as antacids. Common antacids include the following:

- Alka-Seltzer
- Maalox
- Mylanta
- Pepto-Bismol
- Riopan
- Rolaids

Other drugs used to relieve GERD symptoms are antisecretory drugs such as histamine$_2$ (H$_2$) blockers or proton pump inhibitors. Common H$_2$ blockers include the following:

- cimetidine (Tagamet HB)
- famotidine (Pepcid AC)
- nizatidine (Axid AR)
- ranitidine (Zantac 75)

Common proton pump inhibitors include the following:

- esomeprazole (Nexium)
- lansoprazole (Prevacid)
- omeprazole (Prilosec)
- pantoprazole (Protonix)
- rabeprazole (Aciphex)

People who have GERD symptoms frequently should consult a physician. Other diseases can have similar symptoms, and prescription medications in combination with other measures might be needed to reduce reflux. GERD that is untreated over a long period of time can lead to complications, such as an ulcer in the esophagus that could cause bleeding. Another common complication is scar tissue that blocks the movement of swallowed food and drink through the esophagus; this condition is called stricture.

Esophageal reflux may also cause certain less common symptoms, such as hoarseness or chronic cough, and sometimes provokes conditions such as asthma. While most patients find that lifestyle modifications and acid-blocking drugs relieve their symptoms, doctors occasionally recommend surgery. Overall, more than sixty million American adults experience GERD, making it one of the most common medical conditions.

GERD and Barrett Esophagus

The exact causes of Barrett esophagus are not known, but it is thought to be caused in part by the same factors that cause GERD. Although people who do not have heartburn can have Barrett esophagus, it is found about three to five times more often in people with this condition.

Barrett esophagus is uncommon in children. The average age at diagnosis is sixty, but it is usually difficult to determine when the problem started. It is about twice as common in men as in women and much more common in white men than in men of other races.

Barrett Esophagus and Cancer of the Esophagus

Barrett esophagus does not cause symptoms itself and is important only because it seems to precede the development of a particular kind of cancer—esophageal adenocarcinoma. The risk of developing adenocarcinoma is 30 to 125 times higher in people who have Barrett esophagus than in people who do not. This type of cancer is increasing rapidly in white men. This increase may be related to the rise in obesity and GERD.

For people who have Barrett esophagus, the risk of getting cancer of the esophagus is small: less than 1 percent (0.4 percent to 0.5 percent) per year. Esophageal adenocarcinoma is often not curable, partly because the disease is frequently discovered at a late stage and because treatments are not effective.

Diagnosis and Screening

Barrett esophagus can be diagnosed only by an upper GI endoscopy to obtain biopsies of the esophagus. At present, it cannot be diagnosed on the basis of symptoms, physical exam, or blood tests. In an upper GI endoscopy, a flexible tube called an endoscope, which has a light and miniature camera, is passed into the esophagus. If the tissue appears suspicious, then biopsies must be done. A biopsy is the removal of a small piece of tissue using a pincher-like device passed through the endoscope. A pathologist examines the tissue under a microscope to confirm the diagnosis.

Looking for a medical problem in people who do not know whether they have one is called screening. Currently, there are no commonly accepted guidelines on who should have endoscopy to check for Barrett esophagus. Among the many reasons for the lack of firm recommendations about screening are the great expense and occasional risk of side effects of the test. Also, the rate of finding Barrett esophagus is low, and finding the problem early has not been proven to prevent deaths from cancer.

Many physicians recommend that adult patients who are over the age of forty and have had GERD symptoms for a number of years have endoscopy to see whether they have Barrett esophagus. Screening for this condition in people who have no symptoms is not recommended.

Treatment

Barrett esophagus has no cure, short of surgical removal of the esophagus, which is a serious operation. Surgery is recommended only for people who have a high risk of developing cancer or who already have it. Most physicians recommend treating GERD with acid-blocking drugs, since this is sometimes associated with improvement in the extent of the Barrett tissue. However, this approach has not been proven to reduce the risk of cancer. Treating reflux with a surgical procedure for GERD also does not seem to cure Barrett esophagus.

Several different experimental approaches are under study. One attempts to see whether destroying the Barrett tissue by heat or other means through an endoscope can eliminate the condition. This approach, however, has potential risks and unknown effectiveness.

Surveillance for Dysplasia and Cancer

Periodic endoscopic examinations to look for early warning signs of cancer are generally recommended for people who have Barrett esophagus. This approach is called surveillance. When people who have Barrett esophagus develop cancer, the process seems to go through an intermediate stage in which cancer cells appear in the Barrett tissue. This condition is called dysplasia and can be seen only in biopsies with a microscope. The process is patchy and cannot be seen directly through the endoscope, so multiple biopsies must be taken. Even then, the cancer cells can be missed.

The process of change from Barrett to cancer seems to happen in only a few patients, less than 1 percent per year, and over a relatively long period of time. Most physicians recommend that patients with

Barrett esophagus undergo periodic surveillance endoscopy to have biopsies. The recommended interval between endoscopies varies depending on specific circumstances, and the ideal interval has not been determined.

Treatment for Dysplasia or Esophageal Adenocarcinoma

If a person with Barrett esophagus is found to have dysplasia or cancer, the doctor will usually recommend surgery if the person is strong enough and has a good chance of being cured. The type of surgery may vary, but it usually involves removing most of the esophagus and pulling the stomach up into the chest to attach it to what remains of the esophagus. Many patients with Barrett esophagus are elderly and have many other medical problems that make surgery unwise; in these patients, other approaches to treating dysplasia are being investigated.

Points to Remember

- In Barrett esophagus, the cells lining the esophagus change and become similar to the cells lining the intestine.

- Barrett esophagus is associated with gastroesophageal reflux disease or GERD.

- A small number of people with Barrett esophagus may develop esophageal cancer.

- Barrett esophagus is diagnosed by upper gastrointestinal endoscopy and biopsy.

- People who have Barrett esophagus should have periodic esophageal examinations.

- Taking acid-blocking drugs for GERD may result in improvements in Barrett esophagus.

- Removal of the esophagus is recommended only for people who have a high risk of developing cancer or who already have it.

Chapter 14

Gastroesophageal Reflux Disease (GERD) and Associated Conditions

Chapter Contents

Section 14.1

Heartburn, Hiatal Hernia, and Gastroesophageal Reflux Disease

Reprinted from "Heartburn, Hiatal Hernia, and Gastroesophageal
Reflux Disease (GERD)." National Institute of Diabetes and Digestive
and Kidney Diseases, NIH Publication No. 03-0882, June 2003.

Gastroesophageal reflux disease, or GERD, occurs when the lower
esophageal sphincter (LES) does not close properly and stomach contents leak back, or reflux, into the esophagus. The LES is a ring of
muscle at the bottom of the esophagus that acts like a valve between
the esophagus and stomach. The esophagus carries food from the
mouth to the stomach.

When refluxed stomach acid touches the lining of the esophagus,
it causes a burning sensation in the chest or throat called heartburn.
The fluid may even be tasted in the back of the mouth, and this is
called acid indigestion. Occasional heartburn is common but does not
necessarily mean one has GERD. Heartburn that occurs more than
twice a week may be considered GERD, and it can eventually lead to
more serious health problems.

Anyone, including infants, children, and pregnant women, can have
GERD.

What are the symptoms of GERD?

The main symptoms are persistent heartburn and acid regurgitation. Some people have GERD without heartburn. Instead, they experience pain in the chest, hoarseness in the morning, or trouble
swallowing. You may feel like you have food stuck in your throat or
like you are choking or your throat is tight. GERD can also cause a
dry cough and bad breath.

Is GERD found in children?

Studies[1] show that GERD is common and may be overlooked in
infants and children. It can cause repeated vomiting, coughing, and

other respiratory problems. Children's immature digestive systems are usually to blame, and most infants grow out of GERD by the time they are one year old. Still, you should talk to your child's doctor if the problem occurs regularly and causes discomfort. Your doctor may recommend simple strategies for avoiding reflux, like burping the infant several times during feeding or keeping the infant in an upright position for thirty minutes after feeding. If your child is older, the doctor may recommend avoiding these foods and drinks:

- sodas that contain caffeine
- chocolate and peppermint
- spicy foods like pizza
- acidic foods like oranges and tomatoes
- fried and fatty foods

Avoiding food two to three hours before bed may also help. The doctor may recommend that the child sleep with head raised. If these changes do not work, the doctor may prescribe medicine for your child. In rare cases, a child may need surgery.

What causes GERD?

No one knows why people get GERD. A hiatal hernia may contribute. A hiatal hernia occurs when the upper part of the stomach is above the diaphragm, the muscle wall that separates the stomach from the chest. The diaphragm helps the LES keep acid from coming up into the esophagus. When a hiatal hernia is present, it is easier for the acid to come up. In this way, a hiatal hernia can cause reflux. A hiatal hernia can happen in people of any age; many otherwise healthy people over fifty have a small one.

Other factors that may contribute to GERD include the following:

- alcohol use
- being overweight
- pregnancy
- smoking

Also, certain foods can be associated with reflux events, including the following:

- citrus fruits

173

- chocolate
- drinks with caffeine
- fatty and fried foods
- garlic and onions
- mint flavorings
- spicy foods
- tomato-based foods, like spaghetti sauce, chili, and pizza

How is GERD treated?

If you have had heartburn or any of the other symptoms for a while, you should see your doctor. You may want to visit an internist, a doctor who specializes in internal medicine, or a gastroenterologist, a doctor who treats diseases of the stomach and intestines. Depending on how severe your GERD is, treatment may involve one or more of the following lifestyle changes and medications or surgery.

- If you smoke, stop.
- Do not drink alcohol.
- Lose weight if needed.
- Eat small meals.
- Wear loose-fitting clothes.
- Avoid lying down for three hours after a meal.
- Raise the head of your bed six to eight inches by putting blocks of wood under the bedposts—just using extra pillows will not help.

Medications: Your doctor may recommend over-the-counter antacids, which you can buy without a prescription, or medications that stop acid production or help the muscles that empty your stomach.

Antacids, such as Alka-Seltzer, Maalox, Mylanta, Pepto-Bismol, Rolaids, and Riopan, are usually the first drugs recommended to relieve heartburn and other mild GERD symptoms. Many brands on the market use different combinations of three basic salts—magnesium, calcium, and aluminum—with hydroxide or bicarbonate ions to neutralize the acid in your stomach. Antacids, however, have side effects. Magnesium salt can lead to diarrhea, and aluminum salts can cause constipation. Aluminum and magnesium salts are often combined in a single product to balance these effects.

Calcium carbonate antacids, such as Tums, Titralac, and Alka-2, can also be a supplemental source of calcium. They can cause constipation as well.

Foaming agents, such as Gaviscon, work by covering your stomach contents with foam to prevent reflux. These drugs may help those who have no damage to the esophagus.

H_2 blockers, such as cimetidine (Tagamet HB), famotidine (Pepcid AC), nizatidine (Axid AR), and ranitidine (Zantac 75), impede acid production. They are available in prescription strength and over the counter. These drugs provide short-term relief, but over-the-counter H_2 blockers should not be used for more than a few weeks at a time. They are effective for about half of those who have GERD symptoms. Many people benefit from taking H_2 blockers at bedtime in combination with a proton pump inhibitor.

Proton pump inhibitors include omeprazole (Prilosec), lansoprazole (Prevacid), pantoprazole (Protonix), rabeprazole (Aciphex), and esomeprazole (Nexium), which are all available by prescription. Proton pump inhibitors are more effective than H_2 blockers and can relieve symptoms in almost everyone who has GERD.

Another group of drugs, *prokinetics*, helps strengthen the sphincter and makes the stomach empty faster. This group includes bethanechol (Urecholine) and metoclopramide (Reglan). Metoclopramide also improves muscle action in the digestive tract, but these drugs have frequent side effects that limit their usefulness.

Because drugs work in different ways, combinations of drugs may help control symptoms. People who get heartburn after eating may take both antacids and H_2 blockers. The antacids work first to neutralize the acid in the stomach, while the H_2 blockers act on acid production. By the time the antacid stops working, the H_2 blocker will have stopped acid production. Your doctor is the best source of information on how to use medications for GERD.

What if symptoms persist?

If your heartburn does not improve with lifestyle changes or drugs, you may need additional tests.

- **A barium swallow radiograph** uses x-rays to help spot abnormalities such as a hiatal hernia and severe inflammation of the esophagus. With this test, you drink a solution and then x-rays are taken. Mild irritation will not appear on this test, although narrowing of the esophagus—called stricture—ulcers, hiatal hernia, and other problems will.

- **Upper endoscopy** is more accurate than a barium swallow radiograph and may be performed in a hospital or a doctor's office. The doctor will spray your throat to numb it and slide down a thin, flexible plastic tube called an endoscope. A tiny camera in the endoscope allows the doctor to see the surface of the esophagus and to search for abnormalities. If you have had moderate to severe symptoms and this procedure reveals injury to the esophagus, usually no other tests are needed to confirm GERD. The doctor may use tiny tweezers (forceps) in the endoscope to remove a small piece of tissue for biopsy. A biopsy viewed under a microscope can reveal damage caused by acid reflux and rule out other problems if no infecting organisms or abnormal growths are found.

- In an ambulatory **pH monitoring examination**, the doctor puts a tiny tube into the esophagus that will stay there for twenty-four hours. While you go about your normal activities, it measures when and how much acid comes up into your esophagus. This test is useful in people with GERD symptoms but no esophageal damage. The procedure is also helpful in detecting whether respiratory symptoms, including wheezing and coughing, are triggered by reflux.

Surgery: Surgery is an option when medicine and lifestyle changes do not work. Surgery may also be a reasonable alternative to a lifetime of drugs and discomfort.

Fundoplication, usually a specific variation called Nissen fundoplication, is the standard surgical treatment for GERD. The upper part of the stomach is wrapped around the LES to strengthen the sphincter and prevent acid reflux and to repair a hiatal hernia.

This fundoplication procedure may be done using a laparoscope and requires only tiny incisions in the abdomen. To perform the fundoplication, surgeons use small instruments that hold a tiny camera. Laparoscopic fundoplication has been used safely and effectively in people of all ages, even babies. When performed by experienced surgeons, the procedure is reported to be as good as standard fundoplication. Furthermore, people can leave the hospital in one to three days and return to work in two to three weeks.

In 2000, the U.S. Food and Drug Administration (FDA) approved two endoscopic devices to treat chronic heartburn. The Bard EndoCinch system puts stitches in the LES to create little pleats that help strengthen the muscle. The Stretta system uses electrodes to create tiny cuts on the LES. When the cuts heal, the scar tissue helps toughen the muscle. The long-term effects of these two procedures are unknown.

Implant: Recently the FDA approved an implant that may help people with GERD who wish to avoid surgery. Enteryx is a solution that becomes spongy and reinforces the LES to keep stomach acid from flowing into the esophagus. It is injected during endoscopy. The implant is approved for people who have GERD and who require and respond to proton pump inhibitors. The long-term effects of the implant are unknown.

What are the long-term complications of GERD?

Sometimes GERD can cause serious complications. Inflammation of the esophagus from stomach acid causes bleeding or ulcers. In addition, scars from tissue damage can narrow the esophagus and make swallowing difficult. Some people develop Barrett esophagus, where cells in the esophageal lining take on an abnormal shape and color, which over time can lead to cancer.

Also, studies have shown that asthma, chronic cough, and pulmonary fibrosis may be aggravated or even caused by GERD.

Points to Remember

- Heartburn, also called acid indigestion, is the most common symptom of GERD. Anyone experiencing heartburn twice a week or more may have GERD.

- You can have GERD without having heartburn. Your symptoms could be excessive clearing of the throat, problems swallowing, the feeling that food is stuck in your throat, burning in the mouth, or pain in the chest.

- In infants and children, GERD may cause repeated vomiting, coughing, and other respiratory problems. Most babies grow out of GERD by their first birthday.

- If you have been using antacids for more than two weeks, it is time to see a doctor. Most doctors can treat GERD. Or you may want to visit an internist—a doctor who specializes in internal medicine—or a gastroenterologist—a doctor who treats diseases of the stomach and intestines.

- Doctors usually recommend lifestyle and dietary changes to relieve heartburn. Many people with GERD also need medication. Surgery may be an option.

Hope through Research

No one knows why some people who have heartburn develop GERD. Several factors may be involved, and research is under way on many levels. Risk factors—what makes some people get GERD but not others—are being explored, as is GERD's role in other conditions such as asthma and bronchitis.

The role of hiatal hernia in GERD continues to be debated and explored. It is a complex topic because some people have a hiatal hernia without having reflux, while others have reflux without having a hernia.

Much research is needed into the role of the bacterium *Helicobacter pylori*. Our ability to eliminate *H. pylori* has been responsible for reduced rates of peptic ulcer disease and some gastric cancers. At the same time, GERD, Barrett esophagus, and cancers of the esophagus have increased. Researchers wonder whether having *H. pylori* helps prevent GERD and other diseases. Future treatment will be greatly affected by the results of this research.

Notes

1. Jung AD. Gastroesophageal reflux in infants and children. *American Family Physician*. 2001; 64(11): 1853–60.

Section 14.2

Implant for Gastroesophageal Reflux Disease

Reprinted from "FDA Approves an Implant for Gastroesophageal Reflux Disease," FDA Talk Paper, U.S. Food and Drug Administration (FDA), April 22, 2003.

The Food and Drug Administration has approved Enteryx, a permanently implanted device to help patients with symptoms of gastroesophageal reflux disease (GERD), a condition in which some of the stomach's contents—including acid—flows up into the esophagus, causing heartburn or burning pain in the chest or back of the throat. More than sixty million American adults experience GERD, and about twenty-five million of them have daily symptoms.

Inserted through an endoscope procedure, this device prevents the reflux of stomach acid into the throat, potentially allowing patients with chronic GERD to avoid daily medications.

Mild heartburn can be treated by adopting dietary changes such as avoiding foods that cause heartburn and eating smaller portions. Treatment of chronic GERD, however, may also require prescription drugs to help maintain a reduced level of acid secretion in the stomach.

Enteryx, a product of Enteric Medical Technologies, which is a wholly owned subsidary of Boston Scientific, Inc., is approved for use in patients who have GERD symptoms and who require and respond to certain medications. The device is a solution made up of a polymer and a solvent that is implanted by injection during an x-ray guided endoscopic procedure into the wall of the lower esophagus. After the injection, the solvent separates away and the polymer solidifies into a spongy material that is intended to help prevent the reflux.

The device has been found to help eliminate or reduce the need for medications, and to improve the symptoms of GERD. In a twelve-month study of eighty-five patients conducted in the United States, Canada, and Europe, approximately 67 percent of the participants were able to discontinue all of their medications, 9 percent could reduce the dose by at least one-half, and most patients (72 percent) noted an improvement in their symptoms when compared to taking no medications prior to implant.

Although many patients had improvements in their symptoms and medication requirements, objective evaluations of the esophagus performed during the clinical trial showed evidence of persistent acid reflux in 61 percent of patients and low-grade inflammation in 37 percent of patients at twelve months.

The most common side effect observed in patients undergoing Enteryx treatment was pain beneath the breastbone that usually diminished within two weeks. Other common side effects included temporary difficulty with swallowing(20 percent of participants), fever (12 percent), sore throat (11 percent), and gas/bloating/belching (7 percent).

The device should not be used in people who are unable to undergo endoscopy, or who have dilated veins in the esophagus due to liver disease.

Chapter 15

Swallowing Disorders

About Swallowing Disorders

What is a swallowing disorder?

There are numerous types of swallowing disorders, however, many of the symptoms are similar. For example, if one is experiencing any of the following discomforts, a physician should be seen: food sticking in the throat, heartburn, choking on food, inability to swallow liquids, pain when swallowing, persistent cough or sore throat, hoarseness or a gurgly voice during or after eating, a "lump in the throat" sensation, and wheezing without a history of asthma or lung problems.

How does the process of swallowing work?

Swallowing takes place in four stages. Different problems can occur at each stage to disrupt the normal swallowing process.

Stage 1: Biting and chewing food takes place in the mouth. At this stage, lack of strength, control, or feeling in the mouth—which may be due to stroke or muscle or nerve disease—may cause food or liquid to fall directly into the throat and cause choking.

"About Swallowing Disorders" is reprinted with permission from the Cleveland Clinic Department of Gastroenterology and Hepatology, © 2002 The Cleveland Clinic. "Achalasia" is excerpted with permission from the Cleveland Clinic Department of Gastroenterology and Hepatology, © 2002 The Cleveland Clinic.

Stage 2: The tongue pushes the food to the back of the mouth where a structure folds over the top of the windpipe to keep food out. At the back of the mouth, the presence of food triggers muscle contractions. At this stage, the muscle at the back of the mouth that opens to allow food into the esophagus may malfunction and cause aspiration (food passing into the windpipe), which results in choking.

Stage 3: Muscle contractions push food down the esophagus. At this stage, lack of or inadequate muscle contractions may cause food to stick in the chest.

Stage 4: Food moves through the esophagus, and the lower esophageal sphincter muscle opens to let food pass into the stomach. At this stage, weakening of this sphincter muscle at the stomach opening may allow acidic stomach secretions to come back up into the esophagus from the stomach, a condition called reflux.

What causes swallowing disorders and who gets them?

Over fifteen million Americans have a swallowing disorder. They can occur at any age. Swallowing problems may be temporary, or they may be an indication of a serious medical problem. There are many causes including nerve and muscle problems, head and neck injuries, cancer, or they may occur because of a stroke. Certain medications can also contribute to the disorder.

How can specific disorders be diagnosed?

Your family physician or a gastroenterologist (a physician who specializes in treating problems of the digestive system) can determine the location and the extent of the problem based on symptoms, a physical examination, diagnostic tests, and x-rays. One of the most useful tools is the painless barium swallow, a special video x-ray study that shows the entire swallowing process and anatomy. A gastroenterologist, radiologist, and swallowing therapist review the video to pinpoint the specific problem areas and decide on appropriate treatment.

Additional tests may include a motility study, which records movement and pressures of the esophagus; x-rays of the neck, head, or thyroid; twenty-four-hour pH test to determine the amount of acid reflux, endoscopy to view the inside of the esophagus, or an endoscopic ultrasound to determine the nature and extent of tumors and other lesions.

How are swallowing disorders treated?

Sometimes just learning different physical techniques is enough to improve swallowing ability. Other times, and depending on the precise ailment, medical intervention or surgery may be needed.

There are various strategies that are used to have a more comfortable eating and swallowing experience. These are general strategies; a swallowing therapist will be able to help tailor strategies to specific situations.

- Avoid eating when tired or stressed.

- Change head position and posture when swallowing (generally chin to chest is best).

- Minimize head movements.

- Eat smaller, more frequent meals.

- Lubricate dry food by mixing it with a sauce.

- Always swallow all food in mouth before taking another bite.

- Do not eat foods that will stick together—for example, fresh bread.

- Thickened liquids are generally easier to swallow.

Medical interventions are sometimes also needed. For instance, stretching the esophagus can be done in a noninvasive way. Also, medications are effective for some people. Some medications can reduce stomach acid, overcome spasms of the esophagus, or just help the swallowing nerves function better.

And sometimes surgery is an option for people with swallowing disorders. Surgical treatments depend on the location of the swallowing disorder. Surgery may involve strengthening or loosening the upper or lower esophageal valves, or removing obstructions or tumors from the esophagus.

Achalasia

What is achalasia?

Achalasia is a condition in which the esophageal muscle lacks the ability to move food into the stomach. The lower esophageal sphincter (LES), located between the esophagus and stomach, stays closed, resulting in the backup of food. Other symptoms include vomiting undigested food, chest pain, heartburn, and weight loss.

How is achalasia diagnosed?

Three tests are most commonly used to diagnose and evaluate a swallowing problem:

- **Barium swallow.** The patient swallows a barium preparation (liquid or other form) and its movement through the esophagus is evaluated using x-ray technology.

- **Endoscopy.** A flexible, narrow tube called an endoscope is passed into the esophagus and projects images of the inside onto a screen.

- **Manometry.** This test measures the timing and strength of esophageal contractions and muscular valve relaxations.

Does achalasia have to be treated?

If left untreated, achalasia can be debilitating. People experience considerable weight loss that can result in malnutrition. Lung infections and pneumonia due to aspiration of food can result, particularly in the elderly. Although the exact cause of achalasia is unknown, researchers think it may be linked to a virus.

What are the treatment options?

Balloon Dilation: Most often, achalasia can be successfully treated nonsurgically with balloon (pneumatic) dilation. While the patient is under light sedation, the gastroenterologist inserts a specifically designed balloon through the LES and inflates it. The procedure acts to relax and open the muscle.

Some patients may have to undergo several dilation treatments in order to achieve symptom improvement, and the treatment may have to be repeated every few years to ensure long-term results. Up to two-thirds of patients are treated successfully with balloon dilation.

Medication: Other patients, particularly those who are not appropriate candidates for balloon dilation or surgery, benefit from Botox® injections. Botox is a protein made by the bacteria that cause botulism. When injected into muscles in very small quantities, it can relax spastic muscles. It works by preventing nerves from sending signals to the muscles that tell them to contract. A smaller percentage of patients (up to 35 percent) achieve good results using Botox compared to balloon dilation. In addition, the injections must be repeated frequently in order to achieve symptom relief.

Other medications, such as nifedipine and nitroglycerin, may help to relax spastic muscles. Patients who take nifedipine every day may experience satisfactory results for a couple of years.

Minimally Invasive Surgery: For select patients with severe achalasia, a minimally invasive surgical technique called laparoscopic esophagomyotomy or the Heller myotomy may help.

As with all minimally invasive surgery, surgeons use a thin, telescope-like instrument called an endoscope, which is inserted through a small incision. The endoscope is connected to a tiny video camera—smaller than a dime—that projects a view of the operative site onto video monitors located in the operating room. Minimally invasive surgery techniques offer patients a shorter hospital stay, quicker recovery, and less scarring than traditional procedures.

Up to two-third of patients are treated successfully with surgery, though some patients may have to repeat the surgery or undergo balloon dilation to achieve satisfactory long-term results.

Chapter 16

What You Need to Know about Peptic Ulcers

What is a peptic ulcer?

A peptic ulcer is a sore in the lining of your stomach or duodenum. The duodenum is the first part of your small intestine. If peptic ulcers are found in the stomach, they're called gastric ulcers. If they're found in the duodenum, they're called duodenal ulcers. You can have more than one ulcer.

Many people have peptic ulcers. Peptic ulcers can be treated successfully. Seeing your doctor is the first step.

What are the symptoms of peptic ulcers?

A burning pain in the gut is the most common symptom. The pain:

- feels like a dull ache;
- comes and goes for a few days or weeks;
- starts two to three hours after a meal;
- comes in the middle of the night when your stomach is empty;
- usually goes away after you eat.

Other symptoms are:

Reprinted from "What I Need to Know about Peptic Ulcers," National Institute of Diabetes and Digestive and Kidney Diseases, NIH Publication No. 05-5042, October 2004.

- losing weight;
- not feeling like eating;
- having pain while eating;
- feeling sick to your stomach;
- vomiting.

Some people with peptic ulcers have mild symptoms. If you have any of these symptoms, you may have a peptic ulcer and should see your doctor.

What causes peptic ulcers?

Peptic ulcers are caused by:

- bacteria called *Helicobacter pylori*, or *H. pylori* for short;
- nonsteroidal anti-inflammatory drugs (NSAIDs) such as aspirin and ibuprofen;
- other diseases.

Your body makes strong acids that digest food. A lining protects the inside of your stomach and duodenum from these acids. If the lining breaks down, the acids can damage the walls. Both *H. pylori* and NSAIDs weaken the lining so acid can reach the stomach or duodenal wall.

H. pylori causes almost two-thirds of all ulcers. Many people have *H. pylori* infections. But not everyone who has an infection will develop a peptic ulcer.

Most other ulcers are caused by NSAIDs. Only rarely do other diseases cause ulcers.

Do stress or spicy foods cause peptic ulcers?

No, neither stress nor spicy foods cause ulcers. Yet they can make ulcers worse. Drinking alcohol or smoking can make ulcers worse, too.

What increases my risk of getting peptic ulcers?

You're more likely to develop a peptic ulcer if you:

- have an *H. pylori* infection;
- use NSAIDs often;

- smoke cigarettes;
- drink alcohol;
- have relatives who have peptic ulcers;
- are fifty years old or older.

Can peptic ulcers get worse?

Peptic ulcers will get worse if they aren't treated. Call your doctor right away if you have any of these symptoms:

- sudden sharp pain that doesn't go away
- black or bloody stools
- bloody vomit or vomit that looks like coffee grounds

These could be signs that:

- the ulcer has gone through, or perforated, the stomach or duodenal wall;
- the ulcer has broken a blood vessel;
- the ulcer has stopped food from moving from the stomach into the duodenum.

These symptoms must be treated quickly. You may need surgery.

How can I find out whether I have peptic ulcers?

If you have symptoms, see your doctor. Your doctor may:

- take x-rays of your stomach and duodenum, called an upper GI series. You'll drink a liquid called barium to make your stomach and duodenum show up clearly on the x-rays.
- use a thin lighted tube with a tiny camera on the end to look at the inside of your stomach and duodenum. This procedure is called an endoscopy. You'll take some medicine to relax you so your doctor can pass the thin tube through your mouth to your stomach and duodenum. Your doctor may also remove a tiny piece of your stomach to view under a microscope. This procedure is called a biopsy.

If you do have a peptic ulcer, your doctor may test your breath, blood, or tissue to see whether bacteria caused the ulcer.

How are peptic ulcers treated?

Peptic ulcers can be cured. Medicines for peptic ulcers are:

- proton pump inhibitors or histamine receptor blockers to stop your stomach from making acids;
- antibiotics to kill the bacteria.

Depending on your symptoms, you may take one or more of these medicines for a few weeks. They'll stop the pain and help heal your stomach or duodenum.

Ulcers take time to heal. Take your medicines even if the pain goes away. If these medicines make you feel sick or dizzy, or cause diarrhea or headaches, your doctor can change your medicines.

If NSAIDs caused your peptic ulcer, you'll need to stop taking them. If you smoke, quit. Smoking slows healing of ulcers.

Can I use antacids?

Yes. If you have a peptic ulcer, taking antacids will:

- stop the acids from working and reduce the pain;
- help ulcers heal.

You can buy antacids at any grocery store or drugstore. However, you must take them several times a day. Also, antacids don't kill the bacteria, so your ulcer could come back even if the pain goes away.

Can peptic ulcers come back?

Yes. If you stop taking your antibiotic too soon, not all the bacteria will be gone and not all the sores will be healed. If you still smoke or take NSAIDs, your ulcers may come back.

What happens if peptic ulcers don't heal? Will I need surgery?

In many cases, medicine heals ulcers. You may need surgery if your ulcers:

- don't heal;
- keep coming back;
- perforate, bleed, or obstruct the stomach or duodenum.

Surgery can:

- remove the ulcers;
- reduce the amount of acid your stomach makes.

What can I do to prevent peptic ulcers?

- Stop using NSAIDs. Talk with your doctor about other pain relievers.

What can I do to lower my risk of getting peptic ulcers?

- Don't smoke.
- Don't drink alcohol.

Chapter 17

Gastroparesis

What Is Gastroparesis?

Gastroparesis, also called delayed gastric emptying, is a disorder in which the stomach takes too long to empty its contents. It often occurs in people with type 1 diabetes or type 2 diabetes.

Gastroparesis happens when nerves to the stomach are damaged or stop working. The vagus nerve controls the movement of food through the digestive tract. If the vagus nerve is damaged, the muscles of the stomach and intestines do not work normally, and the movement of food is slowed or stopped.

Diabetes can damage the vagus nerve if blood glucose levels remain high over a long period of time. High blood glucose causes chemical changes in nerves and damages the blood vessels that carry oxygen and nutrients to the nerves.

Signs and Symptoms

Signs and symptoms of gastroparesis include the following:

- heartburn
- nausea
- vomiting of undigested food

Excerpted from "Gastroparesis and Diabetes," National Institute of Diabetes and Digestive and Kidney Diseases, NIH Publication No. 04-4348, December 2003.

- an early feeling of fullness when eating
- weight loss
- abdominal bloating
- erratic blood glucose levels
- lack of appetite
- gastroesophageal reflux
- spasms of the stomach wall

These symptoms may be mild or severe, depending on the person.

Complications of Gastroparesis

If food lingers too long in the stomach, it can cause problems like bacterial overgrowth from the fermentation of food. Also, the food can harden into solid masses called bezoars that may cause nausea, vomiting, and obstruction in the stomach. Bezoars can be dangerous if they block the passage of food into the small intestine.

Gastroparesis can make diabetes worse by adding to the difficulty of controlling blood glucose. When food that has been delayed in the stomach finally enters the small intestine and is absorbed, blood glucose levels rise. Since gastroparesis makes stomach emptying unpredictable, a person's blood glucose levels can be erratic and difficult to control.

Major Causes of Gastroparesis

Gastroparesis is most often caused by these conditions:

- diabetes
- postviral syndromes
- anorexia nervosa
- surgery on the stomach or vagus nerve
- medications, particularly anticholinergics and narcotics (drugs that slow contractions in the intestine)
- gastroesophageal reflux disease (rarely)
- smooth muscle disorders such as amyloidosis and scleroderma
- nervous system diseases, including abdominal migraine and Parkinson disease
- metabolic disorders, including hypothyroidism

Diagnosis

The diagnosis of gastroparesis is confirmed through one or more of the following tests.

- **Barium x-ray.** After fasting for twelve hours, you will drink a thick liquid called barium, which coats the inside of the stomach, making it show up on the x-ray. Normally, the stomach will be empty of all food after twelve hours of fasting. If the x-ray shows food in the stomach, gastroparesis is likely. If the x-ray shows an empty stomach but the doctor still suspects that you have delayed emptying, you may need to repeat the test another day. On any one day, a person with gastroparesis may digest a meal normally, giving a falsely normal test result. If you have diabetes, your doctor may have special instructions about fasting.

- **Barium beefsteak meal.** You will eat a meal that contains barium, thus allowing the radiologist to watch your stomach as it digests the meal. The amount of time it takes for the barium meal to be digested and leave the stomach gives the doctor an idea of how well the stomach is working. This test can help detect emptying problems that do not show up on the liquid barium x-ray. In fact, people who have diabetes-related gastroparesis often digest fluid normally, so the barium beefsteak meal can be more useful.

- **Radioisotope gastric-emptying scan.** You will eat food that contains a radioisotope, a slightly radioactive substance that will show up on the scan. The dose of radiation from the radioisotope is small and not dangerous. After eating, you will lie under a machine that detects the radioisotope and shows an image of the food in the stomach and how quickly it leaves the stomach. Gastroparesis is diagnosed if more than half of the food remains in the stomach after two hours.

- **Gastric manometry.** This test measures electrical and muscular activity in the stomach. The doctor passes a thin tube down the throat into the stomach. The tube contains a wire that takes measurements of the stomach's electrical and muscular activity as it digests liquids and solid food. The measurements show how the stomach is working and whether there is any delay in digestion.

- **Blood tests.** The doctor may also order laboratory tests to check blood counts and to measure chemical and electrolyte levels.

To rule out causes of gastroparesis other than diabetes, the doctor may do an upper endoscopy or an ultrasound.

- **Upper endoscopy.** After giving you a sedative, the doctor passes a long, thin tube called an endoscope through the mouth and gently guides it down the esophagus into the stomach. Through the endoscope, the doctor can look at the lining of the stomach to check for any abnormalities.

- **Ultrasound.** To rule out gallbladder disease or pancreatitis as a source of the problem, you may have an ultrasound test, which uses harmless sound waves to outline and define the shape of the gallbladder and pancreas.

Treatment

The primary treatment goal for gastroparesis related to diabetes is to regain control of blood glucose levels. Treatments include insulin, oral medications, changes in what and when you eat, and, in severe cases, feeding tubes and intravenous feeding.

It is important to note that in most cases treatment does not cure gastroparesis—it is usually a chronic condition. Treatment helps you manage the condition so that you can be as healthy and comfortable as possible.

Insulin for Blood Glucose Control

If you have gastroparesis, your food is being absorbed more slowly and at unpredictable times. To control blood glucose, you may need to take these steps:

- take insulin more often
- take your insulin after you eat instead of before
- check your blood glucose levels frequently after you eat and administer insulin whenever necessary

Your doctor will give you specific instructions based on your particular needs.

Medication

Several drugs are used to treat gastroparesis. Your doctor may try different drugs or combinations of drugs to find the most effective treatment.

- **Metoclopramide (Reglan).** This drug stimulates stomach muscle contractions to help empty food. It also helps reduce nausea and vomiting. Metoclopramide is taken twenty to thirty minutes before meals and at bedtime. Side effects of this drug are fatigue, sleepiness, and sometimes depression, anxiety, and problems with physical movement.

- **Erythromycin.** This antibiotic also improves stomach emptying. It works by increasing the contractions that move food through the stomach. Side effects are nausea, vomiting, and abdominal cramps.

- **Domperidone.** The Food and Drug Administration is reviewing domperidone, which has been used elsewhere in the world to treat gastroparesis. It is a promotility agent like metoclopramide. Domperidone also helps with nausea.

- **Other medications.** Other medications may be used to treat symptoms and problems related to gastroparesis. For example, an antiemetic can help with nausea and vomiting. Antibiotics will clear up a bacterial infection. If you have a bezoar, the doctor may use an endoscope to inject medication that will dissolve it.

Meal and Food Changes

Changing your eating habits can help control gastroparesis. Your doctor or dietitian will give you specific instructions, but you may be asked to eat six small meals a day instead of three large ones. If less food enters the stomach each time you eat, it may not become overly full. Or the doctor or dietitian may suggest that you try several liquid meals a day until your blood glucose levels are stable and the gastroparesis is corrected. Liquid meals provide all the nutrients found in solid foods, but can pass through the stomach more easily and quickly.

The doctor may also recommend that you avoid high-fat and high-fiber foods. Fat naturally slows digestion—a problem you do not need if you have gastroparesis—and fiber is difficult to digest. Some high-fiber foods like oranges and broccoli contain material that cannot be digested. Avoid these foods because the indigestible part will remain in the stomach too long and possibly form bezoars.

Feeding Tube

If other approaches do not work, you may need surgery to insert a feeding tube. The tube, called a jejunostomy tube, is inserted through the skin on your abdomen into the small intestine. The feeding tube allows you to put nutrients directly into the small intestine, bypassing the stomach altogether. You will receive special liquid food to use with the tube. A jejunostomy is particularly useful when gastroparesis prevents the nutrients and medication necessary to regulate blood glucose levels from reaching the bloodstream. By avoiding the source of the problem—the stomach—and putting nutrients and medication directly into the small intestine, you ensure that these products are digested and delivered to your bloodstream quickly. A jejunostomy tube can be temporary and is used only if necessary when gastroparesis is severe.

Parenteral Nutrition

Parenteral nutrition refers to delivering nutrients directly into the bloodstream, bypassing the digestive system. The doctor places a thin tube called a catheter in a chest vein, leaving an opening to it outside the skin. For feeding, you attach a bag containing liquid nutrients or medication to the catheter. The fluid enters your bloodstream through the vein. Your doctor will tell you what type of liquid nutrition to use.

This approach is an alternative to the jejunostomy tube and is usually a temporary method to get you through a difficult spell of gastroparesis. Parenteral nutrition is used only when gastroparesis is severe and is not helped by other methods.

New Treatments

A gastric neurostimulator has been developed to assist people with gastroparesis. The battery-operated device is surgically implanted and emits mild electrical pulses that help control nausea and vomiting associated with gastroparesis. This option is available to people whose nausea and vomiting do not improve with medications.

The use of botulinum toxin has been shown to improve stomach emptying and the symptoms of gastroparesis by decreasing the prolonged contractions of the muscle between the stomach and the small intestine (pyloric sphincter). The toxin is injected into the pyloric sphincter.

Points to Remember

- Gastroparesis may occur in people with type 1 diabetes or type 2 diabetes.

- Gastroparesis is the result of damage to the vagus nerve, which controls the movement of food through the digestive system. Instead of the food moving through the digestive tract normally, it is retained in the stomach.

- The vagus nerve becomes damaged after years of poor blood glucose control, resulting in gastroparesis. In turn, gastroparesis contributes to poor blood glucose control.

- Symptoms of gastroparesis include early fullness, nausea, vomiting, and weight loss.

- Gastroparesis is diagnosed through tests such as x-rays, manometry, and scanning.

- Treatments include changes in when and what you eat, changes in insulin type and timing of injections, oral medications, a jejunostomy, parenteral nutrition, gastric neurostimulators, or botulinum toxin.

Chapter 18

Pyloric Stenosis

While you were anticipating your new baby, you probably mentally prepared yourself for the messier aspects of child rearing: poopy diapers, food stains, and of course, spit up. But what's normal and what's not when it comes to spitting up or vomiting in infants?

Pyloric stenosis, a condition that affects the gastrointestinal tract during infancy, isn't normal—it can cause your baby to vomit forcefully and often and may cause other problems such as dehydration and salt and fluid imbalances. Keep reading to understand why getting immediate treatment for pyloric stenosis is so important.

What Is Pyloric Stenosis?

Pyloric stenosis is a narrowing of the pylorus, the lower part of the stomach through which food and other stomach contents pass to enter the small intestine. When an infant has pyloric stenosis, the muscles in the pylorus have become enlarged to the point where food is prevented from emptying out of the stomach.

Also called infantile hypertrophic pyloric stenosis or gastric outlet obstruction, pyloric stenosis is fairly common—it affects about three out of one thousand babies in the United States. Pyloric stenosis is about four times more likely to occur in firstborn male infants. It has also been shown to run in families—if a parent had pyloric stenosis, then an infant has up to a 20 percent risk of developing the condition. Pyloric stenosis occurs more commonly in Caucasian infants than in babies of other ethnic backgrounds, and affected infants are more likely to have blood type B or O.

Most infants who develop pyloric stenosis are usually between two weeks and two months of age—symptoms usually appear during or after the third week of life. It is one of the more common causes of intestinal obstruction during infancy that requires surgery.

What Causes Pyloric Stenosis?

It is believed that babies who develop the condition are not born with pyloric stenosis, but that the progressive thickening of the pylorus occurs after birth. An affected infant begins showing symptoms when the pylorus is so thickened that the stomach can no longer empty properly.

It is not known exactly what causes the thickening of the muscles of the pylorus—it may be a combination of several factors. Some researchers believe that maternal hormones could be a contributing cause. Others believe that the thickening of the muscle is the stomach's response to some type of allergic reaction in the body.

Some scientists believe that babies with pyloric stenosis lack receptors in the pyloric muscle that detect nitric oxide, a chemical in the body that tells the pylorus muscle to relax. As a result, the muscle is in a state of contraction almost continually, which causes it to become larger and thicker over time. It may take some time for this thickening to occur, which is why pyloric stenosis usually appears in babies a few weeks after birth.

Signs and Symptoms

Symptoms of pyloric stenosis generally begin around three weeks of age. They include:

Vomiting

The first symptom of pyloric stenosis is usually vomiting. At first it may seem that the baby is simply spitting up frequently, but then it tends to progress to projectile vomiting, in which the breast milk or formula is ejected forcefully from the mouth, in an arc, sometimes over a distance of several feet. Projectile vomiting usually takes place soon after the end of a feeding, although in some cases it may be delayed for hours. Rarely, the vomit may contain blood.

In some cases, the vomited milk may smell curdled because it has mixed with stomach acid. The vomit will not contain bile, a greenish fluid from the liver that mixes with digested food after it leaves the stomach.

Despite vomiting, a baby with pyloric stenosis is usually hungry again soon after vomiting and will want to eat. The symptoms of pyloric stenosis can be deceptive because even though a baby may seem uncomfortable, he may not appear to be in great pain or at first look very ill.

Changes in Stools

Babies with pyloric stenosis usually have fewer, smaller stools because little or no food is reaching the intestines. Constipation or stools that have mucus in them may also be symptoms.

Failure to Gain Weight and Lethargy

Most babies with pyloric stenosis will fail to gain weight or will lose weight. As the condition worsens, they are at risk for developing fluid and salt abnormalities and becoming dehydrated.

Dehydrated infants are lethargic and less active than usual, and they will develop a sunken "soft spot" on their heads, sunken eyes, and a doughy, softened, or wrinkled appearance of the skin on the belly and upper parts of the arms and legs. Because urine output is decreased, it may be more than four to six hours between wet diapers.

After feeds, increased stomach contractions may make noticeable ripples, or waves of peristalsis, which move from left to right over the infant's belly as the stomach tries to empty itself against the thickened pylorus.

It's important to talk to your child's doctor if your baby experiences any of these symptoms.

Other conditions can have similar symptoms as pyloric stenosis. For instance, gastroesophageal reflux disease (GERD) usually begins before eight weeks of age, with excess spitting up, or reflux—which may resemble vomiting—taking place after feedings. However, most infants with GERD do not experience projectile vomiting, and although they may have poor weight gain, they tend to have normal stools.

In infants, symptoms of gastroenteritis—inflammation in the digestive tract that can be caused from viral or bacterial infection—may also somewhat resemble pyloric stenosis. Vomiting and dehydration are seen with both conditions; however, infants with gastroenteritis usually also have diarrhea with loose, watery, or sometimes bloody stools. Diarrhea usually isn't seen with pyloric stenosis.

Diagnosis and Treatment

Your child's doctor will ask detailed questions about the baby's feeding and vomiting patterns, including the appearance of the vomit. "The most important part of diagnosing pyloric stenosis is a reliable and consistent history and description of the vomiting," says Aviva Katz, M.D., a pediatric surgeon.

The baby will be fully examined, and any weight loss or failure to maintain growth since birth will be noted. During the exam, the doctor will attempt to feel if there is a pyloric mass—a firm, movable lump that feels like an olive and is sometimes detected in the belly of an infant with pyloric stenosis. If the doctor feels this mass, it's a strong indication that the baby has pyloric stenosis; the baby will be referred to a pediatric surgeon and hospitalized for further treatment.

If the baby's feeding history and physical examination suggest pyloric stenosis but no "olive" is felt, then an ultrasound of the baby's abdomen will usually be performed. The enlarged, thickened pylorus can be seen on ultrasound images.

Sometimes instead of an ultrasound, a barium swallow is performed. The baby swallows a small amount of a chalky liquid (barium), and then special x-rays are taken to view the pyloric region of the stomach to see if there is any narrowing or obstruction.

Infants suspected of having pyloric stenosis usually undergo blood tests because the continuous vomiting of stomach acid, as well as the resulting dehydration from fluid losses, can cause salt (electrolyte) imbalances in the blood that need to be corrected.

When an infant is diagnosed with pyloric stenosis, either through physical examination, ultrasound, or barium swallow, the baby will be admitted to the hospital and prepared for surgery. Any dehydration or electrolyte problems in the blood will be corrected with intravenous (IV) fluids, usually within twenty-four hours.

A surgical procedure called pyloromyotomy, which involves cutting through the thickened muscles of the pylorus, is performed to relieve the obstruction from pyloric stenosis. "We examine the pylorus through a very small incision, and spread the muscles that are overgrown and thickened. Nothing is cut out. The stitches are under the skin and there are no stitches or clips to remove," Dr. Katz says.

After surgery, most babies are able to return to normal feedings fairly quickly. "The baby starts feeding again three to four hours after the surgery, and the baby can return to breast-feeding or the formula that he was on prior to the surgery," Dr. Katz says. Because of swelling at the surgery site, the baby may still vomit small amounts for a day or so after surgery. As long as there are no complications, most babies who have undergone pyloromyotomy can return to a normal feeding schedule and be sent home within forty-eight hours of the surgery.

If you are breast-feeding, you may be concerned about being able to continue feeding while your baby is hospitalized. The hospital should be able to provide you with a breast pump and assist you in its use so that you can continue to express milk until your baby can once again feed regularly.

After a successful pyloromyotomy, your infant will not need to follow any special feeding schedules. Your child's doctor will probably want to examine your child at a follow-up appointment to make sure the surgical site is healing properly and that your infant is feeding well and maintaining or gaining weight.

Pyloric stenosis should not recur after a complete pyloromyotomy. If your baby continues to display symptoms weeks after the surgery, it may suggest another medical problem, such as inflammation of the stomach (gastritis) or GERD—or it could indicate that the initial pyloromyotomy was incomplete.

When to Call Your Child's Doctor

Pyloric stenosis is a medical emergency that requires immediate treatment. Call your child's doctor if your baby has any of the following symptoms:

- persistent or projectile vomiting after feeding
- poor weight gain or noted weight loss
- decreased activity or lethargy
- few or no stools over a period of one or two days
- signs of dehydration such as decreased urination (more than four to six hours between wet diapers); wrinkly or doughy appearance of the skin on the arms, legs, or belly; sunken "soft spot" on the head; sunken eyes; or possible jaundice (yellowing of the skin)

Chapter 19

Other Diseases of the Upper Gastrointestinal Tract

Chapter Contents

Section 19.1

Gastritis

Reprinted from "Gastritis," National Institute of Diabetes and Digestive and Kidney Diseases, NIH Publication No. 05-4764, December 2004.

Gastritis is not a single disease, but several different conditions that all have inflammation of the stomach lining. Gastritis can be caused by drinking too much alcohol, prolonged use of nonsteroidal anti-inflammatory drugs (NSAIDs) such as aspirin or ibuprofen, or infection with bacteria such as *Helicobacter pylori* (*H. pylori*). Sometimes gastritis develops after major surgery, traumatic injury, burns, or severe infections. Certain diseases, such as pernicious anemia, autoimmune disorders, and chronic bile reflux, can cause gastritis as well.

The most common symptoms are abdominal upset or pain. Other symptoms are belching, abdominal bloating, nausea, and vomiting or a feeling of fullness or of burning in the upper abdomen. Blood in your vomit or black stools may be a sign of bleeding in the stomach, which may indicate a serious problem requiring immediate medical attention.

Gastritis is diagnosed through one or more medical tests:

- **Upper gastrointestinal endoscopy.** The doctor eases an endoscope, a thin tube containing a tiny camera, through your mouth (or occasionally nose) and down into your stomach to look at the stomach lining. The doctor will check for inflammation and may remove a tiny sample of tissue for tests. This procedure to remove a tissue sample is called a biopsy.

- **Blood test.** The doctor may check your red blood cell count to see whether you have anemia, which means that you do not have enough red blood cells. Anemia can be caused by bleeding from the stomach.

- **Stool test.** This test checks for the presence of blood in your stool, a sign of bleeding. Stool test may also be used to detect the presence of *H. pylori* in the digestive tract.

Treatment usually involves taking drugs to reduce stomach acid and thereby help relieve symptoms and promote healing. (Stomach acid irritates the inflamed tissue in the stomach.) Avoidance of certain foods, beverages, or medicines may also be recommended.

If your gastritis is caused by an infection, that problem may be treated as well. For example, the doctor might prescribe antibiotics to clear up *H. pylori* infection. Once the underlying problem disappears, the gastritis usually does too. Talk to your doctor before stopping any medicine or starting any gastritis treatment on your own.

Section 19.2

Ménétrier Disease

Reprinted from "Ménétrier's Disease," National Institute of Diabetes and Digestive and Kidney Diseases, NIH Publication No. 03-4639, April 2003.

Ménétrier disease causes giant folds of tissue to grow in the wall of the stomach. The tissue may be inflamed and may contain ulcers. The disease also causes glands in the stomach to waste away and causes the body to lose fluid containing a protein called albumin. Ménétrier disease increases a person's risk of stomach cancer. People who have this rare, chronic disease are usually men between ages thirty and sixty. The cause of the disease is unknown.

Ménétrier disease is also called giant hypertrophic gastritis, protein losing gastropathy, or hypertrophic gastropathy.

Symptoms

Symptoms include pain or discomfort and tenderness in the top middle part of the abdomen, loss of appetite, nausea, vomiting, diarrhea, vomiting blood, swelling in the abdomen, and ulcer-like pain after eating.

Diagnosis

Ménétrier disease is diagnosed through x-rays, endoscopy, and biopsy of stomach tissue. Endoscopy involves looking at the inside of the stomach using a long, lighted tube that is inserted through the mouth. Biopsy involves removing a tiny piece of stomach tissue to examine under the microscope for signs of disease.

Treatment

Treatment may include medications to relieve ulcer symptoms and treat inflammation, and a high-protein diet. Part or all of the stomach may need to be removed if the disease is severe.

Section 19.3

Rapid Gastric Emptying

Reprinted from "Rapid Gastric Emptying," National Institute of Diabetes and Digestive and Kidney Diseases, NIH Publication No. 05-4629, December 2004.

Rapid gastric emptying, or dumping syndrome, happens when the lower end of the small intestine (jejunum) fills too quickly with undigested food from the stomach. "Early" dumping begins during or right after a meal. Symptoms of early dumping include nausea, vomiting, bloating, cramping, diarrhea, dizziness, and fatigue. "Late" dumping happens one to three hours after eating. Symptoms of late dumping include hypoglycemia, weakness, sweating, and dizziness. Many people have both types.

Certain types of stomach surgery that allow the stomach to empty rapidly are the main cause of dumping syndrome. Patients with Zollinger-Ellison syndrome may also have dumping syndrome. (Zollinger-Ellison syndrome is a rare disorder involving extreme peptic ulcer disease and gastrin-secreting tumors in the pancreas.)

Doctors diagnose dumping syndrome primarily on the basis of symptoms in patients who have had gastric surgery that causes the syndrome. Tests may be needed to exclude other conditions that have similar symptoms.

Treatment includes changes in eating habits and medication. People who have dumping syndrome need to eat several small meals a day that are low in carbohydrates and should drink liquids between meals, not with them. People with severe cases take medicine to slow their digestion. Doctors may also recommend surgery.

Section 19.4

Zollinger-Ellison Syndrome

Reprinted from "Zollinger-Ellison Syndrome," National Institute of Diabetes and Digestive and Kidney Diseases, NIH Publication No. 04-4692, September 2004.

Zollinger-Ellison syndrome (ZES) is a rare disorder that causes tumors in the pancreas and duodenum and ulcers in the stomach and duodenum. The pancreas is a gland located behind the stomach. It produces enzymes that break down fat, protein, and carbohydrates from food, and hormones like insulin that break down sugar. The duodenum is the first part of the small intestine.

The tumors secrete a hormone called gastrin that causes the stomach to produce too much acid, which in turn causes stomach and duodenal ulcers (peptic ulcers). The ulcers caused by ZES are less responsive to treatment than ordinary peptic ulcers. What causes people with ZES to develop tumors is unknown, but approximately 25 percent of ZES cases are associated with a genetic disorder called multiple endocrine neoplasia type 1, which is associated with additional disorders.

The symptoms of ZES include signs of peptic ulcers: gnawing, burning pain in the abdomen; diarrhea; nausea; vomiting; fatigue; weakness; weight loss; and bleeding. Physicians diagnose ZES through blood tests to measure levels of gastrin and gastric acid secretion. They may check for ulcers by doing an endoscopy, which involves looking at the lining of the stomach and duodenum through a lighted tube.

The primary treatment for ZES is medication to reduce the production of stomach acid. Proton pump inhibitors that suppress acid production and promote healing are the first line of treatment and include lansoprazole, omeprazole, pantoprazole, and rabeprazole. H_2 blockers such as cimetidine, famotidine, and ranitidine may also be used, but are less effective in reducing stomach acid. Surgery to treat peptic ulcers or to remove tumors in the pancreas or duodenum are other treatment options. People who have been treated for ZES should be monitored in case the ulcers or tumors recur.

Part Four

Disorders of the Lower Gastrointestinal Tract

Chapter 20

Irritable Bowel Syndrome

Irritable bowel syndrome (IBS) is a disorder that interferes with the normal functions of the large intestine (colon). It is characterized by a group of symptoms—crampy abdominal pain, bloating, constipation, and diarrhea.

One in five Americans has IBS, making it one of the most common disorders diagnosed by doctors. It occurs more often in women than in men, and it usually begins around age twenty.

IBS causes a great deal of discomfort and distress, but it does not permanently harm the intestines and does not lead to intestinal bleeding or to any serious disease such as cancer. Most people can control their symptoms with diet, stress management, and medications prescribed by their physician. Yet for some people IBS can be disabling. They may be unable to work, go to social events, or travel even short distances.

What causes IBS?

What causes one person to have IBS and not another? No one knows. Symptoms cannot be traced to a single organic cause. Research suggests that people with IBS seem to have a colon that is more sensitive and reactive than usual to a variety of things, including certain foods and stress. Some evidence indicates that the immune system,

Excerpted from "Irritable Bowel Syndrome," National Institute of Diabetes and Digestive and Kidney Diseases, NIH Publication No. 03-693, April 2003.

which fights infection, is also involved. IBS symptoms result from the following:

- The normal motility of the colon may not work properly. It can be spasmodic or can even stop temporarily. Spasms are sudden strong muscle contractions that come and go.

- The lining of the colon (epithelium), which is affected by the immune and nervous systems, regulates the passage of fluids in and out of the colon. In IBS, the epithelium appears to work properly. However, fast movement of the colon's contents can overcome the absorptive capacity of the colon. The result is too much fluid in the stool. In other patients, colonic movement is too slow, too much fluid is absorbed, and constipation develops.

- The colon responds strongly to stimuli (for example, foods or stress) that would not bother most people.

In people with IBS, stress and emotions can strongly affect the colon. It has many nerves that connect it to the brain. Like the heart and the lungs, the colon is partly controlled by the autonomic nervous system, which has been proven to respond to stress. For example, when you are frightened, your heart beats faster, your blood pressure may go up, or you may gasp. The colon responds to stress also. It may contract too much or too little. It may absorb too much water or too little.

Research has shown that very mild or hidden (occult) celiac disease is present in a smaller group of people with symptoms that mimic IBS. People with celiac disease cannot digest gluten, which is present in wheat, rye, barley, and possibly oats. Foods containing gluten are toxic to these people, and their immune system responds by damaging the small intestine. A blood test can determine whether celiac disease is present.

The following have been associated with a worsening of IBS symptoms:

- large meals
- bloating from gas in the colon
- medicines
- wheat, rye, barley, chocolate, milk products, or alcohol
- drinks with caffeine, such as coffee, tea, or colas
- stress, conflict, or emotional upsets

Researchers have also found that women with IBS may have more symptoms during their menstrual periods, suggesting that reproductive hormones can exacerbate IBS problems.

What does the colon do?

The colon, which is about five feet long, connects the small intestine with the rectum and anus. The major function of the colon is to absorb water, nutrients, and salts from the partially digested food that enters from the small intestine. Two pints of liquid matter enter the colon from the small intestine each day. Stool volume is a third of a pint. The difference in volume represents what the colon absorbs each day.

Colon motility (the contraction of the colon muscles and the movement of its contents) is controlled by nerves and hormones and by electrical activity in the colon muscle. Contractions move the contents slowly back and forth but mainly toward the rectum. During this passage, water and nutrients are absorbed into the body. What remains is stool. A few times each day, strong muscle contractions move down the colon, pushing the stool ahead of them. Some of these strong contractions result in a bowel movement. The muscles of the pelvis and anal sphincters have to relax at the right time to allow the stool to be expelled. If the muscles of the colon, sphincters, and pelvis do not contract in a coordinated way, the contents do not move smoothly, resulting in abdominal pain, cramps, constipation or diarrhea, and a sense of incomplete stool movement.

What are the symptoms of IBS?

Abdominal pain or discomfort in association with bowel dysfunction is the main symptom. Symptoms may vary from person to person. Some people have constipation (hard, difficult-to-pass, or infrequent bowel movements); others have diarrhea (frequent loose stools, often with an urgent need to move the bowels); and still others experience alternating constipation and diarrhea. Some people experience bloating, which is gas building up in the intestines and causing the feeling of pressure inside the abdomen.

IBS affects the motility or movement of stool and gas through the colon and how fluids are absorbed. When stool remains in the colon for a long time, too much water is absorbed from it. Then it becomes hard and difficult to pass. Or spasms push the stool through the colon too fast for the fluid to be absorbed, resulting in diarrhea. In addition, with spasms, gas may get trapped in one area or stool may collect in one place, temporarily unable to move forward.

Sometimes people with IBS have a crampy urge to move their bowels but cannot do so or pass mucus with their bowel movements.

Bleeding, fever, weight loss, and persistent severe pain are not symptoms of IBS and may indicate other problems such as inflammation or rarely cancer.

How is IBS diagnosed?

If you think you have IBS, seeing your doctor is the first step. IBS is generally diagnosed on the basis of a complete medical history that includes a careful description of symptoms and a physical examination.

No particular test is specific for IBS. However, diagnostic tests may be performed to rule out other diseases. These tests may include stool or blood tests, x-rays, or endoscopy (viewing the colon through a flexible tube inserted through the anus). If these tests are all negative, the doctor may diagnose IBS based on your symptoms: that is, how often you have had abdominal pain or discomfort during the past year, when the pain starts and stops in relation to bowel function, and how your bowel frequency and stool consistency are altered.

Criteria for IBS Diagnosis

- Abdominal pain or discomfort for at least twelve weeks out of the previous twelve months. These twelve weeks do not have to be consecutive.

- The abdominal pain or discomfort has two of the following three features:
  - It is relieved by having a bowel movement.
  - When it starts, there is a change in how often you have a bowel movement.
  - When it starts, there is a change in the form of the stool or the way it looks.

What is the treatment for IBS?

No cure has been found for IBS, but many options are available to treat the symptoms. Your doctor will give you the best treatments available for your particular symptoms and encourage you to manage stress and make changes to your diet.

Medications are an important part of relieving symptoms. Your doctor may suggest fiber supplements or occasional laxatives for constipation, as well as medicines to decrease diarrhea, tranquilizers to calm you, or drugs that control colon muscle spasms to reduce abdominal pain. Antidepressants may also relieve some symptoms. Medications available to treat IBS specifically are the following:

- Alosetron hydrochloride (Lotronex) has been re-approved by the U.S. Food and Drug Administration (FDA) for women with severe IBS who have not responded to conventional therapy and whose primary symptom is diarrhea. However, even in these patients, it should be used with caution because it can have serious side effects, such as severe constipation or decreased blood flow to the colon.

- Tegaserod maleate (Zelnorm) has been approved by the FDA for the short-term treatment (usually four weeks) of women with IBS whose primary symptom is constipation.

With any medication, even over-the-counter medications such as laxatives and fiber supplements, it is important to follow your doctor's instructions. Laxatives can be habit forming if they are not used carefully or are used too frequently.

It is also important to note that medications affect people differently and that no one medication or combination of medications will work for everyone with IBS. You need to work with your doctor to find the best combination of medicine, diet, counseling, and support to control your symptoms.

How does stress affect IBS?

Stress—feeling mentally or emotionally tense, troubled, angry, or overwhelmed—stimulates colon spasms in people with IBS. The colon has a vast supply of nerves that connect it to the brain. These nerves control the normal rhythmic contractions of the colon and cause abdominal discomfort at stressful times. People often experience cramps or "butterflies" when they are nervous or upset. Yet with IBS, the colon can be overly responsive to even slight conflict or stress. Stress also makes the mind more tuned to the sensations that arise in the colon and makes the stressed person perceive these sensations as unpleasant.

Some evidence suggests that IBS is affected by the immune system, which fights infection in the body. The immune system is also affected by stress. For all these reasons, stress management is an important part of treatment for IBS. Stress management comprises

- stress reduction (relaxation) training and relaxation therapies, such as meditation
- counseling and support
- regular exercise such as walking or yoga
- changes to the stressful situations in your life
- adequate sleep

Can changes in diet help IBS?

For many people, careful eating reduces IBS symptoms. Before changing your diet, keep a journal noting the foods that seem to cause distress. Then discuss your findings with your doctor. You may also want to consult a registered dietitian, who can help you make changes to your diet. For instance, if dairy products cause your symptoms to flare up, you can try eating less of those foods. You might be able to tolerate yogurt better than other dairy products because it contains bacteria that supply the enzyme needed to digest lactose, the sugar found in milk products. Dairy products are an important source of calcium and other nutrients. If you need to avoid dairy products, be sure to get adequate nutrients in the foods you substitute, or take supplements.

In many cases, dietary fiber may lessen IBS symptoms, particularly constipation. However, it may not help pain or diarrhea. Whole-grain breads and cereals, fruits, and vegetables are good sources of fiber. High-fiber diets keep the colon mildly distended, which may help prevent spasms. Some forms of fiber also keep water in the stool, thereby preventing hard stools that are difficult to pass. Doctors usually recommend a diet with enough fiber to produce soft, painless bowel movements. High-fiber diets may cause gas and bloating, but these symptoms often go away within a few weeks as your body adjusts.

Drinking six to eight glasses of plain water a day is important, especially if you have diarrhea. But drinking carbonated beverages, such as sodas, may result in gas and cause discomfort. Chewing gum and eating too quickly can lead to swallowing air, which again leads to gas.

Also, large meals can cause cramping and diarrhea, so eating smaller meals more often or eating smaller portions should help IBS symptoms.

It may also help if your meals are low in fat and high in carbohydrates, such as pasta, rice, whole-grain breads and cereals (unless you have celiac disease), fruits, and vegetables.

Is IBS linked to other diseases?

IBS itself is not a disease. As its name indicates, it is a syndrome— a combination of signs and symptoms. Yet IBS has not been shown to lead to any serious, organic diseases, including cancer. Through the years, IBS has been called by many names, among them colitis, mucous colitis, spastic colon, or spastic bowel. However, no link has been established between IBS and inflammatory bowel diseases such as Crohn disease or ulcerative colitis.

Points to Remember

- IBS is a disorder that interferes with the normal functions of the colon. The symptoms are crampy abdominal pain, bloating, constipation, and diarrhea.

- IBS is a common disorder found more often in women than in men and usually begins around age twenty.

- People with IBS have colons that are more sensitive and react to things that might not bother other people, such as stress, large meals, gas, medicines, certain foods, caffeine, or alcohol.

- IBS is diagnosed by its symptoms and by the absence of other diseases.

- Most people can control their symptoms by taking medicines (laxatives, antidiarrhea medicines, tranquilizers, or antidepressants), reducing stress, and changing their diet.

- IBS does not harm the intestines and does not lead to cancer. It is not related to Crohn disease or ulcerative colitis.

Chapter 21

Inflammatory Bowel Disease

Chapter Contents

Section 21.1

Inflammatory Bowel Disease: An Overview

Reprinted from "Inflammatory Bowel Disease,"
National Women's Health Information Center, August 2002.

What is inflammatory bowel disease?

Inflammatory bowel disease (IBD) is a chronic disorder that causes an inflamed and swollen digestive tract or intestinal wall. When the digestive tract becomes inflamed or swollen with IBD, sores (ulcers) form and bleed. This, in turn, can cause abdominal pain, watery diarrhea, blood in the stool, fatigue, reduced appetite, weight loss, or fever. The two most common forms of IBD are ulcerative colitis (UC) and Crohn disease (CD).

A healthy digestive system removes nutrients from food so they can be absorbed into the bloodstream. It then stores the unwanted waste until it passes out of the body. Food moves from the esophagus to the small intestine, where the nutrients are absorbed. The leftover water and waste move to the large intestine (colon), then through the rectum and out the anus.

Who is affected by IBD?

IBD affects millions of people throughout the world, but is more common in people who live in regions farther away from the equator (like North America, Europe, and Australia). Estimates from 1994 show one million cases in the United States alone. The disease most often develops during the second and third decades of life in both men and women. The average age of diagnosis is twenty-seven. A second, but much smaller, peak of new cases occurs in people after age sixty-five. Overall, women and men are equally affected by IBD. In the past, whites have been shown to have the highest risk for the disease, especially people of Jewish and European descent.

What causes IBD?

No one knows exactly what causes IBD, but these things may all play a role: an unknown virus or bacterium, heredity, and the environment.

Your digestive tract may become inflamed when your body tries to fight off an invading bacterium, or the inflammation can result from the virus or bacterium itself.

The most recent data shows that rates of IBD are similar in whites and Americans of African descent, but the disease is rare in Africa itself, which points to the role of the environment. Some of the environmental factors linked to IBD are a lifestyle with little activity, higher socioeconomic status, and living in a more developed country.

Besides the environment, IBD can also run in families. About 15 to 30 percent of people with IBD have a relative with the disease. Studies are looking at whether a certain gene or group of genes makes a person more likely to get IBD. In 2001, the first gene for CD was found. An abnormal form of the gene known as *Nod2* occurs twice as often in persons with CD as in the general population. In the abnormal form of this gene, some of the body's power to fight bacteria is missing, and it has been known for a long time that there is a link between bacteria in the gut and CD.

Stress does not cause IBD. As with other illnesses though, stress can worsen the symptoms of IBD. There also is no known link between eating certain kinds of foods and getting IBD, but changing your diet can help reduce symptoms and replace lost nutrients.

What is ulcerative colitis (UC)?

Ulcerative colitis (UC) causes inflammation and sores called ulcers in the top layers of the inner lining of the large intestine (colon) or rectum. It most often occurs in the lower part of the colon and rectum, but may affect the whole colon. When it is located only in the rectum, it is called proctitis. It most often occurs in young people between the ages of fifteen and forty.

What are the symptoms of UC?

The most common symptom is diarrhea because the inflammation keeps water from being absorbed into the bloodstream and makes the colon empty often. Inflammation also kills healthy colon lining cells, which causes ulcers to form and bleed, and make pus and mucus. Other symptoms include bloody diarrhea, severe abdominal cramps, nausea, and frequent fever. Most people with UC have times when they feel well (remission) and times when they feel sick (relapse). About half of the people with UC have only mild symptoms. In severe cases, people can become malnourished and may need to have a special diet or be fed fluids through a vein.

What are the complications of UC?

UC also can cause problems like arthritis, inflammation in the eye, liver disease, skin rashes, anemia, and kidney stones. No one knows why these problems occur outside of the colon. They may occur when the immune system triggers inflammation in other parts of the body. These problems are usually mild and go away when the colitis is treated. Osteoporosis can occur due to low calcium and vitamin D intake through dairy products, poor absorption of nutrients in the body, inflammation, and use of corticosteroids (for treatment of UC).

How do I know if I have UC?

In order to find out if you have UC, your doctor will examine you and may order blood tests or samples of a bowel movement to check for blood or germs. He or she also may give you a barium enema, which

Table 21.1. Differences between Ulcerative Colitis (UC) and Crohn Disease (CD)

	UC	CD
Symptoms	Diarrhea	Diarrhea
	Bloody Diarrhea	Rectal bleeding
	Pus or mucus in the stool	Pain and tenderness in abdomen, especially in the lower right side
	Severe abdominal cramps	
		Low-grade fever
	Nausea	
		Anemia
	Frequent fever	
		Sometimes constipation because of a blockage
		Slowed growth and delayed sexual development in some childhood cases
Parts of Digestive System Affected	Only the top layers of the walls of the colon or rectum (most often in the lower part of the colon and rectum)	Deep in the lining of the walls of the colon or small intestine
		Any part of the digestive tract from mouth to anus

is an x-ray of the colon, or a flexible sigmoidoscopy or colonoscopy, screening tests that allow the doctor to see the inside lining of the colon.

What is Crohn disease (CD)?

Crohn disease (CD) most commonly causes inflammation deep in the lining of the walls of the large intestine (colon) or the small intestine, but also can affect any part of the digestive tract from the mouth to the anus. Sometimes CD can affect other parts of the upper digestive tract with ulcers forming in the stomach, upper small intestine, or esophagus. About one-third of cases of CD affect the small bowel, usually involving the ileum (the last portion of the small intestine that connects to the large intestine or colon). Nearly half of all cases involve both small and large bowel. About 20 percent of cases are in the colon alone. Lesions near the anus occur in about one-quarter to one-third of persons with CD but are rarely the only site of CD. Like UC, CD also is an illness that brings periods of remission and relapse.

What are the symptoms of CD?

The earliest most common symptoms are pain in the abdomen, especially the lower right side, tenderness, and often diarrhea. Constipation, weight loss, rectal bleeding, and low-grade fever also may occur. Bleeding may be bad enough to cause anemia or an unhealthy, low level of iron in the blood. Children with CD may have slowed growth and delayed sexual development in some cases.

What are the complications of CD?

The most common problem with CD is blockage of the intestine. Because swelling and scar tissue thicken the bowel wall, the intestine passage can become closed off. Fistulas, or abnormal connections between the intestine and other organs, can form from ulcers in the intestine, breaking through into other parts of the intestines or surrounding tissues of the bladder, vagina, or skin. They often form around the anus and rectum.

Nutrition problems are common with CD. Many people have deficiencies of proteins, calories, and vitamins. These can be caused by not eating enough, loss of protein within the intestine, or poor absorption. Osteoporosis also is a threat because of low calcium and vitamin D intake through dairy products, poor absorption of nutrients in the body, or the use of corticosteroids (for treatment of CD or inflammation itself). Some persons with CD have problems with arthritis, their skin, inflammation in the eyes or mouth, kidney stones, gallstones, or other diseases of the liver. Some of these problems get better during treatment for disease in the digestive system, but some are treated separately.

How do I know if I have CD?

In order to find out if you have CD, your doctor will examine you and may order blood tests to check for anemia (low iron levels) which could be a sign of bleeding in the intestine, or samples of a bowel movement to check for blood or germs. He or she also may do an upper gastrointestinal (GI) series to look at the small intestine. This is an x-ray that can show inflammation or other problems in the intestine. You also could have a barium enema, which is an x-ray of the colon, or the same screenings tests used to diagnose UC, flexible sigmoidoscopy or colonoscopy. These tests allow the doctor to view the lining of the colon. A CT scan may also be used to look for inflammation inside and outside the bowel.

Is IBD related to irritable bowel syndrome (IBS)?

UC and CD are different from irritable bowel syndrome (IBS), which is a condition that includes a group of symptoms mainly affecting the colon, or large intestine. Symptoms of IBS may include crampy pain, bloating, gas, mucus in the stool, and changes in bowel habits. IBS is also called spastic colon or spastic bowel. IBS is not a disease and does not cause inflammation, bleeding, damage to the bowel, or cancer or other serious diseases. It is called a functional disorder, which means that there is no sign of disease when the colon is examined, but the bowel doesn't work as it should. There is no direct relationship between IBS and either UC or CD, although some people with UC or CD also have IBS.

What are the signs of IBD? When should I see my health care provider?

See your health care provider if you see blood in the stool, have a change in bowel habits lasting longer than ten days, or if you have any of the following symptoms that do not improve with over-the-counter medicines.

- Severe abdominal cramps or pain
- Severe diarrhea or bloody diarrhea

- Weight loss
- Unexplained fever lasting more than one or two days
- Extreme fatigue
- Loss of appetite
- Nausea

Although UC and CD usually are not fatal, they can cause serious problems. Sometimes symptoms are bad enough that a person has to be hospitalized. For example, a person may have severe diarrhea that causes dehydration and needs to be treated with fluids through his or her vein.

Can IBD be prevented?

Because no one knows exactly what causes IBD, it is hard to try to prevent. But if you have IBD, you can make changes in your diet and lifestyle to control your symptoms. You might need to limit dairy products, try low-fat foods, experiment with how much protein and fiber you eat, avoid problem "gassy" foods, and eat smaller and more frequent meals. It also is important to get enough rest and avoid stress since being tired or overly upset can make your symptoms worse. Your health care provider can tell you the things to try to make you feel better.

How is IBD treated?

While there is no cure for IBD, treatments can help control symptoms. Besides changing diet and lifestyle to control symptoms, most people with UC and CD are treated with medications. In severe cases of disease, a person may need surgery to remove the diseased colon.

What medications are used to treat IBD?

Treating IBD with drugs is complicated and might require several "trial runs." It is very important to keep track of how well the drugs are working, note what side effects you are having, and report all details to your health care provider.

Most people who have mild to moderate disease are first treated with drugs called aminosalicylates. These medications are aspirin-like medications such as 5-ASA agents (a combination of the drugs sulfonamide, sulfapyridine, and salicylate). They can be given either orally or rectally to help control inflammation. Side effects can include heartburn, nausea, vomiting, diarrhea, and headache. These drugs include mesalamine and sulfasalazine, which have fewer side effects and can relieve symptoms in more than 80 percent of people with UC in the lower colon and rectum. A newer drug form of mesalamine called Colazal is reported to have even fewer side effects.

People with more severe IBD also can be treated with corticosteroids, such as prednisone and hydrocortisone, to reduce inflammation. Side effects of these drugs can include weight gain, acne, facial hair, high blood pressure, mood swings, and a higher risk of infection. A newly approved drug called Entocort EC is a steroid therapy that causes fewer side effects in people with mild to moderate CD in the ileum (the last portion of the small intestine that connects to the large intestine or colon).

Drugs that block the immune system's reaction to inflammation are also used to treat CD. Side effects can include nausea, vomiting, diarrhea, and higher risk of infection. People with moderate to severe CD who do not respond to 5-ASA agents, corticosteroids, or immune system drugs, or who have open, draining fistulas may be given a drug called infliximab (Remicade). This is the first treatment approved for CD and works to remove a protein produced by the immune system that may cause inflammation. Studies are looking at its long-term safety and effectiveness. Azathioprine and 6-mercaptopurine (6-MP) also can be used with steroids, and seem to be the most effective immunosuppressive drugs for the long-term management of both CD and UC. They are proven effective for steroid-dependent, chronically active, and steroid-resistant disease.

Antibiotics also are used to treat disease and heal fistulas in the small intestine.

Drugs like antidiarrheals, laxatives, and pain relievers also can be given to help relieve symptoms. Every person should talk with his or her doctor first before taking these drugs since some may be too harsh for the system or can make symptoms worse.

What types of surgery are used to treat IBD?

There are different types of surgery used to treat IBD. For CD, surgery is necessary at some point in the lifetime of about half of persons with this disease. Surgery can relieve symptoms or correct problems like blockages or bleeding in the intestine. Surgery to remove part of the intestine can help CD but cannot cure it. The inflammation tends to return next to the area of intestine that has been removed. Therefore, people considering surgery should carefully weigh the risks and benefits compared to other treatments.

Types of surgery for CD include:

- **Colectomy (colon removal):** A part of the colon or the entire colon and rectum may be removed. A colostomy or ileostomy may be done after the diseased colon is removed. A colostomy or ileostomy creates an opening on the abdomen (stoma) for the drainage of stool (feces) from the large intestine (colon) or small intestine (ileum) and may be temporary or permanent.

- **Small bowel resection:** The diseased parts of the small bowel can be removed and the two healthy ends sewn back together. If it is necessary to spare the intestine from its normal digestive work while it heals, a temporary opening (stoma) of the intestine onto the abdomen (ileostomy) may be done. A temporary ileostomy will be closed and repaired later. If a large portion of the bowel is removed, the ileostomy may be permanent.

For UC, persons with severe cases of this disease may need surgery to remove the diseased colon. Some of the IBD-related problems that cause health care providers to consider surgery include growth retardation, steroid dependency, serious medication side effects, cancer or pre-cancerous changes, disease that is unresponsive to medication, narrowing of the colon, and extraintestinal disease (disease caused by IBD in areas outside of the digestive tract).

Types of surgery for UC include:

- **Colectomy, or colon removal.** About 25 to 40 percent of people with UC must have surgery to remove the colon because of bleeding, severe illness, rupture of the colon, or risk of cancer. For years, individuals who had colons removed had to wear a "bag" outside their bodies to collect waste from the digestive system. Recent surgical techniques make that no longer necessary in the vast majority of persons with CD.

- **Ileoanal pouch anastomosis:** The colon and interior of the rectum are removed during this surgery. An internal pouch is created from part of the ileum (the end of the small intestine) by pulling a portion of the ileum through the wall of the rectum and attaching it to the anus. This allows a person to continue to eliminate waste through the anus. While some people can have this surgery done all at once, this procedure is usually done in two stages. The colon and interior of the rectum are removed and a temporary ileostomy is created. Once the pouch has healed (about six to eight weeks), the temporary ileostomy is closed, restoring waste elimination through the anus.

If I have IBD and need surgery, have I failed at managing my disease?

Nothing could be further from the truth. Surgery for IBD often is viewed as a "failure" by both the person who has IBD and his or her doctor. Yet surgery, in combination with pre- and postoperative medical therapy, can lead to the best results for the person's health and quality of life.

What research is being done on new treatments for IBD?

Studies are looking at the use of human growth hormone (HGH) combined with a high-protein diet to treat CD. In a clinical trial, people treated this way had fewer symptoms after one month, and the benefits continued. The long-term risks and benefits are still being studied. Studies also are looking at the use of a gene-based drug to help growth of healthy tissue in people with UC, as well as new medications to use against factors that cause or promote inflammation.

Is there a link between IBD and colon cancer?

Having IBD can increase your chances for getting colon cancer. The risk of cancer gets higher the longer and the more the colon is involved. For example, if only the lower colon and rectum are involved, the risk of cancer is not higher than normal. However, if the whole colon is involved, the risk of cancer may be as great as thirty-two times the normal rate.

People who have had IBD throughout their colon for at least eight years, or IBD in only the left colon for at least fifteen years, should have a screening colonoscopy every one to two years to check for precancerous changes in the cells of the colon lining. This screening won't reduce the risk for getting colon cancer, but can help find cancer early, when it is easier to treat.

Does having IBD increase my chances of getting cancer? Is there any way to tell if I am developing cancer?

Some studies have found that persons with IBD have a much higher risk for other cancers for reasons not yet known. For CD, these include skin and bladder cancers. For UC, there have been reports of increased risk for connective-tissue and brain cancers, nonmelanoma skin cancers, and bone and endometrial cancers.

The most widely available test to find pre-cancerous or cancerous tissues at an early, curable stage in persons with IBD is endoscopy with biopsy of the colon. An endoscope is a device with a flexible tube and light that allows your doctor to see parts of your digestive system. The tube is inserted through the mouth or anus while you are sedated. A colonoscopy shows the entire colon, a sigmoidoscopy shows the two feet of the colon closest to the anal opening only. A biopsy is when your doctor takes small samples of tissue during the endoscopy to study under a microscope.

How is fertility affected in women with IBD?

Women with UC or inactive CD do not seem to have related fertility problems, but women with active CD or women with UC who have had an IPAA do experience more problems with fertility. Women who have inactive disease at the time of conception are no more likely to have a flare of their disease during pregnancy than if they were not pregnant. Flares are more likely to occur in the first trimester and right after the baby is born.

Is pregnancy safe for women with IBD?

Pregnancy and delivery can be relatively normal in women with IBD. Even so, women with IBD should discuss their illness with their health care providers before pregnancy. Most medications used for IBD are safe or likely safe in pregnancy. Surgery, if necessary, is safest in the second trimester. Pre-term birth or early delivery has been reported to be increased two- to threefold in women with IBD, although most children born to women with IBD are unaffected.

Section 21.2

Diet and Nutrition with Inflammatory Bowel Disease

Diet and nutrition concerns of patients with inflammatory bowel disease are extremely common, and appropriate. Patients often believe that their disease is caused by, and can be cured by diet. Unfortunately, that seems to be too simplistic an approach, which is not supported by clinical and scientific data. Diet can certainly affect symptoms of these diseases, and may play some role in the underlying inflammatory process, but it appears not to be the major factor in the inflammatory process.

Because Crohn disease and ulcerative colitis are diseases of the digestive tract, it is only natural that you will have many questions about diet and nutrition if you have been diagnosed with one of these disorders. First of all, you may be surprised to learn that there is no evidence that anything in your diet history caused or contributed to these diseases. Once you develop IBD, however, paying special attention to what you eat may go a long way toward reducing symptoms and promoting healing.

The information provided here offers an overall dietary guide for patients and their families. It is based on the results of ongoing studies and the accumulation of knowledge gained in recent years. As this research continues, we will learn even more about the relationship between nutrition and IBD.

How do Crohn disease and ulcerative colitis interfere with digestion?

To get a better idea of how diet affects people with IBD, here's a brief explanation of the way in which the body processes the food you put into it.

The real work of the digestive system takes place in the small intestine, which lies just beyond the stomach. In the small intestine, digestive juices (termed bile) from both the liver and the pancreas mix with food. This mixing is powered by the churning action of the intestinal muscle wall. After digested food is broken down into small molecules, it is absorbed through the surface of the small intestine and distributed to the rest of the body by way of the bloodstream. Watery food residue and secretions that are not digested in the small intestine pass on into the large intestine (the colon). The colon reabsorbs much of the water added to food in the small intestine. This is a kind of water conservation or "recycling" mechanism. Solid, undigested food residue is then passed from the large intestine as a bowel movement.

When the small intestine is inflamed—as it often is with Crohn disease—the intestine becomes less able to fully digest and absorb the nutrients from food. Such nutrients, as well as unabsorbed bile salts, can escape into the large intestine to varying degrees, depending on how extensively the small intestine has been injured by inflammation. This is one reason why people with Crohn disease become malnourished, in addition to just not having much appetite. Furthermore, incompletely digested foods that travel through the large intestine interfere with water conservation, even if the colon itself is not damaged. Thus, when Crohn disease affects the small intestine, it may cause diarrhea as well as malnutrition. Should the large intestine also be inflamed, the diarrhea may become even more extreme.

In ulcerative colitis, only the colon is inflamed; the small intestine continues to work normally. But because the inflamed colon does not recycle water properly, diarrhea can be severe.

Is IBD caused by allergy to food?

No. Although some people do have allergic reactions to certain foods, neither Crohn disease nor ulcerative colitis is related to food allergy. People with IBD may think they are allergic to foods because they associate the symptoms of IBD with eating.

Do any specific foods worsen the inflammation of IBD?

No. Although certain foods may aggravate symptoms of these diseases, there is no evidence that the inflammation of the intestine is directly affected. Obviously, any contaminated food that leads to food poisoning or dysentery will aggravate IBD.

Is there a special diet for people with IBD?

There is no one single diet or eating plan that will do the trick for everyone with IBD. Dietary recommendations must be individualized. They should be tailored just for you—depending on which disease you have and what part of your intestine is affected. Furthermore, these diseases are not static; they change over time, and eating patterns should reflect those changes. The key point is to strive for a well-balanced, healthy diet. Healthy eating habits, of course, are desirable for everyone but they're especially important for people with IBD.

Often, patients have questions regarding the Specific Carbohydrate Diet™ (SCD), popularized by Elaine Gottschall, M.S., author of *Breaking the Vicious Cycle*. At this time, the SCD is supported only by patient testimonials, not by systematic studies. With diseases like ulcerative colitis and Crohn disease, the only way to see if any treatment has widespread value is by appropriate, rigorous testing. The diet itself is not particularly unbalanced, but many patients find it particularly onerous to maintain. Decreasing poorly digestible carbohydrates may decrease symptoms of gas, bloat, cramps, and diarrhea in patients with IBD, but that is not the same thing as decreasing the inflammation, or affecting the disease process. Unlike the gluten-free diet for celiac sprue, which has a well-researched basis and well-demonstrated track record for affecting the underlying mechanisms at work in the disease process, the SCD does not. Bottom line: it may be worth a try (there are plenty of other diets being touted in the marketplace), but do not abandon your conventional treatment, and keep in touch with your doctor.

Which foods should be avoided?

Again, there are no blanket rules or recommendations. If a particular kind of food causes digestive problems, then try to avoid it. Yet it's important to distinguish between an actual allergy to one kind of food and an intolerance. Many people have food intolerances—far more than really have true food allergies. Elimination tests are better at diagnosing which foods must be avoided or modified than the standard allergy skin or blood testing. Many good books discuss the proper way to follow such an "elimination diet," which involves keeping a food and symptom diary over several weeks.

In fact, a food diary can not only help pinpoint which foods are troublesome for you, but it can also reveal whether or not your diet is providing an adequate supply of nutrients. By reviewing your food diary, your dietitian can see if you are getting the recommended daily allowances (RDAs) for a person of your age, sex, and size. If not, the dietitian can suggest ways to amend your diet so that your intake of nutrients is improved. That may mean increasing the amount of food you eat, changing what you eat, or adding supplements to your diet.

It's important to remember that it's not just the amount of food you consume that guarantees a healthy diet. Your daily intake needs to include an adequate amount of calories, proteins, and nutrients. A balanced diet should contain a variety of foods from all food groups. Meat, fish, poultry, and dairy products, if tolerated, are sources of protein; bread, cereal, starches, fruits, and vegetables are sources of carbohydrate; margarine and oils are sources of fat.

Should people with IBD be concerned about fluid intake?

Yes. In a condition with chronic diarrhea, the risk of dehydration always exists. If fluid intake does not keep up with diarrhea, kidney function may be affected. Patients with Crohn and other diarrheal diseases have an increased incidence of kidney stones, which is related to this problem. Furthermore, dehydration and salt loss create a feeling of weakness. For these reasons, people with IBD should consume ample fluids—especially in warm weather when loss of salt and water through the skin may be high. A good rule of thumb is to drink one half ounce per day for every pound of body weight. That means that if you weight 140 pounds, you should drink at least 70 ounces a day—or eight and three-quarters glasses. Sip your beverages, rather than gulp them. By introducing air into the digestive system, gulping can cause discomfort.

Is nutrition of special importance to IBD patients?

Yes, vitally so. IBD patients, especially people with Crohn disease whose small intestine is affected, are prone to becoming malnourished for several reasons:

- Loss of appetite—a result of nausea, abdominal pain, or altered taste sensation—may cause inadequate food intake.

- Chronic disease tends to increase the caloric or energy needs of the body; this is especially true during disease flares.

- IBD—particularly Crohn disease—is often associated with poor digestion and malabsorption of dietary protein, fat, carbohydrates, water, and a wide variety of vitamins and minerals. Thus, much of what a person eats may never truly get into the body.

Good nutrition is one of the ways the body restores itself to health. Therefore, every effort must be made to avoid becoming malnourished. Restoring and maintaining good nutrition is a key principle in the management of IBD for several reasons, including the following:

- Medications tend to be more effective in people with good nutritional status.

- When proteins and other nutrients are lost in IBD, more food must be taken in to compensate for these losses; that may be difficult for many patients when intestinal symptoms are active.

- Lost proteins, calories, and other nutrients may cause growth retardation in children and teenagers.

- Weight loss in women and girls can have an impact on hormonal levels, resulting in menstrual irregularities or even cessation of menstruation.

How does nutrition affect growth?

In young people with IBD who had onset of their disease before puberty, growth may be retarded. Poor food intake may further contribute to poor growth. Thus, good nutritional habits and adequate caloric intake are very important. Control of the disease with drugs or, less often, surgical removal of a particularly diseased region of intestine, is most successful when appropriate dietary intake is maintained.

What's the best way to decrease intestinal cramping after eating?

During periods of disease flares, eating may prompt abdominal discomfort and cramping. Here are some ways to reduce these symptoms:

- Eat smaller meals at more frequent intervals: five small meals (think in terms of "fist-sized" portions) every three or four hours, for example, rather than the traditional three large meals a day.

- Reduce the amount of greasy or fried foods in your diet. Butter, margarine, cream sauces, and pork products may all cause diarrhea and gas if fat absorption is incomplete. These symptoms tend to occur more in people who have had large amounts of small bowel (particularly ileum) removed.

- Limit consumption of milk or milk products if you are lactose intolerant. Some people cannot properly digest lactose, the sugar present in milk and many milk products, regardless of whether they have IBD. This may occur because the inner surface of the small intestine lacks a digestive enzyme, called lactase. Poor lactose digestion may lead to cramping, abdominal pain, gas, diarrhea, and bloating. Because symptoms of lactose intolerance may mimic those of IBD, it may be difficult to recognize lactose intolerance. A simple "lactose tolerance test" can be performed to identify the problem. If there is any question, milk consumption may be limited. Alternatively, lactase supplements may be added to many dairy products so that they no longer cause symptoms. Your dietitian may assist you or your child with this. However, it's desirable to maintain intake of at least some dairy products because they represent such a good source of nutrition, particularly calcium and protein.

- Restrict your intake of certain high-fiber foods such as nuts, seeds, corn, popcorn, and various Chinese vegetables. If there is narrowing of the bowel, these foods may cause cramping. High-fiber foods also provoke contractions once they enter the large intestine. Because they are not completely digested by the small intestine, these foods may also cause diarrhea. That is why a low-fiber, low-residue diet (see following) is often recommended.

However, some people who follow these guidelines may still continue to experience abdominal cramping following eating. In these cases, medication may be helpful. Prednisone and other corticosteroids, for example, may reduce intestinal inflammation—allowing the bowel to work more normally. Taking antispasmodics or antidiarrheal medications fifteen to twenty minutes before eating may also be helpful in reducing symptoms and maintaining good nutrition, particularly when the disease is mild; they should be avoided with more severe disease.

What is a low-fiber with low-residue diet?

About two-thirds of people with small bowel Crohn disease develop a marked narrowing (or stricture) of the lower small intestine, the ileum. For these patients, a low-fiber with low-residue diet or a special liquid diet may be beneficial in minimizing abdominal pain and other symptoms. This diet minimizes the consumption of foods that add "scrapy" residue to the stool. These include raw fruits, vegetables, and seeds, as well as nuts and corn hulls. The registered dietitian associated with your IBD treatment program can assist you in devising such a diet when appropriate. Often, these dietary adjustments are temporary; the patient follows them until the inflammation that caused the narrowing responds either to medical treatment or to a corrective surgical procedure.

It is important, however, to watch out that you do not impose too many food restrictions on yourself or your child. These limit variety in the diet and make a balanced intake of foods more difficult to achieve.

Is there a place for fast or "junk" food?

Children with IBD face special challenges, and eating nutritiously is high up on the list. Parents would like to think that there's no place in a healthy diet for fast food, but this may not be true. Some of these foods provide a valuable supply of nutrients as well as calories. Take pizza, for instance. The cheese offers calcium, protein, and vitamin D; the tomato sauce provides vitamins A and C; and the crust supplies B vitamins. The same is true for other popular favorites such as hamburgers or cheeseburgers, although all of these foods also contain more fat and salt than should be consumed on a regular basis. Milk shakes and ice cream also offer a good source of calcium, proteins, and calories. If lactose intolerance is a problem, that can be overcome by taking commercially available lactase in tablet form before consuming any dairy products.

Do patients with IBD absorb foods normally?

Most often, yes. Patients who have inflammation only in the large intestine absorb food normally. People with Crohn disease may have problems with digestion if their disease involves the small intestine. They may eat enough food but cannot absorb it adequately. In fact, up to 40 percent of people with Crohn disease do not absorb carbohydrates properly. They may experience bloating, gaseousness, and diarrhea as well as a loss in important nutrients. Fat malabsorption is another problem in Crohn disease, affecting at least one-third of patients. At particular risk are people who have had terminal ileal resections. The degree to which digestion is impaired depends on how much of the small intestine is diseased and whether any intestine has been removed during surgery. If only the last foot or two of the ileum is inflamed, the absorption of all nutrients except vitamin B_{12} will probably be normal. If more than two or three feet of ileum is diseased, significant malabsorption of fat may occur. If the upper small intestine is also inflamed, the degree of malabsorption in Crohn disease is apt to be much worse, and deficiencies of many nutrients, minerals, and more vitamins are likely. Some IBD therapies—especially the 5-ASA medications (e.g., Asacol®, Pentasa®)—cause interference with the absorption of folate, which is essential in helping to prevent cancer and birth defects, so it should be taken in supplement form.

Should supplemental vitamins be taken? If so, which ones?

Again, that depends on the extent and location of the disease. As noted previously, vitamin B_{12} is absorbed in the lower ileum. That means that people who have ileitis (Crohn disease that affects the ileum) or those who have undergone small bowel surgery may have a vitamin B_{12} deficiency because they are unable to absorb enough of this vitamin from their diet or from oral supplements. To correct this deficiency (which can be determined by measuring the amount of this vitamin in the blood), a monthly intramuscular injection of vitamin B_{12} may be required. Folic acid (another B vitamin) deficiency is also quite common in patients who are on the drug sulfasalazine. They should take a folate tablet, 1 mg daily, as a supplement. For most people with chronic IBD, it is worthwhile to take a multivitamin preparation regularly. If you suffer from maldigestion or have undergone intestinal surgery, other vitamins—particularly vitamin D—may be required. Affecting as many as 68 percent of people, vitamin D deficiency is one of the most common nutritional deficiencies seen in association with Crohn disease. Vitamin D is essential for good bone formation and for the metabolism of calcium. Supplementation of this vitamin should be in the range of 800 I.U./day, especially in the non-sunny areas of the country, and particularly for those with active disease. Together with vitamins A, E, and K, vitamin D is a fat-soluble vitamin; these tend to be less easily absorbed than water-soluble vitamins. Consequently, they may be absorbed better in liquid rather than pill form.

Are any special minerals recommended?

In most IBD patients, there is no obvious lack of minerals. However, iron deficiency is fairly common in people with ulcerative colitis and Crohn colitis and less common in those with small intestine disease. It results from blood loss following inflammation and ulceration of the colon. Blood iron levels are easily measured, and if a deficiency is found (otherwise known as anemia), oral iron tablets or liquid may be given. The usual dose is 300 mg, taken one to three times a day—depending on the extent of the deficiency and the patient's tolerance.

Oral iron turns the stool black, which can be mistaken for intestinal bleeding.

Other mineral deficiencies include potassium and magnesium. People may develop potassium deficiencies with diarrhea or vomiting, or as a result of prednisone therapy. Potassium supplements are available in tablet and other forms. Oral supplements of magnesium oxide may prove necessary for people who have magnesium deficiency caused by chronic diarrhea or extensive small intestinal disease, or those who have had substantial lengths of intestine removed through surgery.

Trace elements are nutrients that are absorbed in the body in minute quantities. Still, they are essential for some important biologic functions. Deficiencies in trace elements are noted in people with advanced Crohn disease—mainly those with poor nutritional intake and extensive small intestine disease.

What about calcium deficiency and bone disease in IBD?

One of the more important deficiencies seen in association with IBD is calcium deficiency—either alone or in conjunction with vitamin D deficiency. People with IBD may have limited intake of calcium in their diet, avoiding dairy products because they have a lactose intolerance or because they think they have one. Other people may consume enough calcium in their diet but not absorb it properly because of small-intestine disease or resection. Then, too, certain medications used in IBD may have an adverse effect on bone health. Long-term use of prednisone and other steroids, for example, slows the process of new bone formation and accelerates the breakdown of old bone. It also interferes with calcium absorption. In addition to steroid use, Crohn' disease itself has been shown to be linked with bone thinning and osteoporosis, so screening with bone density studies is suggested for those at risk.

If prednisone cannot be discontinued altogether, a reduction in dosage or an alternate-day dosing may help prevent IBD-related bone loss. Patients should aim for at least 1,500 mg of calcium daily, either in dietary form or as supplements taken in three divided doses during the day. Vitamin D supplements are also recommended.

Research is currently under way to determine whether other therapies for bone disease—such as those used in people with postmenopausal osteoporosis—might be appropriate for IBD-related bone loss. These include the bisphosphonates (such as Fosamax®), calcitonin, and fluoride.

What is nutritional support?

Because IBD, especially Crohn disease, may improve with nutritional support, it may be necessary to provide nutrition by delivering a nutrient-rich liquid formula directly into the stomach or small bowel. Known as enteral nutrition, this type of feeding is given overnight through a tube, most commonly from the nose to the stomach. This is called a nasogastric (NG) tube. This method ensures that patients receive nutrition while sleeping. In the morning, they remove the tube and go to work or school and generally pursue their normal activities. In this way, patients receive all the nutrition they need and are free to eat normally—or not—throughout the day.

Enteral feedings can also be given through a gastrostomy tube (G-tube). A gastrostomy is a surgically created opening through the abdominal wall, leading directly into the stomach. The feeding tube is passed through this opening. The feedings are most commonly given overnight, but they can also be given intermittently throughout the day. Some patients prefer this approach because it avoids the discomfort of passing a tube down through the nose.

Total parenteral nutrition (TPN) is delivered through a catheter placed into a large blood vessel, usually one in the chest. Although it bypasses the intestine and thereby allows the bowel to rest, parenteral nutrition may create more complications than enteral nutrition. It is also more expensive than the other methods of nutritional support and requires more specialized training to use.

What's new in nutritional therapy for IBD?

Eating to help the gut heal itself is one of the new concepts in IBD treatment, and numerous experimental studies are being conducted in this area. Fish or flaxseed oils, in the diet or as supplements, have been used to help fight the inflammation in IBD. The complex carbohydrates that are not digested by the small bowel, such as psyllium, stimulate the bacteria in the colon to produce short-chain fatty acids. These fatty acids help the mucosa (the lining) of the colon to heal itself.

Another approach is the use of probiotics, which are just beginning to be appreciated as a therapeutic aid in IBD. Probiotics are "good" bacteria that restore balance to the enteric microflora—bacteria that live in everybody's intestine. Lactobacillus preparations and live-culture yogurt can be very helpful in aiding recovery of the intestine. There is much work being done in the use of diet and supplements to aid in the healing of IBD and much more to be learned.

Cancer chemoprevention with minerals (selenium, calcium), vitamins (folic acid), and medications (the 5-ASA drugs seem to fulfill this role for many with IBD) is a developing field, and there will be more about this as new research studies are published.

In summary, while diet and nutrition do not play a role in causing IBD, maintaining a well-balanced diet that is rich in nutrients can help you to live a healthier life. Proper nutrition depends, in large part, on whether you have Crohn disease or ulcerative colitis, and what part of your intestine is affected. It's important to talk to your doctor (and it also can be helpful to ask your physician to recommend a dietitian) to develop a diet that works for you.

Section 21.3

Introduction to Crohn Disease

"Living with Crohn's Disease," © 2005 Crohn's and Colitis Foundation of America, Inc. (CCFA). Reprinted with permission.

Understanding the Diagnosis

Your doctor has just told you that you have a disease called Crohn disease. Quite possibly, you have never even heard of this condition before. (Most people, in fact, are unfamiliar with Crohn disease.) And now you have it. And, to make matters worse, your doctor has said that Crohn disease doesn't go away.

If you feel overwhelmed and scared right now, that's only natural. You probably have a ton of questions, starting with "Just what is Crohn disease?" But you're also wondering how you got it and, more important, how it will affect you—both now and down the road. For example, you'll want to know:

• Will I be able to work, travel, and exercise?

• Should I be on a special diet?

• Will I need surgery?

• How will Crohn disease change my life?

That's the purpose of this section: to answer those questions and to walk you through the key points about Crohn disease and what you may expect in the future. You won't become an expert overnight, but gradually you'll learn more and more. And the more you know, the better you'll be able to cope with the disease and become an active member of your own health care team.

What Is Crohn Disease?

The disease is named after Dr. Burrill B. Crohn, who published a landmark paper with colleagues Oppenheimer and Ginsburg in 1932, describing the features of what is known today as Crohn disease. Crohn and a related disease, ulcerative colitis, are the two main disease categories that belong to a larger group of illnesses called inflammatory bowel disease (IBD).

Both Crohn disease and ulcerative colitis cause diarrhea (sometimes bloody), as well as abdominal pain. Because the symptoms of these two illnesses are so similar, it is sometimes difficult for doctors to make a definitive diagnosis. In fact, approximately 10 percent of cases are unable to be pinpointed as either Crohn disease or ulcerative colitis.

While ulcerative colitis is limited to the colon (also called the large intestine), Crohn disease may involve any part of the gastrointestinal (GI) tract from the mouth to the anus. However, it may also include most of the intestine (the ileum) and the beginning of the colon. All layers of the intestine may be involved, and there can be normal healthy bowel in between patches of diseased bowel. These are the so-called skip areas. In contrast, ulcerative colitis moves in a more even and continuous distribution and affects only the superficial layers of the colon.

What Does "Chronic" Mean?

No one knows exactly what causes either Crohn disease or ulcerative colitis. Also, no one can predict how the disease—once it is diagnosed—will affect a particular person. Some people go for years without having any symptoms, while others have more frequent flare-ups of disease. However, one thing is sure: Crohn disease—like ulcerative colitis—is a chronic condition.

Chronic conditions are ongoing situations. They can be controlled with treatment but cannot be cured. That means that the disease is long-term, but it does *not* mean that it is fatal. It isn't. Most people who have Crohn disease lead full and productive lives.

A Brief Introduction to the GI Tract

Most of us aren't very familiar with the gastrointestinal (GI) tract, even though it occupies a lot of "real estate" in our bodies.

Here's a quick tour:

The GI tract actually starts at the mouth. It follows a twisting and turning course and ends, many yards later, at the rectum. In between are a number of organs that all play a part in processing food and transporting it through the body. The first is the esophagus, a narrow tube that connects the mouth to the stomach. After that comes the stomach itself. Moving downward, the next organ is the small intestine. That leads to the colon, or large intestine, which connects to the rectum.

Types of Crohn Disease and Associated Symptoms

The symptoms and potential complications of Crohn disease differ, depending on what part of the GI tract is inflamed. That's why it is important for you to know which part of your intestine is affected by Crohn disease. Your doctor also may refer to your illness by various names based on the main area involved. The following are five types of Crohn disease:

- **Ileocolitis:** The most common form of Crohn, affecting the ileum and colon. Symptoms include diarrhea and cramping or pain in the right lower part or middle of the abdomen. Often accompanied by significant weight loss.

- **Ileitis:** Affects the ileum. Symptoms are the same as ileocolitis. Complications may include fistulas or inflammatory abscess in the right lower quadrant of the abdomen.

- **Gastroduodenal Crohn disease:** Affects the stomach and duodenum (the first part of the small intestine). Symptoms include loss of appetite, weight loss, and nausea. Vomiting may indicate that narrowed segments of the bowel are obstructed.

- **Jejunoileitis:** Produces patchy areas of inflammation in the jejunum (upper half of the small intestine). Symptoms include abdominal pain, ranging from mild to intense, and cramps following meals, as well as diarrhea. Fistulas may form. These are tunnels leading from one loop of intestine to another or between the intestine and another part of the body.

- **Crohn (granulomatous) colitis:** Affects the colon only. Symptoms include diarrhea, rectal bleeding, and disease around the anus (abscess, fistulas, ulcers). Skin lesions and joint pains are more common in this form of Crohn than in others.

Who Gets Crohn Disease?

Up to 1.4 million Americans have either Crohn disease or ulcerative colitis. That number is almost evenly split between the two conditions.

Here are some quick facts and figures:

- About thirty thousand new cases of Crohn and colitis are diagnosed each year.

- Most people diagnosed with Crohn disease are young, between the ages of fifteen and thirty-five.

- However, Crohn disease can also occur in people who are seventy or older and in young children as well. In fact, 10 percent of those affected—or an estimated one hundred thousand—are under the age of eighteen.

- Males and females appear to be affected equally.

- More Caucasians than people from other racial groups develop ulcerative colitis.

- The disease tends to occur more often in Jews (largely of Eastern European ancestry) than in people of non-Jewish descent.

- Both Crohn disease and ulcerative colitis are diseases found mainly in developed countries, more commonly in urban areas rather than rural ones, and more in northern climates than in southern ones.

The Genetic Connection

Researchers have discovered that Crohn disease tends to run in certain families. In fact, up to 20 percent of people with Crohn disease have a first-degree relative (first cousin or closer) with either Crohn disease or ulcerative colitis.

So genetics clearly plays a role. Investigators have been working actively for some time to find a link to specific genes that control the transmission of Crohn disease. Recently, a team of IBD researchers made a major breakthrough when they identified the first gene for Crohn disease. They discovered an abnormal mutation or alteration in a gene known as NOD2. This mutation, which limits the ability to fight bacteria, occurs twice as frequently in Crohn patients as in the general population. Currently, there's no method to screen people for this gene. And there is no way to predict which, if any, family members will develop Crohn disease. It also appears that more than one gene may be involved. Thanks to new technologies, though, researchers may soon close in on those genes.

What Causes Crohn Disease?

As we noted before, no one knows the exact cause or causes. One thing is clear, though. Nothing that you did made you get Crohn disease. You didn't catch it from anyone. It wasn't anything that you ate or drank or smoked. And leading a stressful lifestyle didn't bring it on. So, above all, don't blame yourself!

Now, what are some of the likely causes? Most experts think there is a multifactorial explanation. This simply means that it takes a number of circumstances working together to bring about Crohn disease—including these top three suspects:

- Genes
- An inappropriate reaction by the immune system
- Something in the environment

It's likely that one or more genes of the disease a person has inherited set the stage for the development of Crohn disease. Then it requires some kind of "trigger" in the environment to enter the scene. For example, the trigger could be a virus or a bacterium, but not necessarily. Whatever it is, it prompts the person's immune system to "turn on" and launch an attack against the foreign substance. That's when the inflammation begins. Unfortunately, the immune system doesn't "turn off." So the inflammation continues, damaging the lining of the colon and causing the symptoms of ulcerative colitis.

What Are the Signs and Symptoms of Crohn Disease?

Persistent diarrhea (loose, watery, or frequent bowel movements), crampy abdominal pain, fever, and, at times, rectal bleeding. These are the hallmark symptoms of Crohn disease, but they vary from person to person and may change over time. Loss of appetite and subsequent weight loss also may occur. Fatigue is another common complaint. Children who have Crohn disease may suffer delays in both growth and sexual development.

Some patients may develop tears (fissures) in the lining of the anus, which may cause pain and bleeding, especially during bowel movements. Inflammation may also cause a fistula to develop. A fistula is a tunnel that leads from one loop of intestine to another, or that connects the intestine to the bladder, vagina, or skin. Fistulas occur most commonly around the anal area. If this complication arises, you may notice drainage of mucus, pus, or stool from this opening.

Symptoms may range from mild to severe. Because Crohn disease is a chronic disease, patients will go through periods in which the disease flares up, is active, and causes symptoms. These episodes are followed by times of remission—periods in which symptoms disappear or decrease and good health returns. In general, though, people with Crohn disease lead full, active, and productive lives.

Beyond the Intestine

In addition to having symptoms in the GI tract, some people also may experience Crohn disease in other parts of the body. Signs and symptoms of the disease may be evident in:

- eyes (redness and itchiness);
- mouth (sores);
- joints (swelling and pain);
- skin (bumps and other lesions);
- bones (osteoporosis);
- kidney (stones);
- liver (hepatitis and cirrhosis)—a rare development.

All of these are known as extraintestinal manifestations of Crohn disease because they occur outside of the intestine. In some people these may actually be the first signs of Crohn disease, appearing even before the bowel symptoms. In others, they may occur right before a flare-up of the disease.

The Range of Symptoms

Approximately half of all patients with Crohn disease have relatively mild symptoms. However, others may suffer from severe abdominal cramping, bloody diarrhea, nausea, and fever. The symptoms of Crohn disease do tend to come and go. In between flare-ups, people may experience no distress at all. These disease-free periods can span months or even years, although symptoms do eventually return. The unpredictable course of Crohn disease may make it difficult for doctors to evaluate whether a particular course of treatment has been effective or not.

Making the Diagnosis

How does a doctor establish the diagnosis of Crohn disease? The path toward diagnosis begins by taking a complete family and personal medical history, including full details regarding the symptoms described previously. A physical examination is next.

A number of other conditions can cause diarrhea and abdominal pain, even rectal bleeding. That's why your doctor relies on various medical tests to rule out other sources, such as infection. Stool tests can eliminate the possibility of bacterial, viral, and parasitic causes of diarrhea. They also can reveal the presence of blood. Blood tests may be performed to check for anemia, which could suggest bleeding in the colon or rectum. Blood tests also may detect a high white blood cell count, which indicates the presence of inflammation somewhere in the body.

Looking Inside the Colon

The next step is an examination of the colon itself, either through a sigmoidoscopy or a colonoscopy. With a sigmoidoscopy, the doctor inserts a flexible instrument into the rectum and the lower part of the colon. This permits visualization of those areas to see if there is inflammation and, if so, how much. A colonoscopy is similar, but the advantage is that it allows visualization of the entire colon.

Using these techniques, your physician can detect inflammation, bleeding, or ulcers on the colon wall, as well as determine the extent of disease. During either of these procedures, the examining doctor may take a sample of the colon lining (a biopsy) to send to a pathologist for further study. In that way, Crohn disease can be distinguished from other diseases of the colon that cause rectal bleeding—such as ulcerative colitis, diverticular disease, and cancer.

Treatment

As we mentioned earlier, there is no medical cure for Crohn disease. Yet there are treatments available that can control it. They work by quieting the abnormal inflammation in the lining of the intestines.

This permits them to heal. It also relieves the symptoms of diarrhea, rectal bleeding, and abdominal pain.

The two basic goals of treatment are to achieve remission (the absence of symptoms) and, once that is accomplished, to maintain remission. Some of the medications used for these two aims may be the same, but they are given in different dosages and for different lengths of time. There is no "one-size-fits-all" treatment for everyone with Crohn disease. The treatment approach must be tailored to the individual because each person's disease is different.

Some medications used to treat Crohn disease have been around for years. Others are recent breakthroughs. The most commonly prescribed drugs fall into three basic categories:

- **Aminosalicylates:** These include aspirin-like compounds that contain 5-aminosalicylate acid (5-ASA). Examples are sulfasalazine, mesalamine, olsalazine, and balsalazide. These drugs, which can be given either orally or rectally, alter the body's ability to launch and maintain an inflammatory process. They are effective in treating mild-to-moderate episodes of Crohn disease. They also are useful in preventing relapses of the disease.

- **Corticosteroids:** These medications, which include prednisone and prednisolone, also affect the body's ability to launch and maintain an inflammatory process. In addition, they work to suppress the immune system. Corticosteroids are used for people with moderate-to-severe Crohn disease. They can be administered orally, rectally, or intravenously. They are also effective for short-term control of acute episodes (that is, flare-ups); however, they are not recommended for long-term or maintenance use because of their side effects. Budesonide is a nonsystemic steroid used to treat mild-to-moderate Crohn disease. Budesonide causes fewer side effects. If you cannot come off steroids without suffering a relapse of your symptoms, your doctor may need to add some other medications to help manage your disease.

- **Immunomodulators:** These include azathioprine, 6-mercaptopurine (6-MP), and cyclosporine. This class of medications basically overrides the body's immune system so it cannot cause ongoing inflammation. Usually given orally, immunomodulators generally are used in people in whom aminosalicylates and corticosteroids haven't been effective or have been only partially effective. They may be useful in reducing or eliminating dependency on corticosteroids. They also may be effective in maintaining remission in people who haven't responded to other medications given for this purpose. Immunomodulators may take up to three months to begin to work.

- **Biologic therapies:** The newest class of drugs to be used in IBD includes infliximab. It is indicated for people with moderately to severely active Crohn disease who haven't responded well to conventional therapy. It also is effective for reducing the number of fistulas. Infliximab is an antibody that binds to tumor necrosis factor alpha (TNF-alpha), a protein in the immune system that plays a role in inflammation. The drug may be an effective strategy for tapering people off steroids, as well as for maintaining remission.

  Other biologic drugs are currently undergoing clinical trials for Crohn disease. Adalimumab has already been approved for use in treating rheumatoid arthritis and natalizumab has been approved for use in treating multiple sclerosis.

- **Antibiotics:** Metronidazole, ciprofloxacin, and other antibiotics may be used when infections, such as abscesses, occur in Crohn disease. This is just an overview of the medications commonly used in the treatment of Crohn disease.

Surgery

Many individuals with Crohn disease respond well to medical treatment and never have to undergo surgery. However, two-thirds to three-quarters of people will require surgery at some point during their lives.

Surgery may become necessary in Crohn disease when medications are no longer effective in controlling symptoms. It may also be performed to repair a fistula or fissure. Another indication for surgery is the presence of an intestinal obstruction or other complication, such as an intestinal abscess. In most cases, the diseased segment of bowel and any associated abscess is removed. This is called a resection. The two ends of healthy bowel are then joined together in a procedure called an anastomosis. While resection and anastomosis may allow many symptom-free years, this surgery is not considered a cure for Crohn disease, because the disease frequently recurs at or near the site of anastomosis.

An ileostomy also may be required when surgery is performed for Crohn disease of the colon. After surgeons remove the colon, they bring the small bowel to the skin so that waste products may be emptied into a pouch attached to the abdomen. This procedure is needed if the rectum is diseased and cannot be used for an anastomosis.

The overall goal of surgery in Crohn disease is to conserve bowel and return the individual to the best possible quality of life. Unlike surgery for ulcerative colitis, though, surgery for Crohn disease does not represent a cure.

The Role of Nutrition

You may wonder if eating any particular foods caused or contributed to Crohn disease. The answer is no. However, once the disease has developed, paying some attention to diet may help you reduce the symptoms, replace lost nutrients, and promote healing. For example, when your disease is active, you may find that bland, soft foods may cause less discomfort than spicy or high-fiber foods. Smaller, more frequent meals also may help.

Maintaining proper nutrition is important in the management of Crohn disease. Good nutrition is essential in any chronic disease but especially in this illness. Abdominal pain and fever can cause loss of appetite and weight loss. Diarrhea and rectal bleeding can rob the body of fluids, nutrients, and electrolytes. These are minerals in the body that must remain in proper balance for the body to function properly.

But that doesn't mean that you must eat certain foods or avoid others. Except for restricting milk products in lactose-intolerant people or restricting caffeine when severe diarrhea occurs, most doctors simply recommend a well-balanced diet to prevent nutritional deficiency. A healthy diet should contain a variety of foods from all food groups. Meat, fish, poultry, and dairy products (if tolerated) are sources of protein; bread, cereal, starches, fruits, and vegetables are sources of carbohydrates; margarine and oils are sources of fat. A dietary supplement, like a multivitamin, can help fill the gaps.

Probiotics and Prebiotics

Researchers have been looking at other forms of intestinal protection for people with Crohn disease. That's where probiotics and prebiotics come in.

What are these substances? Probiotics, also known as "beneficial" or "friendly" bacteria, are microscopic organisms that assist in maintaining a healthy GI tract. Approximately four hundred different types of good bacteria live within the human digestive system, where they keep the growth of harmful bacteria in check. A proper balance between good and bad bacteria is key. If beneficial bacteria become depleted or the balance is otherwise thrown off, that's when harmful bacteria can overgrow—causing diarrhea and other digestive problems. In people with already damaged GI tracts, like those with Crohn disease, symptoms may be particularly severe. Mounting evidence suggests the use of probiotics—available in capsules, powders, liquids, and wafers—may represent another therapeutic option for people with IBD, particularly in helping to maintain remission.

Prebiotics are nondigestible food ingredients that provide nutrients that allow beneficial bacteria in the gut to multiply. They also stimulate the growth of probiotics.

The Role of Stress and Emotional Factors

Some people think it takes a certain personality type to develop Crohn disease or other inflammatory bowel diseases. They're wrong. But because body and mind are so closely interrelated, emotional stress can influence the symptoms of Crohn disease—or, for that matter, any chronic illness. Although the disease occasionally recurs after a person has been experiencing emotional problems, there is no proof that stress causes Crohn disease.

It is much more likely that the emotional distress that people sometimes feel is a reaction to the symptoms of the disease itself. Individuals with Crohn disease should receive understanding and emotional support from their families and doctors. Although formal psychotherapy is generally not necessary, some people are helped considerably by speaking with a therapist who is knowledgeable about IBD or about chronic illness in general. CCFA offers local support groups to help patients and their families cope with Crohn disease and ulcerative colitis.

Plan Ahead

You'll learn that there are numerous strategies that can make living with Crohn disease easier. Coping techniques for dealing with the disease may take many forms. For example, attacks of diarrhea or abdominal pain may make people fearful of being in public places. But that isn't necessary. All it takes is some practical advance planning. Find out where the restrooms are in restaurants, shopping areas, theaters, and on public transportation. Carrying along extra underclothing or toilet paper is another smart maneuver. When venturing further away or for longer periods of time, speak to your doctor first. Travel plans should include a large enough supply of your medication, its generic name in case you run out or lose it, and the names of doctors in the area you will be visiting.

Living a Normal Life with Crohn Disease

Perhaps the most difficult period for you is right now, when you have just learned you have this chronic illness called Crohn disease. As time goes on, though, this fact will not always occupy the top spot on your mind. In the meantime, don't hide your condition from family, friends, and co-workers. Discuss it with them and let them help and support you.

Try to go about your daily life as normally as possible, pursuing activities as you did before your diagnosis. There's no reason for you to sit out on things that you have always enjoyed or have dreamed of doing one day. Learn coping strategies from others—your local CCFA chapter offers support groups as well as informational meetings—and share what you know with others, too. Follow your doctor's instructions about taking medication (even when you are feeling perfectly well) and maintain a positive outlook. That's the basic—and best—prescription.

While Crohn disease is a serious chronic disease, it is not a fatal one. There's no doubt that living with this illness is challenging—you have to take medication and, occasionally, may be hospitalized. Yet it's important to remember that most people with Crohn disease are able to lead rich and productive lives.

Remember, also, that taking maintenance medication can significantly decrease flare-ups of Crohn disease. In between disease flares, most people are free of symptoms and feel well.

Hope for the Future

Laboratories all over the world are devoted to the scientific investigation of Crohn disease. That's good news when it comes to the development of new therapies for this disease. CCFA-sponsored research has led to huge strides in the fields of immunology, the study of the body's immune defense system; microbiology, the study of microscopic organisms with the power to cause disease; and genetics. Through CCFA's continuing research efforts, much more will be learned and eventually a cure will be found.

Section 21.4

Introduction to Ulcerative Colitis

"Living with Ulcerative Colitis," © 2005 Crohn's and Colitis Foundation of America, Inc. (CCFA). Reprinted with permission.

Understanding the Diagnosis

Your doctor has just told you that you have a disease called ulcerative colitis. Quite possibly, you have never even heard of this condition before. (Most people, in fact, are unfamiliar with ulcerative colitis.) And now you have it. And, to make matters worse, your doctor has said that ulcerative colitis doesn't go away.

If you feel overwhelmed and scared right now, that's only natural. You probably have a ton of questions, starting with "Just what is ulcerative colitis?" But you're also wondering how you got it and, more important, how it will affect you—both now and down the road. For example, you'll want to know:

- Will I be able to work, travel, exercise?
- Should I be on a special diet?
- Will I need surgery?
- How will ulcerative colitis change my life?

That's the purpose of this section: to answer those questions and to walk you through the key points about ulcerative colitis and what you may expect in the future. You won't become an expert overnight, but gradually you'll learn more and more. And the more you know, the better you'll be able to cope with the disease and become an active member of your own health care team.

What Is Ulcerative Colitis?

Ulcerative colitis belongs to a group of conditions known as inflammatory bowel disease (IBD). Another illness in this group is Crohn disease. Both conditions cause diarrhea (sometimes bloody), as well as abdominal pain. Because the symptoms of these two illnesses are so similar, it is sometimes difficult for doctors to make a definitive diagnosis. In fact, approximately 10 percent of cases are unable to be pinpointed as either ulcerative colitis or Crohn disease.

While Crohn disease may involve any part of the gastrointestinal (GI) tract, ulcerative colitis is limited to the colon—also called the large intestine. The inflammation begins at the rectum and extends up the colon in a continuous manner. There are no areas of normal intestine between the areas of diseased intestine. In contrast, such so-called skip areas may occur in Crohn disease. And whereas Crohn disease can affect the entire thickness of the bowel wall, ulcerative colitis involves only the innermost lining of the colon—causing it to become inflamed. Tiny open sores or ulcers form on the surface of the lining, where they bleed and produce pus and mucus. In short, ulcerative colitis is an inflammatory disease of the lining of the colon.

What Does "Chronic" Mean?

No one knows exactly what causes either ulcerative colitis or Crohn disease. Also, no one can predict how the disease—once it is diagnosed—will affect a particular person. Some people go for years without having any symptoms, while others have more frequent flare-ups of disease. However, one thing is sure: ulcerative colitis—like Crohn disease—is a chronic condition.

Chronic conditions are ongoing situations. They can be controlled with treatment but cannot be cured. That means that the disease is long-term, but it does *not* mean that it is fatal. It isn't. Most people who have ulcerative colitis lead full and productive lives.

A Brief Introduction to the GI Tract

Most of us aren't very familiar with the gastrointestinal tract (GI), even though it occupies a lot of "real estate" in our bodies.

Here's a quick tour:

The GI tract actually starts at the mouth. It follows a twisting and turning course and ends, many yards later, at the rectum. In between are a number of organs that all play a part in processing food and transporting it through the body.

The first is the esophagus, a narrow tube that connects the mouth to the stomach. After that comes the stomach itself. Moving downward, the next organ is the small intestine. That leads to the colon, or large intestine, which connects to the rectum.

The principal function of the colon is to absorb excess water and salts from the waste material (what's left after food has been digested). It also stores the solid waste, converting it to stool, and excretes it through the anus.

The inflammation in ulcerative colitis usually begins in the rectum and lower colon, but it also may involve the entire colon. Ulcerative colitis may be called by other names, depending on where the disease is located in the colon.

- **Ulcerative proctitis:** involves only the rectum
- **Proctosigmoiditis:** affects the rectum and sigmoid colon (the lower segment of the colon before the rectum)
- **Distal colitis:** involves only the left side of the colon
- **Pancolitis:** affects the entire colon

Who Gets Ulcerative Colitis?

Up to 1.4 million Americans have either ulcerative colitis or Crohn disease. That number is almost evenly split between the two conditions. Here are some quick facts and figures:

- About thirty thousand new cases of Crohn and colitis are diagnosed each year.
- Ulcerative colitis can occur at any age.
- On average, people are diagnosed with ulcerative colitis in their mid-thirties.
- Men are more likely than women to be diagnosed with ulcerative colitis in their fifties and sixties.
- More Caucasians than people from other racial groups develop ulcerative colitis.
- The disease tends to occur more often in Jews (largely of Eastern European ancestry) than in people of non-Jewish descent.
- Both ulcerative colitis and Crohn disease are diseases found mainly in developed countries, more commonly in urban areas rather than rural ones, and more in northern climates than southern ones.

The Genetic Connection

Researchers have discovered that ulcerative colitis tends to run in certain families.

In fact, up to 20 percent of people with ulcerative colitis have a first-degree relative (first cousin or closer) with either ulcerative colitis or Crohn disease. So genetics clearly plays a role, although no specific pattern of inheritance has been identified. That means there is no way to predict which, if any, family members will develop ulcerative colitis or Crohn disease.

What Causes Ulcerative Colitis?

As we noted before, no one knows the exact cause or causes. One thing is clear, though: Nothing that you did made you get ulcerative colitis. You didn't catch it from anyone. It wasn't anything that you ate or drank or smoked. And leading a stressful lifestyle didn't bring it on. So, above all, don't blame yourself!

Now, what are some of the likely causes? Most experts think there is a multifactorial explanation. This simply means that it takes a number of circumstances working together to bring about ulcerative colitis—including these top three suspects:

- Genes
- An inappropriate reaction by the body's immune system
- Something in the environment

It's likely that one or more genes of the disease a person has inherited sets the stage for the development of ulcerative colitis. Then it takes some kind of "trigger" in the environment to enter the scene. For example, the trigger could be a virus or a bacterium, but not necessarily. Whatever it is, it prompts the person's immune system to "turn on" and launch an attack against the foreign substance. That's when the inflammation begins. Unfortunately, the immune system doesn't "turn off." So the inflammation continues, damaging the lining of the colon and causing the symptoms of ulcerative colitis.

What Are the Signs and Symptoms of Ulcerative Colitis?

As the intestinal lining becomes more inflamed and ulcerated, it loses its ability to absorb water from the waste material that passes through the colon. That, in turn, leads to a progressive loosening of the stool—in other words, diarrhea. The damaged intestinal lining also can produce a lot of mucus in the stool. Moreover, ulceration in the lining can cause bleeding so the stool also may be bloody. Eventually, that blood loss may lead to anemia.

Most people with ulcerative colitis experience an urgency to have a bowel movement as well as crampy abdominal pain. The pain may be stronger on the left side. That's because the colon descends on the left.

Together, diarrhea and abdominal pain may result in loss of appetite and subsequent weight loss. These symptoms also can produce fatigue, which is a side effect of anemia as well. Children with ulcerative colitis may fail to develop or grow properly.

Beyond the Intestine

In addition to having symptoms in the GI tract, some people may also experience ulcerative colitis in other parts of the body. Signs and symptoms of the disease may be evident in:

- eyes (redness and itchiness);
- mouth (sores);
- joints (swelling and pain);
- skin (bumps and other lesions);
- bones (osteoporosis);
- kidney (stones);
- liver (hepatitis and cirrhosis)—a rare development.

All of these are known as extraintestinal manifestations of ulcerative colitis because they occur outside of the intestine. In some people, these actually may be the first signs of ulcerative colitis, appearing even before the bowel symptoms. In others, they may occur right before a flare-up of the disease.

People who have had ulcerative colitis for eight to ten years have a higher risk of getting colon cancer. You should talk to your doctor about what you can do to help prevent cancer and lower your risk.

The Range of Symptoms

Approximately half of all patients with ulcerative colitis have relatively mild symptoms.

However, others may suffer from severe abdominal cramping, bloody diarrhea, nausea, and fever. The symptoms of ulcerative colitis do tend to come and go. In between flare-ups, people may experience no distress at all. These disease-free periods can span months or even years, although symptoms do eventually return. The unpredictable course of ulcerative colitis may make it difficult for doctors to evaluate whether a particular treatment program has been effective or not.

Making the Diagnosis

How does a doctor establish the diagnosis of ulcerative colitis? The path toward diagnosis begins by taking a complete family and personal medical history, including full details regarding symptoms. A physical examination is next.

A number of other conditions can cause diarrhea, abdominal pain, and rectal bleeding. That's why your doctor relies on various medical tests to rule out other potential sources, such as infection.

Stool tests can eliminate the possibility of bacterial, viral, and parasitic causes of diarrhea. They also can reveal the presence of blood. Blood tests may be performed to check for anemia, which could suggest bleeding in the colon or rectum.

Blood tests also may detect a high white blood cell count, which indicates the presence of inflammation somewhere in the body.

Looking Inside the Colon

The next step is an examination of the colon itself, through either a sigmoidoscopy or a colonoscopy. With a sigmoidoscopy, the doctor inserts a flexible instrument into the rectum and the lower part of the colon. This permits visualization of those areas to see if there is inflammation and, if so, how much. A colonoscopy is similar, but the advantage is that it allows visualization of the entire colon.

Using these techniques, your physician can detect inflammation, bleeding, or ulcers on the colon wall, as well as determine the extent of disease.

During either of these procedures, the examining doctor may take a sample of the colon lining (a biopsy) to send to a pathologist for further study. In that way, ulcerative colitis can be distinguished from other diseases of the colon that cause rectal bleeding—such as Crohn disease of the colon, diverticular disease, and cancer.

Treatment

As we mentioned earlier, there is no medical cure for ulcerative colitis. Yet there are treatments available that can control it. They work by quieting the abnormal inflammation in the lining of the colon.

This permits the colon to heal. It also relieves the symptoms of diarrhea, rectal bleeding, and abdominal pain.

The two basic goals of treatment are to achieve remission (the absence of symptoms) and, once that is accomplished, to maintain remission. Some of the medications used for these two aims may be the same, but they are given in different dosages and for different lengths of time.

There is no "one-size-fits-all" treatment for everyone with ulcerative colitis. The treatment approach must be tailored to the individual because each person's disease is different.

Some medications used to treat ulcerative colitis have been around for years. Others are recent breakthroughs. The most commonly prescribed drugs fall into three basic categories:

- **Aminosalicylates:** These include aspirin-like compounds that contain 5-aminosalicylate acid (5-ASA). Examples are sulfasalazine, mesalamine, olsalazine, and balsalazide. These drugs, which can be given either orally or rectally, alter the body's ability to launch and maintain an inflammatory process. They are effective in treating mild-to-moderate episodes of ulcerative colitis. They also are useful in preventing relapses of the disease.

- **Corticosteroids:** These medications, which include prednisone and prednisolone, also affect the body's ability to launch and maintain an inflammatory process. In addition, they work to suppress the immune system. Corticosteroids are used for people with moderate-to-severe disease. They can be administered orally, rectally, or intravenously. They are also effective for short-term control of acute episodes (that is, flare-ups); however, they are not recommended for long-term or maintenance use because of their side effects. If you cannot come off steroids without suffering a relapse of your symptoms, your doctor may need to add some other medications to help manage your disease.

- **Immunomodulators:** These include azathioprine, 6-mercaptopurine (6-MP), and cyclosporine. This class of medications basically overrides the body's immune system so it cannot cause ongoing inflammation. Usually given orally, immunomodulators generally are used in people in whom aminosalicylates and corticosteroids haven't been effective or have been only partially effective. They may be useful in reducing or eliminating dependency on corticosteroids. They also may be effective in maintaining remission in people who haven't responded to other medications given for this purpose. Immunomodulators may take up to three months to begin to work.

Surgery

Most people with ulcerative colitis respond well to medical treatment and never have to undergo surgery. However, between 25 percent and 33 percent of individuals may require surgery at some point.

Sometimes surgery is indicated to take care of various complications related to ulcerative colitis. These include severe bleeding from deep ulcerations, perforation (rupture) of the bowel, and a condition called toxic megacolon. Caused by severe inflammation, this is extreme abdominal distension accompanied by fever and constipation. If medical intervention aimed at controlling inflammation and restoring fluid loss doesn't bring about rapid improvement, surgery may become necessary to avoid rupture of the bowel.

Surgery may be considered to remove the entire colon. This is called a colectomy. It may be a desirable option when medical therapies no longer control the disease well or when precancerous changes are found in the colon. Unlike Crohn disease, which can recur after surgery, ulcerative colitis actually is "cured" once the colon is removed.

Depending on a number of factors—including the extent of disease and the person's age and overall health—one of two surgical approaches may be recommended. The first involves the removal of the entire colon and rectum, with the creation of an ileostomy (an opening on the abdomen through which wastes are emptied into a pouch).

Today, many people can take advantage of new surgical techniques that offer another option. This procedure also calls for removal of the colon, but it avoids an ileostomy. By creating an internal pouch from the small bowel and attaching it to the anal sphincter muscle, the surgeon preserves bowel function and eliminates the need for an external ostomy appliance.

The Role of Nutrition

You may wonder if eating any particular foods caused or contributed to your ulcerative colitis. The answer is "no." However, once the disease has developed, paying some attention to diet may help you reduce your symptoms, replace lost nutrients, and promote healing. For example, when your disease is active, you may find that bland, soft foods may cause less discomfort than spicy or high-fiber foods. Smaller, more frequent meals also may help.

Maintaining proper nutrition is important in the management of ulcerative colitis. Good nutrition is essential in any chronic disease, but especially in this illness. Abdominal pain and fever can cause loss of appetite and weight loss. Diarrhea and rectal bleeding can rob the body of fluids, nutrients, and electrolytes. These are minerals in the body that must remain in proper balance for the body to function properly.

But that doesn't mean that you must eat certain foods or avoid others. Except for restricting milk products in lactose-intolerant people, or restricting caffeine when severe diarrhea occurs, most doctors simply recommend a well-balanced diet to prevent nutritional deficiency. A healthy diet should contain a variety of foods from all food groups. Meat, fish, poultry, and dairy products (if tolerated) are sources of protein; bread, cereal, starches, fruits, and vegetables are sources of carbohydrates; margarine and oils are sources of fat. A dietary supplement, like a multivitamin, can help fill the gaps.

Probiotics and Prebiotics

Researchers have been looking at other forms of intestinal protection for people with ulcerative colitis and Crohn disease. That's where probiotics and prebiotics come in.

What are these substances? Probiotics, also known as "beneficial" or "friendly" bacteria, are microscopic organisms that assist in maintaining a healthy GI tract.

Approximately four hundred different types of good bacteria live within the human digestive system, where they keep the growth of harmful bacteria in check. A proper balance between good and bad bacteria is key. If beneficial bacteria drop in number or the balance is otherwise thrown off, that's when harmful bacteria can overgrow—causing diarrhea and other digestive problems. In people with already damaged GI tracts, like those with ulcerative colitis, symptoms may be particularly severe. Mounting evidence suggests the use of probiotics—available in capsules, powders, liquids, and wafers—may represent another therapeutic option for people with IBD, particularly in helping to maintain remission.

Prebiotics are nondigestible food ingredients that provide nutrients to allow beneficial bacteria in the gut to multiply. They also stimulate the growth of probiotics.

The Role of Stress and Emotional Factors

Some people think it takes a certain personality type to develop ulcerative colitis or other inflammatory bowel disease. They're wrong. Yet because body and mind are so closely interrelated, emotional stress can influence the symptoms of ulcerative colitis—or, for that matter, any chronic illness. Although the disease occasionally recurs after a person has been experiencing emotional problems, there is no proof that stress causes ulcerative colitis.

It is much more likely that the emotional distress that people sometimes feel is a reaction to the symptoms of the disease itself. Individuals with ulcerative colitis should receive understanding and emotional support from their families and doctors. Although formal psychotherapy usually isn't necessary, some people are helped considerably by speaking with a therapist who is knowledgeable about IBD or about chronic illness in general. CCFA offers local support groups to help patients and their families cope with ulcerative colitis and Crohn disease.

Plan Ahead

You'll learn that there are numerous strategies that can make living with ulcerative colitis easier. Coping techniques for dealing with the disease may take many forms. For example, attacks of diarrhea or abdominal pain may make people fearful of being in public places. But that isn't necessary. All it takes is some practical advance planning.

Find out where the restrooms are in restaurants, shopping areas, and theaters, and on public transportation. Carrying along extra underclothing or toilet paper is another smart maneuver. When venturing further away or for longer periods of time, speak to your doctor first. Travel plans should include a large enough supply of your medication, its generic name in case you run out or lose it, and the names of doctors in the area you will be visiting.

Living a Normal Life with Ulcerative Colitis

Perhaps the most difficult period for you is right now, when you have just learned you have this chronic illness called ulcerative colitis. As time goes on, though, this fact will not always occupy the top spot on your mind. In the meantime, don't hide your condition from family, friends, and co-workers. Discuss it with them and let them help and support you.

Try to go about your daily life as normally as possible, pursuing activities as you did before your diagnosis. There's no reason for you to sit out on things that you have always enjoyed or have dreamed of doing one day. Learn coping strategies from others—your local CCFA chapter offers support groups as well as educational meetings —and share what you know with others, too. Follow your doctor's instructions about taking medication (even when you are feeling perfectly well) and maintain a positive outlook. That's the basic—and best— prescription.

While ulcerative colitis is a serious chronic disease, it is not a fatal one. There's no doubt that living with this illness is challenging— you have to take medication and, occasionally, may be hospitalized. Yet it's important to remember that most people with ulcerative colitis are able to lead rich and productive lives.

Remember, also, that taking maintenance medication can significantly decrease flare-ups of ulcerative colitis. In between disease flares, most people are free of symptoms and feel well.

Hope for the Future

Laboratories all over the world are devoted to the scientific investigation of ulcerative colitis. That's good news when it comes to the development of new therapies for this disease. CCFA-sponsored research has led to huge strides in the fields of immunology, the study of the body's immune defense system; microbiology, the study of microscopic organisms with the power to cause disease; and genetics. Through CCFA's continuing research efforts, much more will be learned and eventually a cure will be found.

Section 21.5

Collagenous Colitis and Lymphocytic Colitis

Reprinted from "Collagenous Colitis and Lymphocytic Colitis,"
National Institute of Diabetes and Digestive and Kidney Diseases,
NIH Publication No. 03-5036, April 2003.

Inflammatory bowel disease is a general name for diseases that cause inflammation in the intestines. Collagenous colitis and lymphocytic colitis are two types of bowel inflammation that affect the colon (large intestine). They are not related to Crohn disease or ulcerative colitis, which are more severe forms of inflammatory bowel disease (IBD).

Collagenous colitis and lymphocytic colitis are referred to as microscopic colitis because colonoscopy usually shows no signs of inflammation on the surface of the colon. Instead, tissue samples from the colon must be examined under a microscope to make the diagnosis.

No precise cause has been found for collagenous colitis or lymphocytic colitis. Possible causes of damage to the lining of the colon are bacteria and their toxins, viruses, or nonsteroidal anti-inflammatory drugs (NSAIDs). Some researchers have suggested that collagenous colitis and lymphocytic colitis result from an autoimmune response, which means that the body's immune system destroys cells for no known reason.

Symptoms

The symptoms of collagenous colitis and lymphocytic colitis are similar—chronic watery, nonbloody diarrhea. The diarrhea may be continuous or episodic. Abdominal pain or cramps may also be present.

Diagnosis

The diagnosis of collagenous colitis or lymphocytic colitis is made after tissue samples taken during colonoscopy or flexible sigmoidoscopy are examined under a microscope. Collagenous colitis is characterized by a larger-than-normal band of protein called collagen inside the lining of the colon. The thickness of the band varies, so multiple tissue samples from different areas of the colon may need to be examined. In lymphocytic colitis, tissue samples show inflammation with white blood cells known as lymphocytes between the cells that line the colon, and in contrast to collagenous colitis, there is no abnormality of the collagen.

People with collagenous colitis are most often diagnosed in their fifties, although some cases have been reported in adults younger than forty-five years and in children aged five to twelve. It is diagnosed more frequently in women than in men.

People with lymphocytic colitis are also generally diagnosed in their fifties. Both men and women are equally affected.

Treatment

Treatment for collagenous colitis and lymphocytic colitis varies depending on the symptoms and severity of the cases. The diseases have been known to resolve spontaneously, but most patients have recurrent symptoms.

Lifestyle changes aimed at improving diarrhea are usually tried first. Recommended changes include reducing the amount of fat in the diet, eliminating foods that contain caffeine or lactose, and not using NSAIDs.

If lifestyle changes alone are not enough, medications are often used to control the symptoms of collagenous colitis and lymphocytic colitis.

- Antidiarrheal medications such as bismuth subsalicylate and bulking agents reduce diarrhea.

- Anti-inflammatory medications, such as mesalamine, sulfasalazine, and steroids including budesonide, reduce inflammation.

- Immunosuppressive agents, which reduce the autoimmune response, are rarely needed.

For very extreme cases of collagenous colitis and lymphocytic colitis, bypass of the colon or surgery to remove all or part of the colon has been done in a few patients. This is rarely recommended.

Collagenous colitis and lymphocytic colitis do not increase the risk of colon cancer.

Chapter 22

Appendicitis

The appendix is a small, tube-like structure attached to the first part of the large intestine, also called the colon. The appendix is located in the lower right portion of the abdomen. It has no known function. Removal of the appendix appears to cause no change in digestive function.

Appendicitis is an inflammation of the appendix. Once it starts, there is no effective medical therapy, so appendicitis is considered a medical emergency. When treated promptly, most patients recover without difficulty. If treatment is delayed, the appendix can burst, causing infection and even death. Appendicitis is the most common acute surgical emergency of the abdomen. Anyone can get appendicitis, but it occurs most often between the ages of ten and thirty.

Causes

The cause of appendicitis relates to blockage of the inside of the appendix, known as the lumen. The blockage leads to increased pressure, impaired blood flow, and inflammation. If the blockage is not treated, gangrene and rupture (breaking or tearing) of the appendix can result.

Most commonly, feces blocks the inside of the appendix. Also, bacterial or viral infections in the digestive tract can lead to swelling of lymph nodes, which squeeze the appendix and cause obstruction. This swelling of lymph nodes is known as lymphoid hyperplasia. Traumatic injury to the abdomen may lead to appendicitis in a small number of people.

Excerpted from "Appendicitis," National Institute of Diabetes and Digestive and Kidney Diseases, NIH Publication No. 04-4547, June 2004.

Genetics may be a factor in others. For example, appendicitis that runs in families may result from a genetic variant that predisposes a person to obstruction of the appendiceal lumen.

Symptoms

Symptoms of appendicitis may include the following:

- pain in the abdomen, first around the belly button, then moving to the lower right area
- loss of appetite
- nausea
- vomiting
- constipation or diarrhea
- inability to pass gas
- low fever that begins after other symptoms
- abdominal swelling

Not everyone with appendicitis has all the symptoms. The pain intensifies and worsens when moving, taking deep breaths, coughing,

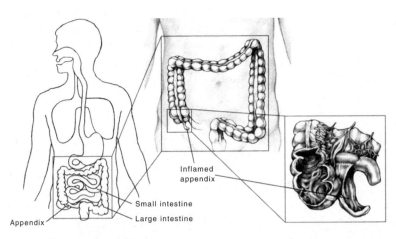

Figure 22.1. The appendix is a small, tube-like structure attached to the first part of the large intestine, also called the colon. The appendix is located in the lower right portion of the abdomen, near where the small intestine attaches to the large intestine.

or sneezing. The area becomes very tender. People may have a sensation called "downward urge," also known as "tenesmus," which is the feeling that a bowel movement will relieve their discomfort. Laxatives and pain medications should not be taken in this situation. Anyone with these symptoms needs to see a qualified physician immediately.

People with Special Concerns

Patients with special conditions may not have the set of symptoms listed here and may simply experience a general feeling of being unwell. Patients with these conditions include:

- people who use immunosuppressive therapy such as steroids;
- people who have received a transplanted organ;
- people infected with the HIV virus;
- people with diabetes;
- people who have cancer or who are receiving chemotherapy;
- obese people.

Pregnant women, infants and young children, and the elderly have particular issues.

Abdominal pain, nausea, and vomiting are more common during pregnancy and may or may not be the signs of appendicitis. Many women who develop appendicitis during pregnancy do not experience the classic symptoms. Pregnant women who experience pain on the right side of the abdomen need to contact a doctor. Women in their third trimester are most at risk.

Infants and young children cannot communicate their pain history to parents or doctors. Without a clear history, doctors must rely on a physical exam and less specific symptoms, such as vomiting and fatigue. Toddlers with appendicitis sometimes have trouble eating and may seem unusually sleepy. Children may have constipation, but may also have small stools that contain mucus. Symptoms vary widely among children. If you think your child has appendicitis, contact a doctor immediately.

Older patients tend to have more medical problems than young patients. The elderly often experience less fever and less severe abdominal pain than other patients do. Many older adults do not know that they have a serious problem until the appendix is close to rupturing. A slight fever and abdominal pain on one's right side are reasons to call a doctor right away.

All patients with special concerns and their families need to be particularly alert to a change in normal functioning, and patients should see their doctors sooner, rather than later, when a change occurs.

Diagnosis

Medical History and Physical Examination

Asking questions to learn the history of symptoms and a careful physical examination are key in the diagnosis of appendicitis. The doctor will ask many questions—much like a reporter—trying to understand the nature, timing, location, pattern, and severity of pain and symptoms. Any previous medical conditions and surgeries, family history, medications, and allergies are important information to the doctor. Use of alcohol, tobacco, and any other drugs should also be mentioned. This information is considered confidential and cannot be shared without the permission of the patient.

Before beginning a physical examination, a nurse or doctor will usually measure vital signs: temperature, pulse rate, breathing rate, and blood pressure. Usually the physical examination proceeds from head to toe. Many conditions such as pneumonia or heart disease can cause abdominal pain. Generalized symptoms such as fever, rash, or swelling of the lymph nodes may point to diseases that wouldn't require surgery.

Examination of the abdomen helps narrow the diagnosis. Location of the pain and tenderness is important. Pain is a symptom described by a patient; tenderness is the response to being touched. Two signs, called peritoneal signs, suggest that the lining of the abdomen is inflamed and surgery may be needed: rebound tenderness and guarding. Rebound tenderness is when the doctor presses on a part of the abdomen and the patient feels more tenderness when the pressure is released than when it is applied. Guarding refers to the tensing of muscles in response to touch. The doctor may also move the patient's legs to test for pain on flexion of the hip (psoas sign), pain on internal rotation of the hip (obturator sign), or pain on the right side when pressing on the left (Rovsing sign). These are valuable indicators of inflammation but not all patients have them.

Laboratory Tests

Blood tests are used to check for signs of infection, such as a high white blood cell count. Blood chemistries may also show dehydration or fluid and electrolyte disorders. Urinalysis is used to rule out a urinary tract infection. Doctors may also order a pregnancy test for women of childbearing age (those who have regular periods).

Imaging Tests

X-rays, ultrasound, and computed tomography (CT) scans can produce images of the abdomen. Plain x-rays can show signs of obstruction, perforation (a hole), foreign bodies, and in rare cases, an appendicolith, which is hardened stool in the appendix. Ultrasound may show appendiceal inflammation and can diagnose gall bladder disease and pregnancy. By far the most common test used, however, is the CT scan. This test provides a series of cross-sectional images of the body and can identify many abdominal conditions and facilitate diagnosis when the clinical impression is in doubt. All women of childbearing age should have a pregnancy test before undergoing any testing with x-rays.

In selected cases, particularly in women when the cause of the symptoms may be either the appendix or an inflamed ovary or fallopian tube, laparoscopy may be necessary. This procedure avoids radiation, but requires general anesthesia. A laparoscope is a thin tube with a camera attached that is inserted into the body through a small cut, allowing doctors to see the internal organs. Surgery can then be performed laparoscopically if the condition present requires it.

Treatment

Surgery

Acute appendicitis is treated by surgery to remove the appendix. The operation may be performed through a standard small incision in the right lower part of the abdomen, or it may be performed using a laparoscope, which requires three to four smaller incisions. If other conditions are suspected in addition to appendicitis, they may be identified using laparoscopy. In some patients, laparoscopy is preferable to open surgery because the incision is smaller, recovery time is quicker, and less pain medication is required. The appendix is almost always removed, even if it is found to be normal. With complete removal, any later episodes of pain will not be attributed to appendicitis.

Recovery from appendectomy takes a few weeks. Doctors usually prescribe pain medication and ask patients to limit physical activity. Recovery from laparoscopic appendectomy is generally faster, but limiting strenuous activity may still be necessary for four to six weeks after surgery. Most people treated for appendicitis recover excellently and rarely need to make any changes in their diet, exercise, or lifestyle.

Antibiotics and Other Treatments

If the diagnosis is uncertain, people may be watched and sometimes treated with antibiotics. This approach is taken when the doctor suspects that the patient's symptoms may have a nonsurgical or medically treatable cause. If the cause of the pain is infectious, symptoms resolve with intravenous antibiotics and intravenous fluids. In general, however, appendicitis cannot be treated with antibiotics alone and will require surgery.

Occasionally the body is able to control an appendiceal perforation by forming an abscess. An abscess occurs when an infection is walled off in one part of the body. The doctor may choose to drain the abscess and leave the drain in the abscess cavity for several weeks. An appendectomy may be scheduled after the abscess is drained.

Complications

The most serious complication of appendicitis is rupture. The appendix bursts or tears if appendicitis is not diagnosed quickly and goes untreated. Infants, young children, and older adults are at highest risk. A ruptured appendix can lead to peritonitis and abscess. Peritonitis is a dangerous infection that happens when bacteria and other contents of the torn appendix leak into the abdomen. In people with appendicitis, an abscess usually takes the form of a swollen mass filled with fluid and bacteria. In a few patients, complications of appendicitis can lead to organ failure and death.

Points to Remember

- The appendix is a small, tube-like structure attached to the first part of the colon. Appendicitis is an inflammation of the appendix.

- Appendicitis is considered a medical emergency.

- Symptoms of appendicitis include pain in the abdomen, loss of appetite, nausea, vomiting, constipation or diarrhea, inability to pass gas, low-grade fever, and abdominal swelling. Not everyone with appendicitis has all the symptoms.

- Physical examination, laboratory tests, and imaging tests are used to diagnose appendicitis.

- Acute appendicitis is treated by surgery to remove the appendix.

- The most serious complication of appendicitis is rupture, which can lead to peritonitis and abscess.

Chapter 23

Gallstones

What are gallstones?

Gallstones form when liquid stored in the gallbladder hardens into pieces of stone-like material. The liquid, called bile, is used to help the body digest fats. Bile is made in the liver, then stored in the gallbladder until the body needs to digest fat. At that time, the gallbladder contracts and pushes the bile into a tube—called the common bile duct—that carries it to the small intestine, where it helps with digestion.

Bile contains water, cholesterol, fats, bile salts, proteins, and bilirubin. Bile salts break up fat, and bilirubin gives bile and stool a yellowish color. If the liquid bile contains too much cholesterol, bile salts, or bilirubin, under certain conditions it can harden into stones.

The two types of gallstones are cholesterol stones and pigment stones. Cholesterol stones are usually yellow-green and are made primarily of hardened cholesterol. They account for about 80 percent of gallstones. Pigment stones are small, dark stones made of bilirubin. Gallstones can be as small as a grain of sand or as large as a golf ball. The gallbladder can develop just one large stone, hundreds of tiny stones, or almost any combination.

Gallstones can block the normal flow of bile if they lodge in any of the ducts that carry bile from the liver to the small intestine. That includes the hepatic ducts, which carry bile out of the liver; the cystic

Reprinted from "Gallstones," National Institute of Diabetes and Digestive and Kidney Diseases, NIH Publication No. 05-2897, November 2004.

duct, which takes bile to and from the gallbladder; and the common bile duct, which takes bile from the cystic and hepatic ducts to the small intestine. Bile trapped in these ducts can cause inflammation in the gallbladder, the ducts, or, rarely, the liver. Other ducts open into the common bile duct, including the pancreatic duct, which carries digestive enzymes out of the pancreas. If a gallstone blocks the opening to that duct, digestive enzymes can become trapped in the pancreas and cause an extremely painful inflammation called gallstone pancreatitis.

If any of these ducts remain blocked for a significant period of time, severe—possibly fatal—damage or infections affecting the gallbladder, liver, or pancreas can occur. Warning signs of a serious problem are fever, jaundice, and persistent pain.

What causes gallstones?

Cholesterol Stones: Scientists believe cholesterol stones form when bile contains too much cholesterol, too much bilirubin, or not enough bile salts, or when the gallbladder does not empty as it should for some other reason.

Pigment Stones: The cause of pigment stones is uncertain. They tend to develop in people who have cirrhosis, biliary tract infections,

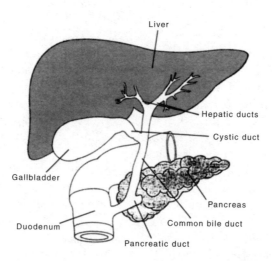

Figure 23.1. *The gallbladder and the ducts that carry bile and other digestive enzymes from the liver, gallbladder, and pancreas to the small intestine are called the biliary system.*

and hereditary blood disorders, such as sickle cell anemia, in which too much bilirubin is formed.

Other Factors: It is believed that the mere presence of gallstones may cause more gallstones to develop. However, other factors that contribute to gallstones have been identified, especially for cholesterol stones.

- *Obesity.* Obesity is a major risk factor for gallstones, especially in women. A large clinical study showed that being even moderately overweight increases the risk for developing gallstones. The most likely reason is that obesity tends to reduce the amount of bile salts in bile, resulting in more cholesterol. Obesity also decreases gallbladder emptying.

- *Estrogen.* Excess estrogen from pregnancy, hormone replacement therapy, or birth control pills appears to increase cholesterol levels in bile and decrease gallbladder movement, both of which can lead to gallstones.

- *Ethnicity.* Native Americans have a genetic predisposition to secrete high levels of cholesterol in bile. In fact, they have the highest rate of gallstones in the United States. A majority of Native American men have gallstones by age sixty. Among the Pima Indians of Arizona, 70 percent of women have gallstones by age thirty. Mexican American men and women of all ages also have high rates of gallstones.

- *Gender.* Women between twenty and sixty years of age are twice as likely to develop gallstones as men.

- *Age.* People over age sixty are more likely to develop gallstones than younger people.

- *Cholesterol-lowering drugs.* Drugs that lower cholesterol levels in blood actually increase the amount of cholesterol secreted in bile. This in turn can increase the risk of gallstones.

- *Diabetes.* People with diabetes generally have high levels of fatty acids called triglycerides. These fatty acids increase the risk of gallstones.

- *Rapid weight loss.* As the body metabolizes fat during rapid weight loss, it causes the liver to secrete extra cholesterol into bile, which can cause gallstones.

- *Fasting.* Fasting decreases gallbladder movement, causing the bile to become over-concentrated with cholesterol, which can lead to gallstones.

Who is at risk for gallstones?

- women
- people over age sixty
- Native Americans
- Mexican Americans
- overweight men and women
- people who fast or lose a lot of weight quickly
- pregnant women, women on hormone replacement therapy, and women who use birth control pills

What are the symptoms?

Symptoms of gallstones are often called a gallstone "attack" because they occur suddenly. A typical attack can cause the following symptoms:

- steady pain in the upper abdomen that increases rapidly and lasts from thirty minutes to several hours
- pain in the back between the shoulder blades
- pain under the right shoulder
- nausea or vomiting

Gallstone attacks often follow fatty meals, and they may occur during the night. Other gallstone symptoms include the following:

- abdominal bloating
- recurring intolerance of fatty foods
- colic
- belching
- gas
- indigestion

People who also have the preceding and any of following symptoms should see a doctor right away:

- chills
- low-grade fever

- yellowish color of the skin or whites of the eyes
- clay-colored stools

Many people with gallstones have no symptoms. These patients are said to be asymptomatic, and these stones are called "silent stones." They do not interfere with gallbladder, liver, or pancreas function, and do not need treatment.

How are gallstones diagnosed?

Many gallstones, especially silent stones, are discovered by accident during tests for other problems. Yet when gallstones are suspected to be the cause of symptoms, the doctor is likely to do an ultrasound exam. Ultrasound uses sound waves to create images of organs. Sound waves are sent toward the gallbladder through a handheld device that a technician glides over the abdomen. The sound waves bounce off the gallbladder, liver, and other organs such as a pregnant uterus, and their echoes make electrical impulses that create a picture of the organ on a video monitor. If stones are present, the sound waves will bounce off them, too, showing their location. Ultrasound is the most sensitive and specific test for gallstones.

Other tests may also be used.

- *Computed tomography (CT) scan.* This test may show the gallstones or complications.

- *Magnetic resonance cholangiogram.* This test may diagnose blocked bile ducts.

- *Cholescintigraphy (HIDA scan).* This test is used to diagnose abnormal contraction of the gallbladder or obstruction. The patient is injected with a radioactive material that is taken up in the gallbladder, which is then stimulated to contract.

- *Endoscopic retrograde cholangiopancreatography (ERCP).* The patient swallows an endoscope—a long, flexible, lighted tube connected to a computer and TV monitor. The doctor guides the endoscope through the stomach and into the small intestine. The doctor then injects a special dye that temporarily stains the ducts in the biliary system. ERCP is used to locate and remove stones in the ducts.

- *Blood tests.* Blood tests may be used to look for signs of infection, obstruction, pancreatitis, or jaundice.

Gallstone symptoms are similar to those of heart attack, appendicitis, ulcers, irritable bowel syndrome, hiatal hernia, pancreatitis, and hepatitis, so accurate diagnosis is important.

What is the treatment?

Surgery: Surgery to remove the gallbladder is the most common way to treat symptomatic gallstones. (Asymptomatic gallstones usually do not need treatment.) Each year more than five hundred thousand Americans have gallbladder surgery. The surgery is called cholecystectomy.

The most common operation is called laparoscopic cholecystectomy. For this operation, the surgeon makes several tiny incisions in the abdomen and inserts surgical instruments and a miniature video camera into the abdomen. The camera sends a magnified image from inside the body to a video monitor, giving the surgeon a close-up view of the organs and tissues. While watching the monitor, the surgeon uses the instruments to carefully separate the gallbladder from the liver, ducts, and other structures. Then the cystic duct is cut and the gallbladder removed through one of the small incisions.

Because the abdominal muscles are not cut during laparoscopic surgery, patients have less pain and fewer complications than they would have had after surgery using a large incision across the abdomen. Recovery usually involves only one night in the hospital, followed by several days of restricted activity at home.

If the surgeon discovers any obstacles to the laparoscopic procedure, such as infection or scarring from other operations, the operating team may have to switch to open surgery. In some cases the obstacles are known before surgery, and an open surgery is planned. It is called "open" surgery because the surgeon has to make a five- to eight-inch incision in the abdomen to remove the gallbladder. This is a major surgery and may require about a two- to seven-day stay in the hospital and several more weeks at home to recover. Open surgery is required in about 5 percent of gallbladder operations.

The most common complication in gallbladder surgery is injury to the bile ducts. An injured common bile duct can leak bile and cause a painful and potentially dangerous infection. Mild injuries can sometimes be treated nonsurgically. Major injury, however, is more serious and requires additional surgery.

If gallstones are in the bile ducts, the physician (usually a gastroenterologist) may use endoscopic retrograde cholangiopancreatography (ERCP) to locate and remove them before or during the gallbladder surgery. In ERCP, the patient swallows an endoscope—a long, flexible, lighted tube connected to a computer and TV monitor. The doctor guides the endoscope through the stomach and into the small intestine. The doctor then injects a special dye that temporarily stains the ducts in the biliary system. Then the affected bile duct is located and an instrument on the endoscope is used to cut the duct. The stone is captured in a tiny basket and removed with the endoscope.

Occasionally, a person who has had a cholecystectomy is diagnosed with a gallstone in the bile ducts weeks, months, or even years after the surgery. The two-step ERCP procedure is usually successful in removing the stone.

Nonsurgical Treatment: Nonsurgical approaches are used only in special situations—such as when a patient has a serious medical condition preventing surgery—and only for cholesterol stones. Stones usually recur after nonsurgical treatment.

- *Oral dissolution therapy.* Drugs made from bile acid are used to dissolve the stones. The drugs ursodiol (Actigall) and chenodiol (Chenix) work best for small cholesterol stones. Months or years of treatment may be necessary before all the stones dissolve. Both drugs cause mild diarrhea, and chenodiol may temporarily raise levels of blood cholesterol and the liver enzyme transaminase.

- *Contact dissolution therapy.* This experimental procedure involves injecting a drug directly into the gallbladder to dissolve stones. The drug—methyl tertbutyl ether—can dissolve some stones in one to three days, but it must be used very carefully because it is a flammable anesthetic that can be toxic. The procedure is being tested in patients with symptomatic, noncalcified cholesterol stones.

Don't people need their gallbladder?

Fortunately, the gallbladder is an organ that people can live without. Losing it won't even require a change in diet. Once the gallbladder is removed, bile flows out of the liver through the hepatic ducts into the common bile duct and goes directly into the small intestine, instead of being stored in the gallbladder. However, because the bile isn't stored in the gallbladder, it flows into the small intestine more frequently, causing diarrhea in about 1 percent of people.

Points to Remember

- Gallstones form when substances in the bile harden.

- Gallstones are more common among older adults, women, Native Americans, Mexican Americans, and people who are overweight.

- Gallstone attacks often occur after eating a meal.

- Symptoms can mimic those of other problems, including heart attack, so accurate diagnosis is important.

- Gallstones can cause serious problems if they become trapped in the bile ducts.

- Laparoscopic surgery to remove the gallbladder is the most common treatment.

Chapter 24

Diverticulosis and Diverticulitis

Many people have small pouches in their colons that bulge outward through weak spots, like an inner tube that pokes through weak places in a tire. Each pouch is called a diverticulum. Pouches (plural) are called diverticula. The condition of having diverticula is called diverticulosis. About 10 percent of Americans over the age of forty have diverticulosis. The condition becomes more common as people age. About half of all people over the age of sixty have diverticulosis.

When the pouches become infected or inflamed, the condition is called diverticulitis. This happens in 10 to 25 percent of people with diverticulosis. Diverticulosis and diverticulitis are also called diverticular disease.

What causes diverticular disease?

Although not proven, the dominant theory is that a low-fiber diet is the main cause of diverticular disease. The disease was first noticed in the United States in the early 1900s. At about the same time, processed foods were introduced into the American diet. Many processed foods contain refined, low-fiber flour. Unlike whole-wheat flour, refined flour has no wheat bran.

Diverticular disease is common in developed or industrialized countries—particularly the United States, England, and Australia—where

Reprinted from "Diverticulosis and Diverticulitis," National Institute of Diabetes and Digestive and Kidney Diseases, NIH Publication No. 04-1163, August 2004.

low-fiber diets are common. The disease is rare in countries of Asia and Africa, where people eat high-fiber vegetable diets.

Fiber is the part of fruits, vegetables, and grains that the body cannot digest. Some fiber dissolves easily in water (soluble fiber). It takes on a soft, jelly-like texture in the intestines. Some fiber passes almost unchanged through the intestines (insoluble fiber). Both kinds of fiber help make stools soft and easy to pass. Fiber also prevents constipation.

Constipation makes the muscles strain to move stool that is too hard. It is the main cause of increased pressure in the colon. This excess pressure might cause the weak spots in the colon to bulge out and become diverticula.

Diverticulitis occurs when diverticula become infected or inflamed. Doctors are not certain what causes the infection. It may begin when stool or bacteria are caught in the diverticula. An attack of diverticulitis can develop suddenly and without warning.

What are the symptoms?

Diverticulosis: Most people with diverticulosis do not have any discomfort or symptoms. However, symptoms may include mild cramps, bloating, and constipation. Other diseases such as irritable bowel syndrome (IBS) and stomach ulcers cause similar problems, so these symptoms do not always mean a person has diverticulosis. You should visit your doctor if you have these troubling symptoms.

Diverticulitis: The most common symptom of diverticulitis is abdominal pain. The most common sign is tenderness around the left side of the lower abdomen. If infection is the cause, fever, nausea, vomiting, chills, cramping, and constipation may occur as well. The severity of symptoms depends on the extent of the infection and complications.

What are the complications?

Diverticulitis can lead to bleeding, infections, perforations or tears, or blockages. These complications always require treatment to prevent them from progressing and causing serious illness.

Bleeding: Bleeding from diverticula is a rare complication. When diverticula bleed, blood may appear in the toilet or in your stool. Bleeding can be severe, but it may stop by itself and not require treatment. Doctors believe bleeding diverticula are caused by a small blood vessel in a diverticulum that weakens and finally bursts. If you have bleeding from the rectum, you should see your doctor. If the bleeding does not stop, surgery may be necessary.

Abscess, Perforation, and Peritonitis: The infection causing diverticulitis often clears up after a few days of treatment with antibiotics. If the condition gets worse, an abscess may form in the colon.

An abscess is an infected area with pus that may cause swelling and destroy tissue. Sometimes the infected diverticula may develop small holes, called perforations. These perforations allow pus to leak out of the colon into the abdominal area. If the abscess is small and remains in the colon, it may clear up after treatment with antibiotics. If the abscess does not clear up with antibiotics, the doctor may need to drain it.

To drain the abscess, the doctor uses a needle and a small tube called a catheter. The doctor inserts the needle through the skin and drains the fluid through the catheter. This procedure is called percutaneous catheter drainage. Sometimes surgery is needed to clean the abscess and, if necessary, remove part of the colon.

A large abscess can become a serious problem if the infection leaks out and contaminates areas outside the colon. Infection that spreads into the abdominal cavity is called peritonitis. Peritonitis requires immediate surgery to clean the abdominal cavity and remove the damaged part of the colon. Without surgery, peritonitis can be fatal.

Fistula: A fistula is an abnormal connection of tissue between two organs or between an organ and the skin. When damaged tissues come into contact with each other during infection, they sometimes stick together. If they heal that way, a fistula forms. When diverticulitis-related infection spreads outside the colon, the colon's tissue may stick to nearby tissues. The organs usually involved are the bladder, small intestine, and skin.

The most common type of fistula occurs between the bladder and the colon. It affects men more than women. This type of fistula can result in a severe, long-lasting infection of the urinary tract. The problem can be corrected with surgery to remove the fistula and the affected part of the colon.

Intestinal Obstruction: The scarring caused by infection may cause partial or total blockage of the large intestine. When this happens, the colon is unable to move bowel contents normally. When the obstruction totally blocks the intestine, emergency surgery is necessary. Partial blockage is not an emergency, so the surgery to correct it can be planned.

How does the doctor diagnose diverticular disease?

To diagnose diverticular disease, the doctor asks about medical history, does a physical exam, and may perform one or more diagnostic tests. Because most people do not have symptoms, diverticulosis is often found through tests ordered for another ailment.

When taking a medical history, the doctor may ask about bowel habits, symptoms, pain, diet, and medications. The physical exam usually involves a digital rectal exam. To perform this test, the doctor inserts a gloved, lubricated finger into the rectum to detect tenderness, blockage, or blood. The doctor may check stool for signs of bleeding and test blood for signs of infection. The doctor may also order x-rays or other tests.

What is the treatment for diverticular disease?

A high-fiber diet and, occasionally, mild pain medications will help relieve symptoms in most cases. Sometimes an attack of diverticulitis is serious enough to require a hospital stay and possibly surgery.

Diverticulosis: Increasing the amount of fiber in the diet may reduce symptoms of diverticulosis and prevent complications such as diverticulitis. Fiber keeps stool soft and lowers pressure inside the colon so that bowel contents can move through easily. The American Dietetic Association recommends twenty to thirty-five grams of fiber each day. Table 24.1 shows the amount of fiber in some foods that you can easily add to your diet.

The doctor may also recommend taking a fiber product such as Citrucel or Metamucil once a day. These products are mixed with water and provide about 2 to 3.5 grams of fiber per tablespoon, mixed with eight ounces of water.

Until recently, many doctors suggested avoiding foods with small seeds such as tomatoes or strawberries because they believed that particles could lodge in the diverticula and cause inflammation. However, it is now generally accepted that only foods that may irritate or get caught in the diverticula cause problems. Foods such as nuts, popcorn hulls, and sunflower, pumpkin, caraway, and sesame seeds should be avoided. The seeds in tomatoes, zucchini, cucumbers, strawberries, and raspberries, as well as poppy seeds, are generally considered harmless. People differ in the amounts and types of foods they can eat. Decisions about diet should be made based on what works best for each person. Keeping a food diary may help identify individual items in one's diet.

Table 24.1. Amount of Fiber in Some Foods

Fruits

Apple, raw, with skin	1 medium	=	3.3 grams
Peach, raw	1 medium	=	1.5 grams
Pear, raw	1 medium	=	5.1 grams
Tangerine, raw	1 medium	=	1.9 grams

Vegetables

Asparagus, fresh, cooked	4 spears	=	1.2 grams
Broccoli, fresh, cooked	1/2 cup	=	2.6 grams
Brussels sprouts, fresh, cooked	1/2 cup	=	2 grams
Cabbage, fresh, cooked	1/2 cup	=	1.5 grams
Carrot, fresh, cooked	1/2 cup	=	2.3 grams
Cauliflower, fresh, cooked	1/2 cup	=	1.7 grams
Romaine lettuce	1 cup	=	1.2 grams
Spinach, fresh, cooked	1/2 cup	=	2.2 grams
Summer squash, cooked	1 cup	=	2.5 grams
Tomato, raw	1	=	1 gram
Winter squash, cooked	1 cup	=	5.7 grams

Starchy Vegetables

Baked beans, canned, plain	1/2 cup	=	6.3 grams
Kidney beans, fresh, cooked	1/2 cup	=	5.7 grams
Lima beans, fresh, cooked	1/2 cup	=	6.6 grams
Potato, fresh, cooked	1	=	2.3 grams

Grains

Bread, whole-wheat	1 slice	=	1.9 grams
Brown rice, cooked	1 cup	=	3.5 grams
Cereal, bran flake	3/4 cup	=	5.3 grams
Oatmeal, plain, cooked	3/4 cup	=	3 grams
White rice, cooked	1 cup	=	0.6 grams

Source: United States Department of Agriculture (USDA). USDA Nutrient Database for Standard Reference Release 15. Available at www.nal.usda.gov/fnic/cgi-bin/nut_search.pl. Accessed April 5, 2004.

If cramps, bloating, and constipation are problems, the doctor may prescribe a short course of pain medication. However, many medications affect emptying of the colon, an undesirable side effect for people with diverticulosis.

Diverticulitis: Treatment for diverticulitis focuses on clearing up the infection and inflammation, resting the colon, and preventing or minimizing complications. An attack of diverticulitis without complications may respond to antibiotics within a few days if treated early.

To help the colon rest, the doctor may recommend bed rest and a liquid diet, along with a pain reliever.

An acute attack with severe pain or severe infection may require a hospital stay. Most acute cases of diverticulitis are treated with antibiotics and a liquid diet. The antibiotics are given by injection into a vein. In some cases, however, surgery may be necessary.

When is surgery necessary?

If attacks are severe or frequent, the doctor may advise surgery. The surgeon removes the affected part of the colon and joins the remaining sections. This type of surgery, called colon resection, aims to keep attacks from coming back and to prevent complications. The doctor may also recommend surgery for complications of a fistula or intestinal obstruction.

If antibiotics do not correct an attack, emergency surgery may be required. Other reasons for emergency surgery include a large abscess, perforation, peritonitis, or continued bleeding.

Emergency surgery usually involves two operations. The first surgery will clear the infected abdominal cavity and remove part of the colon. Because of infection and sometimes obstruction, it is not safe to rejoin the colon during the first operation. Instead, the surgeon creates a temporary hole, or stoma, in the abdomen. The end of the colon is connected to the hole, a procedure called a colostomy, to allow normal eating and bowel movements. The stool goes into a bag attached to the opening in the abdomen. In the second operation, the surgeon rejoins the ends of the colon.

Points to Remember

- Diverticulosis occurs when small pouches, called diverticula, bulge outward through weak spots in the colon (large intestine).

- The pouches form when pressure inside the colon builds, usually because of constipation.

- Most people with diverticulosis never have any discomfort or symptoms.

- The most likely cause of diverticulosis is a low-fiber diet because it increases constipation and pressure inside the colon.

- For most people with diverticulosis, eating a high-fiber diet is the only treatment needed.

- You can increase your fiber intake by eating these foods: whole-grain breads and cereals; fruit like apples and peaches; vegetables like broccoli, cabbage, spinach, carrots, asparagus, and squash; and starchy vegetables like kidney beans and lima beans.

- Diverticulitis occurs when the pouches become infected or inflamed and cause pain and tenderness around the left side of the lower abdomen.

Additional Readings

Diverticular disease. In: Corman ML, Allison SI, Kuehne JP. *Handbook of Colon and Rectal Surgery*. Hagerstown, MD: Lippincott, Williams & Wilkins; 2002: 637–53.

Diverticular disease. In: King JE, ed. *Mayo Clinic on digestive Health*. Rochester, MN: Mayo Clinic; 2000: 125–32.

Marcello PW. Understanding diverticular disease. *Ostomy Quarterly*. 2002; 39(2): 56–57.

Chapter 25

What You Need to Know about Colon Polyps

What are colon polyps?

A polyp is extra tissue that grows inside your body. Colon polyps grow in the large intestine. The large intestine, also called the colon, is part of your digestive system. It's a long, hollow tube at the end of your digestive tract where your body makes and stores stool.

Are polyps dangerous?

Most polyps are not dangerous. Most are benign, which means they are not cancer. But over time, some types of polyps can turn into cancer. Usually, polyps that are smaller than a pea aren't harmful, but larger polyps could someday become cancer or may already be cancer. To be safe, doctors remove all polyps and test them.

Who gets polyps?

Anyone can get polyps, but certain people are more likely than others. You may have a greater chance of getting polyps if:

- you're over fifty. The older you get, the more likely you are to develop polyps.

- you've had polyps before.

Reprinted from "What I Need to Know about Colon Polyps," National Institute of Diabetes and Digestive and Kidney Diseases, NIH Publication No. 03-4977, April 2003.

- someone in your family has had polyps.
- someone in your family has had cancer of the large intestine.

You may also be more likely to get polyps if you:

- eat a lot of fatty foods;
- smoke;
- drink alcohol;
- don't exercise;
- weigh too much.

What are the symptoms?

Most small polyps don't cause symptoms. Often, people don't know they have one until the doctor finds it during a regular checkup or while testing them for something else.

However some people do have symptoms like these:

- bleeding from the anus. You might notice blood on your underwear or on toilet paper after you've had a bowel movement.
- constipation or diarrhea that lasts more than a week.
- blood in the stool. Blood can make stool look black, or it can show up as red streaks in the stool.

If you have any of these symptoms, see a doctor to find out what the problem is.

How does the doctor test for polyps?

The doctor can use four tests to check for polyps:

- **Digital rectal exam.** The doctor wears gloves and checks your rectum, the last part of the large intestine, to see if it feels normal. This test would find polyps only in the rectum, so the doctor may need to do one of the other tests listed here to find polyps higher up in the intestine.
- **Barium enema.** The doctor puts a liquid called barium into your rectum before taking x-rays of your large intestine. Barium makes your intestine look white in the pictures. Polyps are dark, so they're easy to see.

- **Sigmoidoscopy.** With this test, the doctor can see inside your large intestine. The doctor puts a thin flexible tube into your rectum. The device is called a sigmoidoscope, and it has a light and a tiny video camera in it. The doctor uses the sigmoidoscope to look at the last third of your large intestine.

- **Colonoscopy.** This test is like sigmoidoscopy, but the doctor looks at all of the large intestine. It usually requires sedation.

Who should get tested for polyps?

Talk to your doctor about getting tested for polyps if:

- you have symptoms;
- you're fifty years old or older;
- someone in your family has had polyps or colon cancer.

How are polyps treated?

The doctor will remove the polyp. Sometimes, the doctor takes it out during sigmoidoscopy or colonoscopy. Or the doctor may decide to operate through the abdomen. The polyp is then tested for cancer.

If you've had polyps, the doctor may want you to get tested regularly in the future.

How can I prevent polyps?

Doctors don't know of any one sure way to prevent polyps. However you might be able to lower your risk of getting them if you:

- eat more fruits and vegetables and less fatty food;
- don't smoke;
- avoid alcohol;
- exercise every day;
- lose weight if you're overweight.

Eating more calcium and folate can also lower your risk of getting polyps. Some foods that are rich in calcium are milk, cheese, and broccoli. Some foods that are rich in folate are chickpeas, kidney beans, and spinach.

Some doctors think that aspirin might help prevent polyps. Studies are under way.

Points to Remember

- A polyp is extra tissue that grows inside the body. Most polyps are not harmful.

- Symptoms may include constipation or diarrhea for more than a week or blood on your underwear, on toilet paper, or in your stool.

- Many polyps do not cause symptoms.

- Doctors remove all polyps and test them for cancer.

- Talk to your doctor about getting tested for polyps if:
  - you have any symptoms;
  - you're fifty years old or older;
  - someone in your family has had polyps or colon cancer.

Chapter 26

Congenital and Pediatric Disorders of the Lower Gastrointestinal Tract

Chapter Contents

Section 26.1

Hirschsprung Disease

Reprinted from "What I Need to Know about Hirschsprung Disease,"
National Institute of Diabetes and Digestive and Kidney Diseases,
NIH Publication No. 05-4384, October 2004.

What is Hirschsprung disease?

Hirschsprung disease, or HD, is a disease of the large intestine.

The large intestine is also sometimes called the colon. The word *bowel* can refer to the large and small intestines. HD usually occurs in children. It causes constipation, which means that bowel movements are difficult. Some children with HD can't have bowel movements at all. The stool creates a blockage in the intestine.

If HD is not treated, stool can fill up the large intestine. This can cause serious problems like infection, bursting of the colon, and even death.

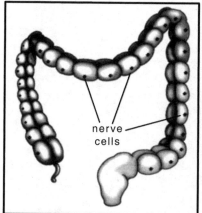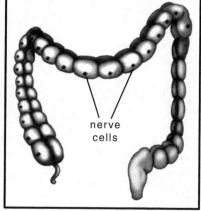

Figure 26.1. *Left: Healthy large intestine; nerve cells are found throughout the intestine. Right: HD large intestine; Nerve cells are missing from the last part of the intestine.*

Most parents feel frightened when they learn that their child has a serious disease. This section will help you understand HD and how you and the doctor can help your child.

Why does HD cause constipation?

Normally, muscles in the intestine push stool to the anus, where stool leaves the body. Special nerve cells in the intestine, called ganglion cells, make the muscles push. A person with HD does not have these nerve cells in the last part of the large intestine.

In a person with HD, the healthy muscles of the intestine push the stool until it reaches the part without the nerve cells. At this point, the stool stops moving. New stool then begins to stack up behind it.

Sometimes the ganglion cells are missing from the whole large intestine and even parts of the small intestine before it. When the diseased section reaches to or includes the small intestine, it is called long-segment disease. When the diseased section includes only part of the large intestine, it is called short-segment disease.

What causes HD?

HD develops before a child is born. Normally, nerve cells grow in the baby's intestine soon after the baby begins to grow in the womb. These nerve cells grow down from the top of the intestine all the way to the anus. With HD, the nerve cells stop growing before they reach the end.

No one knows why the nerve cells stop growing. But we do know that it's not the mother's fault. HD isn't caused by anything the mother did while she was pregnant.

Some children with HD have other health problems, such as Down syndrome and other rare disorders.

If I have more children, will they have HD too?

In some cases, HD is hereditary, which means mothers and fathers could pass it to their children. This can happen even if the parents don't have HD. If you have one child with HD, you could have more children with the disease. Talk to your doctor about the risk.

What are the symptoms?

Symptoms of HD usually show up in very young children, but sometimes they don't appear until the person is a teenager or an adult. The symptoms are a little different for different ages.

Symptoms in Newborns: Newborns with HD don't have their first bowel movement when they should. These babies may also throw up a green liquid called bile after eating, and their abdomens may swell. Discomfort from gas or constipation might make them fussy. Sometimes, babies with HD develop infections in their intestines.

Symptoms in Young Children: Most children with HD have always had severe problems with constipation. Some also have more diarrhea than usual. Children with HD might also have anemia, a shortage of red blood cells, because blood is lost in the stool. Also, many babies with HD grow and develop more slowly than they should.

Symptoms in Teenagers and Adults: Like younger children, teenagers and adults with HD usually have had severe constipation all their lives. They might also have anemia.

How does the doctor find out if HD is the problem?

To find out if a person has HD, the doctor will do one or more tests:

- barium enema x-ray
- manometry
- biopsy

Barium Enema X-ray: An x-ray is a black-and-white picture of the inside of the body. The picture is taken with a special machine that uses a small amount of radiation. For a barium enema x-ray, the doctor puts barium through the anus into the intestine before taking the picture. Barium is a liquid that makes the intestine show up better on the x-ray.

In some cases, instead of barium another liquid, called Gastrografin, may be used. Gastrografin is also sometimes used in newborns to help remove a hard first stool. Gastrografin causes water to be pulled into the intestine, and the extra water softens the stool.

In places where the nerve cells are missing, the intestine looks too narrow. If a narrow large intestine shows on the x-ray, the doctor knows HD might be the problem. More tests will help the doctor know for sure.

Other tests used to diagnose HD are manometry and biopsy.

Manometry: The doctor inflates a small balloon inside the rectum. Normally, the anal muscle will relax. If it doesn't, HD may be the problem. This test is most often done in older children and adults.

Biopsy: This is the most accurate test for HD. The doctor removes and looks at a tiny piece of the intestine under a microscope. If the nerve cells are missing, HD is the problem.

The doctor may do one or all of these tests. It depends on the child.

What is the treatment?

Pull-through Surgery: HD is treated with surgery. The surgery is called a pull-through operation. There are three common ways to do a pull-through, and they are called the Swenson, the Soave, and the Duhamel procedures. Each is done a little differently, but all involve taking out the part of the intestine that doesn't work and connecting the healthy part that's left to the anus. After pull-through surgery, the child has a working intestine.

Colostomy and Ileostomy: Often, the pull-through can be done right after the diagnosis. However, children who have been very sick may first need surgery called an ostomy. This surgery helps the child get healthy before having the pull-through. Some doctors do an ostomy in every child before doing the pull-through.

In an ostomy, the doctor takes out the diseased part of the intestine. Then the doctor cuts a small hole in the baby's abdomen. The hole is called a stoma. The doctor connects the top part of the intestine to

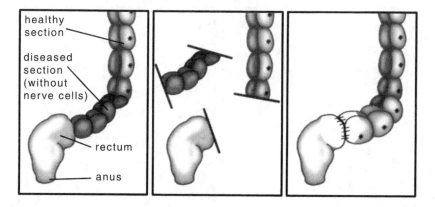

Figure 26.2. Pull-through Surgery. Left: Before surgery—the diseased section is the part of the intestine that doesn't work. Middle: Step 1—the doctor removes the diseased section. Right: Step 2—the healthy section is attached to the rectum or anus.

the stoma. Stool leaves the body through the stoma while the bottom part of the intestine heals. Stool goes into a bag attached to the skin around the stoma. You will need to empty this bag several times a day.

If the doctor removes the entire large intestine and connects the small intestine to the stoma, the surgery is called an ileostomy. If the doctor leaves part of the large intestine and connects that to the stoma, the surgery is called a colostomy.

Later, the doctor will do the pull-through. The doctor disconnects the intestine from the stoma and attaches it just above the anus. The stoma isn't needed any more, so the doctor either sews it up during surgery or waits about six weeks to make sure that the pull-through worked.

What will my child's life be like after surgery?

Ostomy: Most babies are more comfortable after having an ostomy because they can pass gas more easily and aren't constipated anymore.

Older children will be more comfortable, too, but they may have some trouble getting used to an ostomy. They will need to learn how to take care of the stoma and how to change the bag that collects stool. They may be worried about being different from their friends. Most children can lead a normal life after surgery.

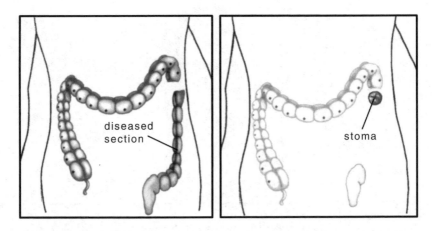

Figure 26.3. Ostomy surgery. Left: Step 1—the doctor takes out most of the diseased part of the intestine. Right: Step 2—the doctor attaches the healthy part of the intestine to the stoma (a hole in the abdomen).

Adjusting after Pull-through: After a pull-through, nine out of ten children pass stool normally. Some children may have diarrhea for a while, and babies may develop a nasty diaper rash. Eventually the stool will become more solid and the child will need to go to the bathroom less often. Toilet training may be delayed, as the child learns how to use the bottom muscles only after pull-through surgery. Older children might stain their underwear for a while after the surgery. It is not their fault. They can't control this problem, but it improves with time.

Some children become constipated, because one in ten children with HD has difficulty moving stool through the part of the colon without nerve cells. A mild laxative may also be helpful. Ask your doctor for suggestions.

Diet and Nutrition: One job of the large intestine is to collect the water and salts the body needs. Since your child's intestine is shorter now, it absorbs less. Your child will need to drink more to make sure his body gets enough fluids.

An infant who has long-segment disease requiring an ileostomy may need special tube feedings. The shortened intestine does not allow the bloodstream enough time to absorb nutrients from food before it is pushed out of the body as stool. Tube feedings that deliver nutrients can make up for what is lost.

Eating high-fiber foods like cereal and bran muffins can help reduce constipation and diarrhea.

Infection: Infections can be very dangerous for a child with Hirschsprung disease. Infection of the large and small intestines is called enterocolitis. It can happen before or after surgery to treat Hirschsprung disease. Here are some of the signs to look for:

- fever
- swollen abdomen
- vomiting
- diarrhea
- bleeding from the rectum
- sluggishness

Call your doctor immediately if your child shows any of these signs. If the problem is enterocolitis, your child may be admitted to the hospital. In the hospital, an intravenous (I.V.) line may be needed to keep body fluids up and to deliver antibiotics to fight the infection. The large intestine will be rinsed regularly with a mild saltwater solution until all remaining stool has been removed. The rinse may also contain antibiotics to kill bacteria.

When the child has recovered from the infection, the doctor may advise surgery. If the child has not had the pull-through surgery yet, the doctor may prepare for it by doing a colostomy or ileostomy before the child leaves the hospital. If the child has already had a pull-through operation, the doctor may correct the obstruction with surgery.

Enterocolitis can be life threatening, so watch for the signs and call your doctor immediately if they occur.

Long-Segment HD: Sometimes HD affects most or all of the large intestine, plus some of the small intestine. Children with long-segment HD can be treated with pull-through surgery, but there is a risk of complications such as infection, diarrhea, and diaper rash afterward. Parents need to pay close attention to their child's health. Also, since some, most, or all of the intestine is removed, drinking a lot of fluid is important.

Points to Remember

- HD is a disease of the large intestine.
- HD develops in children before they are born. It is not caused by anything the mother did while pregnant.
- Symptoms of HD include:
  - delayed first bowel movement in newborns;
  - swollen abdomen and vomiting;
  - constipation since birth;
  - slow growth and development;
  - anemia.
- Children with HD may get an infection, called enterocolitis, which can cause fever and diarrhea.
- HD is a serious disease that needs to be treated right away. HD is treated with pull-through surgery or, sometimes, ostomy.
- After treatment, most children with HD lead normal lives.

Section 26.2

Intussusception

This information was provided by KidsHealth, one of the largest resources online for medically reviewed health information written for parents, kids, and teens. For more articles like this one, visit www.KidsHealth.org, or www.TeensHealth.org. © 2004 The Nemours Center for Children's Health Media, a division of The Nemours Foundation.

Justin cried loudly and drew his tiny legs up to his chest as his bewildered parents tried to soothe him. Their seven-month-old had been colicky before, but this was something new—his crying was more urgent, his mood much more irritable. As the afternoon wore on, Justin's dad noticed that his son's small belly was distended, and when it was time to change the baby's diaper, he suspected that something was wrong.

After speaking with Justin's doctor, Justin's dad bundled him up and took him to the emergency department, where he was diagnosed with and successfully treated for intussusception (pronounced: in-tuh-suh-sep-shun), the most common abdominal emergency to affect children under two years of age. Keep reading to learn about intussusception, its symptoms, its treatment, and more.

What Is Intussusception?

Intussusception occurs when one portion of the bowel slides into the next, much like the pieces of a telescope. When this occurs, it creates an obstruction in the bowel, with the walls of the intestines pressing against one another. This, in turn, leads to swelling, inflammation, and decreased blood flow to the intestines involved.

The most common cause of intestinal obstruction in children between the ages of three months and six years, intussusception:

- occurs most often in children between five and ten months of age (80 percent occur before a child is twenty-four months old);
- affects between one and four infants out of one thousand;
- is three to four times more common in boys than in girls.

Signs and Symptoms

Children with an intussusception have intense abdominal pain, which often begins so suddenly that it causes loud, anguished crying and causes the child to draw the knees up to the chest. The pain is usually intermittent, but recurs and becomes stronger. As the pain subsides, a child with an intussusception may stop crying and seem fine.

Other common symptoms include:

- abdominal swelling or distension
- passing stools (or poop) mixed with blood and mucus, known as currant jelly stool (60 percent of infants with an intussusception will pass currant jelly stool)
- vomiting
- vomiting up bile, a bitter-tasting fluid secreted by the liver that's often golden-brown to greenish in color
- lethargy (i.e., drowsiness or sluggishness)
- shallow breathing
- grunting

As the illness progresses, a child will become progressively weaker and may develop a fever and appear to go into shock. Symptoms of shock include lethargy, rapid heartbeat, weak pulse, low blood pressure, and rapid breathing.

Causes of Intussusception

In infants, the causes of intussusception are unknown, although there are some theories about why it occurs. Because intussusception is seen most often in spring and fall, this seems to suggest a possible connection to the kinds of viruses that children catch during these seasons, including upper respiratory infections.

In some cases, intussusception may follow a recent bout of gastroenteritis (sometimes called stomach flu). Gastrointestinal infections may cause swelling of the infection-fighting lymph tissue that lines the intestine, which may pull one part of the intestine into the other. Intussusception is most common around the age that infants are being introduced to solid foods. It has been suggested that the introduction of new foods may also cause some swelling of the lymph tissue in the intestines, increasing the chance of developing an intussusception.

Recently, there has also been some investigation into the rotavirus vaccine and its possible connection to intussusception, although the number of reported cases of intussusception among babies who received the vaccine is quite small. According to the U.S. Centers for Disease Control and Prevention (CDC), it has not been established that the vaccine causes intussusception, but the CDC and the U.S. Food and Drug Administration have suspended the vaccine until they're able to gather more information. Babies who received the rotavirus vaccine before its suspension have no increased risk of developing intussusception now.

Usually when an adult or a child older than three develops an intussusception, it's often the result of enlarged lymph nodes, a tumor, or a polyp in the intestine.

Diagnosis and Treatment

The doctor will then perform a physical exam on the child, paying special attention to the abdomen. Often, the doctor can feel the part of the intestine that's involved, which is swollen and tender and often is described as a "sausage-shaped mass." Symptoms like pain, drawing up the legs, vomiting, lethargy, and passing bloody or currant jelly stool are meaningful in helping the doctor reach a diagnosis. In addition to doing a physical examination, the doctor will ask the parent about any concerns and symptoms their child has, the child's past health, your family's health, any medications the child is taking, any allergies the child may have, and other issues. This is called the medical history.

If the doctor thinks an intussusception may be the cause of the child's pain, a pediatric surgeon will be consulted to examine the child and decide about treatment. The doctor may order an abdominal x-ray, which may or may not show an obstruction. An ultrasound examination may also help make the diagnosis. If the child appears very ill, suggesting damage to the intestine, the surgeon may opt to take the child immediately to the operating room to correct the bowel obstruction.

A barium or air enema is often used to both diagnose and treat a suspected intussusception. During a barium enema, a liquid mixture containing barium is given through a catheter tube into the child's rectum, and special x-rays are taken. Barium outlines the bowels on the x-rays and, if an intussusception is present, shows the doctors the telescoping piece of intestine.

In many instances, the barium enema not only shows the intussusception, but the pressure from putting it in the bowel may also unfold the bowel that has been turned inside out, instantly curing the obstruction. An air enema, given rectally in a similar way as barium, can also be used to diagnosis and treat an intussusception.

The radiologist usually decides which test is most appropriate to perform. Both procedures are very safe and usually well tolerated by the child, although there is a very small risk of infection or bowel perforation. There's a 10 percent risk of recurrence, which usually occurs within seventy-two hours following the procedure.

If the barium or air enema procedures aren't successful or the child is too ill to attempt the enema, the child will undergo surgery. Enemas are less successful in older children, and they're more likely to require surgery to treat intussusception. Surgeons will try to fix the obstruction but if too much damage has been done, that part of the bowel will be removed.

Some babies with intussusception may be given antibiotics to prevent infection. Babies who have been treated for intussusception will be kept in the hospital and given intravenous feedings until they're able to eat and have normal bowel function.

Complications of Intussusception

If left untreated, intussusception can cause severe complications. Complications are directly related to the amount of time that passes from when the intussusception occurred until it's treated. Most infants who are treated within the first twenty-four hours recover completely from an intussusception with no problems. Further delay increases the risk of complications, which include irreversible tissue damage, perforation of the bowel, infection, and death.

When to Call Your Child's Doctor

Intussusception is a medical emergency. If you're concerned that your child has some or all of the symptoms of intussusception, such as abdominal pain, vomiting, or passing of currant jelly stool, call your child's doctor or emergency medical services immediately.

The outcome for most infants with intussusception is very good, and with early treatment, complications are much less likely to develop. Do not delay, though—in many cases, early diagnosis can mean a child can be successfully treated without surgery.

Section 26.3

Intestinal Malrotation

This information was provided by KidsHealth, one of the largest resources online for medically reviewed health information written for parents, kids, and teens. For more articles like this one, visit www.KidsHealth.org, or www.TeensHealth.org. © 2004 The Nemours Center for Children's Health Media, a division of The Nemours Foundation.

Any blockage of the digestive tract that prevents the proper passage of food is known as an intestinal obstruction. Some causes of intestinal obstruction include a congenital (present at birth) malformation of the digestive tract, hernias, abnormal scar tissue growth after an abdominal operation, and inflammatory bowel disease. These blockages are also called mechanical obstructions because they physically block a portion of the intestine or another part of the digestive tract.

Malrotation is a type of mechanical obstruction caused by abnormal development of the intestines while a fetus is in the mother's womb. It occurs in one out of every five hundred births in the United States and accounts for approximately 5 percent of all intestinal obstructions. Some children with malrotation have other congenital malformations including:

- defects of the digestive system;
- heart defects;
- abnormalities of other organs, including the spleen or liver.

Some people who have malrotation never experience complications and are never diagnosed. But most children with this condition develop symptoms during infancy, often during the first month of life, and the majority are diagnosed by the time they reach one year of age. Although surgery is required to repair malrotation, most children experience normal growth and development once the condition and any problems associated with it are treated and corrected.

What Is Malrotation?

The small and large intestines are the longest part of the digestive system. If stretched out to their full length, they would measure more than twenty feet long by adulthood, but because they are coiled up, they fit into the relatively small space of the abdominal cavity. Malrotation occurs when the intestines don't "coil" properly during fetal development. The exact cause is unknown.

When a fetus is developing in the womb, the intestines start out as a small, straight tube between the stomach and the rectum. As this tube develops into separate organs, the intestines move for a time into the umbilical cord, which supplies nutrients to the developing embryo.

Around the tenth week of pregnancy, the intestine moves from the umbilical cord into the abdomen. It fits in by making two turns that allow it to lie in a specific position within the abdomen. When the intestine does not make these turns properly, malrotation has occurred.

Malrotation in itself may not cause any problems. However, it may be accompanied by additional complications:

- Bands of tissue called Ladd bands may form, obstructing the first part of the small intestine (the duodenum).

- After birth, volvulus may occur. This is when the intestine twists on itself, causing a lack of blood flow to the tissue and leading to tissue death. Malrotation is often diagnosed when volvulus occurs, frequently during the first weeks of life.

Obstruction caused by volvulus or Ladd bands are both life-threatening problems. The intestines can stop functioning and intestinal tissue can die from lack of blood supply if an obstruction isn't recognized and treated.

Signs and Symptoms

One of the earliest signs of malrotation and volvulus is abdominal pain and cramping caused by the inability of the bowel to push food past the obstruction. Infants cannot tell you when their stomachs hurt, but you may notice the following pattern of behavior:

- pulling up the legs and crying
- stopping crying suddenly
- behaving normally for fifteen to thirty minutes
- repeating this behavior when the next cramp happens

Infants may also be irritable, lethargic, or have irregular stools.

Vomiting is another symptom of malrotation, and it can help your child's doctor determine where the obstruction is located. Vomiting that happens soon after your baby starts to cry often means the obstruction is in the small intestine; if it's delayed, it's usually in the large intestine. The vomit may be bilious (this means it contains bile, which is yellow or green in color) or may resemble your child's feces.

Additional symptoms of malrotation and volvulus may include:

- a swollen abdomen that's tender to the touch;
- diarrhea and/or bloody stools (or sometimes no stools at all);
- irritability or crying in pain, with nothing seeming to help;
- rapid heart rate and breathing;
- little or no urine because of fluid loss;
- fever.

Diagnosis and Treatment

If your child's doctor suspects volvulus or another intestinal blockage, he or she will order x-rays, a computed tomography (CT) scan, or an ultrasound of the abdominal area.

Your doctor may use barium to see the x-ray or scan more clearly. Barium provides a contrast that can show if the intestine has a malformation and can usually determine where a blockage is located. Adults and older children usually drink barium in a liquid form. Infants may need to be given barium through a tube inserted from their nose into the stomach, or sometimes are given a barium enema, in which the liquid barium is inserted through the rectum.

The specific treatment of malrotation will depend on your child's age and other health problems. Because malrotation is usually only recognized after a blockage occurs because of volvulus or Ladd bands, your child's doctor will order corrective treatment immediately.

Any child with bowel obstruction will need to be hospitalized. A tube called a nasogastric (NG) tube is usually inserted through the nose and down into the stomach to remove the contents of the stomach and upper intestines. This keeps fluid and gas from building up in the abdomen. Your child may also be given intravenous (IV) fluids to help prevent dehydration and antibiotics to prevent infection.

Surgery to correct bowel obstruction from malrotation is always necessary and is often performed as an emergency procedure to prevent irreversible, life-threatening injury to the bowel. During surgery, which is called a Ladd procedure, the intestine is straightened out, the Ladd bands are divided, the small intestine is coiled on the right side of the abdomen, and the colon is placed on the left side. Because the appendix is usually found on the left side of the abdomen in cases of malrotation (it is normally found on the right), it is removed. Its altered position would make symptoms of appendicitis difficult to determine in the future.

If the doctor suspects that blood may still not be flowing properly to the intestines (because they don't look pink and healthy after being untwisted), he or she may perform a second surgery within forty-eight hours of the first. If the intestine still looks unhealthy at this time, the damaged portion may be removed.

If the baby is seriously ill at the time of surgery, an ileostomy or colostomy will usually be performed. In this procedure, the diseased bowel is completely removed, and the end of the normal, healthy intestine is brought out through an opening on the skin of the abdomen (called a stoma). Fecal matter passes through this opening and into a bag that is taped or attached with adhesive to the child's belly. In young children, depending on how much bowel was removed, ileostomy or colostomy is often a temporary condition that can later be reversed with another operation.

The doctor will monitor your child's progress after surgery to make sure she's developing normally. The majority of these surgeries are successful, although some children have recurring problems after surgery. Recurrent volvulus is rare, but a second bowel obstruction due to adhesions (scar tissue build-up after any type of abdominal surgery) could occur later.

Children who require removal of a large portion of the small intestine can have too little bowel to maintain adequate nutrition (a condition known as short bowel syndrome). They may be dependent on intravenous nutrition for a time after surgery and may require a special diet afterward. Most children in whom the volvulus and malrotation are identified early, before permanent injury to the bowel has occurred, do well and develop normally.

When to Call the Doctor

If you suspect any kind of intestinal obstruction because your child has bilious vomiting, a swollen abdomen, or bloody stools, take her to the emergency room immediately.

Section 26.4

Meckel Diverticulum

Definition

A Meckel diverticulum is a common congenital (present from before birth) pouch on the wall of the small bowel. The diverticulum may contain stomach or pancreatic tissue.

Causes, Incidence, and Risk Factors

A Meckel diverticulum is a remnant of structures within the fetal digestive tract that were not fully reabsorbed before birth. Approximately 2 percent of the population has a Meckel diverticulum, but only a few develop symptoms.

Symptoms include diverticulitis or bleeding in the intestine. Symptoms often occur during the first few years of life but may occur in adults as well.

Symptoms

- Passing of blood in the stool
- Abdominal discomfort or pain ranging from mild to severe

Signs and Tests

- Visible blood in stool
- Occult (invisible) blood in the stool on multiple tests
- Iron deficiency anemia

Tests

- Stool smear for occult blood (stool guaiac)
- Hematocrit

- Hemoglobin
- Technetium scan to demonstrate diverticulum

Treatment

Surgery to remove the diverticulum is recommended if bleeding develops. In rare cases, the segment of small intestine which contains the diverticulum is surgically removed, and the ends of intestine sewn back together. Iron replacement may be needed to correct anemia. If bleeding is significant, blood transfusion may be necessary.

Expectations (Prognosis)

Full recovery can be expected with surgery.

Complications

- Hemorrhage
- Perforation of the bowel at the diverticulum
- Peritonitis
- Intussusception with resultant obstruction

Calling Your Health Care Provider

See your health care provider promptly if your child passes blood or bloody stool or complains repeatedly of abdominal discomfort.

Section 26.5

Necrotizing Enterocolitis

What is necrotizing enterocolitis (NEC)?

Necrotizing enterocolitis (NEC) affects mainly premature babies. It is the most common surgical emergency in newborns. NEC accounts for 15 percent of deaths in premature babies weighing less than 1,500 grams. Overall death from those babies with NEC is 25 percent.

What causes NEC?

No single factor has been established as the cause of NEC. It is now thought that NEC is the result of a combination of several factors. The two consistent findings are prematurity and feedings. The premature intestine reacts abnormally and develops an acute inflammatory response to feedings, leading to intestinal necrosis (death). Some postnatal issues including heart abnormalities, obstruction of circulation in the bowel, infection, or gastroschisis are also associated with NEC.

In the premature infant, NEC usually occurs a week to ten days after the initiation of feedings. In the term baby, NEC occurs within one to four days of life if feeding is started on day one. The risk of NEC is less with later gestational age. Very few unfed infants develop NEC. One theory that connects feeding to bowel mucosa damage involves the overgrowth of bacteria when provided with a carbohydrate source. The digestion of the lactose in formula by premature infants is incomplete and the residual ferments (has a chemical change) that encourages growth of bacteria that cause inflammation.

What are the signs and symptoms of NEC?

NEC is difficult to diagnose. The baby may have lethargy, poor feeding, bilious vomiting, distended abdomen, and blood in stools. Physical examination may show the baby to have abdominal tenderness, periumbilical darkening or erythema (redness), or a fixed loop of bowel that can be felt.

How is NEC diagnosed?

Abdominal x-rays are done frequently if NEC is suspected. These films will show the neonatal team if there are any fixed or distended loops of bowel that may indicate an ileus (obstruction). Pneumatosis intestinalis (air in the bowel wall) can be seen early in NEC and can resolve over a number of hours. Pneumoperitoneum (air in the abdomen) is an indicator for immediate surgery. Air in the abdomen shows that the bowel has perforated (torn).

How is NEC managed?

Medical management consists of stopping feeds, nasogastric drainage to suction (tube in baby's stomach to "suck out" contents), seven to fourteen days of antibiotics, and I.V. nutrition. Close monitoring of fluid status, electrolytes, coagulation, and oxygen requirements are also necessary. 60–80 percent of babies with NEC are managed medically and symptoms resolve without surgery. Feedings postoperatively are started slowly.

What if surgery is needed?

Surgery is necessary if medical management fails or the bowel is perforated (torn). After opening the abdomen, the surgeon may find a swollen, purple bowel with areas of necrosed (dead) bowel. The usual areas involved are the terminal ileum, cecum, and right colon, but the whole bowel may be involved. The goal is to remove only that bowel that is fully necrosed (dead) and to leave any marginal areas in the hope that they will survive. This may require an ostomy or another operation within twenty-four to forty-eight hours to evaluate any surviving bowel. The nutritional outcome is roughly based on the remaining intestinal length, and the medical and surgical team will discuss this with you.

A Note to Parents

Having a baby with NEC is confusing and frightening. Feeding your child is a basic bonding parental experience and a child that can't be fed probably makes you feel helpless and frustrated. We know that soul searching is inevitable with questions like "What did we do wrong?" The frustration and anxiety are increased with the realization that there is nothing to do but "wait and watch." Your nurse and any other members of the team are here to help you. Ask questions. We are here to support you through this difficult time.

Chapter 27

Anorectal Disorders

Chapter Contents

Section 27.1

Proctitis

Reprinted from "Proctitis," National Institute of Diabetes and Digestive and Kidney Diseases, NIH Publication No. 05-4627, March 2005.

Proctitis is inflammation of the lining of the rectum, called the rectal mucosa. Proctitis can be short term (acute) or long term (chronic). Proctitis has many causes. It may be a side effect of medical treatments like radiation therapy or antibiotics. Sexually transmitted diseases like gonorrhea, herpes, and chlamydia may also cause proctitis. Inflammation of the rectal mucosa may be related to ulcerative colitis or Crohn disease, autoimmune conditions that cause inflammation in the colon or small intestine. Other causes include rectal injury, bacterial infection, allergies, and malfunction of the nerves in the rectum.

The most common symptom is a frequent or continuous sensation or urge to have a bowel movement. Other symptoms include constipation, a feeling of rectal fullness, left-sided abdominal pain, passage of mucus through the rectum, rectal bleeding, and anorectal pain.

Physicians diagnose proctitis by looking inside the rectum with a proctoscope or a sigmoidoscope. A biopsy (a tiny piece of tissue from the rectum) may be removed and tested for diseases or infections. A stool sample may also reveal infecting bacteria. If the physician suspects Crohn disease or ulcerative colitis, colonoscopy or barium enema x-rays may be used to examine areas of the intestine.

Treatment depends on the cause of proctitis. For example, the physician may prescribe antibiotics for proctitis caused by bacterial infection. If the inflammation is caused by Crohn disease or ulcerative colitis, the physician may recommend the drug 5-aminosalicylic acid (5ASA) or corticosteroids applied directly to the area in enema or suppository form, or taken orally in pill form. Enema and suppository applications are usually more effective, but some patients may require a combination of oral and rectal applications.

Section 27.2

Rectocele

When the rectum can be seen or felt bulging toward the outside through the back wall of the vagina, the condition is called a rectocele.

Rectoceles occur because weakness in the normal support system between the vagina and the rectum allows the rectum to bulge outward. The skin of the vagina can stretch very much, which is why these bulges can sometimes be seen or felt well beyond the opening of the vagina.

Common Symptoms

Since prolapse (including rectoceles) usually occurs slowly over time, the symptoms can be hard to recognize. Most women don't seek treatment until they actually feel (or see) something protruding outside of their vagina. The very first signs can be subtle—such as pain during intercourse or an inability to keep a tampon inside the vagina. As the prolapse gets worse, some women complain of a bulging or heavy sensation in the vagina that worsens by the end of the day or during bowel movements. Some women with severe prolapse even have to push stool out of the rectum by placing their fingers into the vagina during bowel movements.

Treatment

As with any prolapse problem, the two main treatment options are:

- use a pessary;
- have reconstructive surgery.

The specific type of surgery performed for a rectocele is called a "posterior repair." This surgery may be done alone or in combination with repairs of other forms of pelvic prolapse, urinary incontinence, or bowel incontinence.

Section 27.3

Rectal Prolapse

What Is a Prolapse?

A prolapse is a protrusion of some part of the bowel through and outside the anus. It may occur in childhood or in the elderly. There are three types of prolapse:

1. Incomplete (internal) prolapse, where the rectum is not yet protruding through the anus

2. Mucosal prolapse involving only the inner lining of the rectum

3. Complete (external) prolapse of the rectum

What Causes Prolapse?

The exact cause is not known. Possible explanations are excessive straining at defecation, a weak pelvic floor and anal sphincter muscles, or a lack of fixation of the lower bowel (rectum) to adjacent pelvic structures. Rectal prolapse is six times more common in women than in men, but is not related to childbirth. It is common in early childhood and usually resolves without surgery in this age group.

Symptoms

Protrusion of the bowel occurs during defecation which at first goes back by itself. Later it needs to be reduced by hand. There may be discomfort, bleeding, and the passage of mucus. Incontinence or poor control of the bowel is a very common complaint. This becomes more severe as the prolapse increases in size. A feeling of constipation or incomplete emptying of the rectum may be an associated symptom.

Diagnosis

Inspection by the doctor is often all that is required after asking the patient to strain. Sometimes it is necessary for the patient to sit on the toilet and strain to produce a prolapse. If a prolapse is suspected but the patient cannot induce it, a special x-ray called a proctogram may be required. If incontinence has been a problem there are tests of sphincter muscle function that can be performed.

Treatment

In children treatment of constipation is usually all that is necessary to correct the prolapse. In adults mucosal prolapse is treated either by rubber banding or by surgery. An incomplete prolapse of the rectum in adults may be treated with bulk laxatives in an attempt to reduce straining with defecation. If a complete prolapse of the rectum occurs then surgery is usually required. There are several operations available that may be performed either via the abdomen or via the anus. Abdominal operations involve securing the bowel to the lower spine (sacrum) and may include removal of a part of the bowel if constipation is a special feature. Laparoscopic (key hole) surgery is currently being evaluated to treat this condition. If the results prove to be as successful as those achieved by major surgery this may become the preferred operation for this condition.

Results

The choice of which procedure is best needs to be made on an individual basis. Success rates for surgery are very good but vary for each type of operation. Some alteration in bowel habit after operation may occur. This is variable, usually not severe, and improves with time.

Section 27.4

Pruritus Ani

What Causes Pruritus Ani?

Many patients have had an itchy anus sometime or other. The skin around the anus is sensitive and difficult to keep clean. Seepage of feces and moisture are the most common factors that cause this condition. Hair near the anus may aggravate the problem. The skin becomes irritated, causing itchiness, and the urge to scratch leads to skin damage, more irritation, and a persistent cycle develops.

Several common complaints such as allergies, diabetes, and inflammatory bowel disease may involve the skin around the anus causing pruritus. Hemorrhoids with associated mucous discharge may also be associated with this problem. In children, threadworms may be the cause.

Symptoms

Itch, a raw feeling, and occasional bleeding (caused by scratching) are the common symptoms. The urge to scratch is sometimes uncontrollable. Stress, a change of living circumstances, or a change in diet may make the condition worse. Diarrhea necessitating frequent cleaning of the anus will irritate pruritus.

Diagnosis

Don't be embarrassed about seeing a doctor. This condition is very common. Your doctor will want to examine your anus and an "internal" as well as an "external" examination will be necessary. Swabs or scrapings of the skin near the anus are sometimes taken for pathology examination. More complex bowel tests are usually not necessary.

Treatment

Surgery is not necessary. The important thing to do is to keep your anal skin clean and dry with good anal hygiene. A medication that reduces the itch and has sedative effects may be prescribed by the doctor. The condition has a tendency to recur.

The ten golden rules of treatment are:

1. After a bowel action use only the softest toilet tissue to clean the anus. It is better to use a dabbing technique rather than rubbing across the anus as most people do. You may prefer to use small moistened cotton wool pads rather than toilet paper.

2. To remove any small particles, the area can be kept thoroughly clean by washing with warm water (after each bowel action or before retiring at night).

3. Avoid rubbing with soap or applying antiseptics as this may increase irritation.

4. Ensure the skin around the anus is dry by gently dabbing with soft tissues, towel or cotton wool or using a hair dryer.

5. If an ointment is not being used, a drying powder or baby powder can be applied, but avoid perfumed talcum powder.

6. Do not use ointment unless prescribed by your doctor. Note that ointments containing cortisone should be used in small amounts and not for prolonged periods.

7. Choose sensible clothing (e.g., cotton underwear rather than nylon briefs and generally avoid tight fitting garments).

8. Keep your bowels regular with a high-fiber diet or fiber supplement.

9. Improvement follows diligence. If it recurs be patient and continue with the preceding measures.

10. If these measures do not solve the problem you may need to see a skin specialist after consultation with your family doctor.

Section 27.5

Anal Fissure

Several muscles encircle the anal canal and work together to control bowel movements. The inner muscle, just beneath the lining of the anal canal, is called the internal (involuntary) anal sphincter. This muscle is usually covered by skin. When a bowel movement occurs, the muscle relaxes to allow the stool to pass.

Tears that occur along the anal canal are called anal fissures. When a tear occurs, pain makes the muscle fibers contract, stopping the stool from passing. The fissure pulls apart when the muscle contracts (anal spasm). In turn, this affects the small blood vessels that carry nutrients and oxygen to the torn tissues. As a result, healing is slowed.

Symptoms

The pain and discomfort of an anal fissure usually gets worse when a person has a bowel movement. The pain tends to linger a long time afterward. There may be bleeding from the tear as well. Constipation may also occur as the condition gets worse.

Causes and Risk Factors

A fissure can occur from:

- Passing a hard stool or prolonged episode of diarrhea;
- Lack of fiber in the diet or water with that fiber;
- Food that creates a rough passage through the digestive system, such as popcorn, nuts, or tortilla chips.

Diagnosis

Diagnosis of this condition is usually done on the basis of the symptoms and a physical examination.

Treatment

Most fissures can heal by following good elimination habits:

- Take plenty of water and fiber
- Avoid foods such as popcorn, nuts, or tortilla chips
- Avoid constipating foods

Additionally, the following measures can help:

- Warm baths (sitz baths)
- Use a topical anesthetic cream
- Avoid using hemorrhoid suppositories. These hard, bullet-like medications are painful to insert and sometimes tear the fissure even more.

If pain persists, consult a colorectal surgeon. The surgeon will numb the anus and gently try to dilate it with an instrument called an anoscope. This allows the surgeon to see the fissure and any hemorrhoids around it. The surgeon will treat the internal hemorrhoids to shrink them so the anal canal is larger and doesn't stretch during bowel movements. In addition, the surgeon may prescribe medications (such as topical nitroglycerin ointment or diltiazem) that relax the anal spasm, improve blood supply to the anus, and promote healing.

If common treatments fail, a simple outpatient surgery usually cures the problem. In this surgery, a colorectal surgeon relaxes the internal sphincter and resurfaces the fissure.

Section 27.6

Anal Abscess (Fistula)

Reprinted with permission from the Cleveland Clinic Department of
Colorectal Surgery. © 2005 The Cleveland Clinic.

An abscess results from an acute infection of a small gland just inside the anus, when bacteria or foreign matter enters the tissue through the gland. Certain conditions—colitis or other inflammation of the intestine, for example—can sometimes make these infections more likely.

After an abscess has been drained, a tunnel may persist connecting the anal gland from which the abscess arose to the skin. If this occurs, persistent drainage from the outside opening may indicate the persistence of this tunnel. If the outside opening of the tunnel heals, recurrent abscesses may develop.

Symptoms

Symptoms of both ailments include constant pain, sometimes accompanied by swelling, that is not necessarily related to bowel movements. Other symptoms include irritation of skin around the anus, drainage of pus (which often relieves the pain), fever, and feeling poorly in general.

A fistula develops in about 50 percent of all abscess cases and there is really no way to predict if this will occur.

Treatment

An abscess is treated by draining the pus from the infected cavity, making an opening in the skin near the anus to relieve the pressure. Often, this can be done in the doctor's office using a local anesthetic. A large or deep abscess may require hospitalization and use of a different anesthetic method. Hospitalization may also be necessary for patients prone to more serious infections, such as diabetics or people with decreased immunity. Antibiotics are not usually an alternative to draining the pus because antibiotics are carried by the bloodstream and do not penetrate the fluid within an abscess.

Surgery is necessary to cure an anal fistula. Although fistula surgery is usually relatively straightforward, the potential for complication still exists and the procedure should be performed by a specialist in colon and rectal surgery. It may be performed at the same time as the abscess surgery, although fistulae often develop four to six weeks after an abscess is drained, sometimes even months or years later. Fistula surgery usually involves cutting a small portion of the anal sphincter muscle to open the tunnel, joining the external and internal openings, and converting the tunnel into a groove that will then heal from within. Most of the time, fistula surgery can be performed on an outpatient basis—or with a short hospital stay.

Recovery

Discomfort after fistula surgery can be mild to moderate for the first week and can be controlled with pain pills. The amount of time lost from work or school is usually minimal.

Treatment of an abscess or fistula is followed by a period of time at home, when soaking the affected area in warm water (sitz bath) is recommended three or four times a day. Stool softeners may also be recommended. It may be necessary to wear a gauze pad or mini-pad to prevent the drainage from soiling clothes. Bowel movements will not affect healing.

Prognosis

If properly healed, the problem will usually not return. However, it is important to follow the directions of a colon and rectal surgeon to prevent recurrence.

Chapter 28

Hemorrhoids

What are hemorrhoids?

The term *hemorrhoids* refers to a condition in which the veins around the anus or lower rectum are swollen and inflamed.

Hemorrhoids may result from straining to move stool. Other contributing factors include pregnancy, aging, chronic constipation or diarrhea, and anal intercourse.

Hemorrhoids are either inside the anus (internal) or under the skin around the anus (external).

What are the symptoms of hemorrhoids?

Many anorectal problems, including fissures, fistulae, abscesses, or irritation and itching (pruritus ani), have similar symptoms and are incorrectly referred to as hemorrhoids.

Hemorrhoids usually are not dangerous or life threatening. In most cases, hemorrhoidal symptoms will go away within a few days.

Although many people have hemorrhoids, not all experience symptoms. The most common symptom of internal hemorrhoids is bright red blood covering the stool, on toilet paper, or in the toilet bowl. However, an internal hemorrhoid may protrude through the anus outside the body, becoming irritated and painful. This is known as a protruding hemorrhoid.

Reprinted from "Hemorrhoids," National Institute of Diabetes and Digestive and Kidney Diseases, NIH Publication No. 05-3021, November 2004.

Symptoms of external hemorrhoids may include painful swelling or a hard lump around the anus that results when a blood clot forms. This condition is known as a thrombosed external hemorrhoid.

In addition, excessive straining, rubbing, or cleaning around the anus may cause irritation with bleeding or itching, which may produce a vicious cycle of symptoms. Draining mucus may also cause itching.

How common are hemorrhoids?

Hemorrhoids are very common in both men and women. About half of the population has hemorrhoids by age fifty. Hemorrhoids are also common among pregnant women. The pressure of the fetus in the abdomen, as well as hormonal changes, cause the hemorrhoidal vessels to enlarge. These vessels are also placed under severe pressure during childbirth. For most women, however, hemorrhoids caused by pregnancy are a temporary problem.

How are hemorrhoids diagnosed?

A thorough evaluation and proper diagnosis by the doctor is important any time bleeding from the rectum or blood in the stool occurs. Bleeding may also be a symptom of other digestive diseases, including colorectal cancer.

The doctor will examine the anus and rectum to look for swollen blood vessels that indicate hemorrhoids and will also perform a digital rectal exam with a gloved, lubricated finger to feel for abnormalities.

Closer evaluation of the rectum for hemorrhoids requires an exam with an anoscope, a hollow, lighted tube useful for viewing internal hemorrhoids, or a proctoscope, useful for more completely examining the entire rectum.

To rule out other causes of gastrointestinal bleeding, the doctor may examine the rectum and lower colon (sigmoid) with sigmoidoscopy or the entire colon with colonoscopy. Sigmoidoscopy and colonoscopy are diagnostic procedures that also involve the use of lighted, flexible tubes inserted through the rectum.

What is the treatment?

Medical treatment of hemorrhoids is aimed initially at relieving symptoms. Measures to reduce symptoms include the following:

- tub baths several times a day in plain, warm water for about ten minutes

- application of a hemorrhoidal cream or suppository to the affected area for a limited time

Preventing the recurrence of hemorrhoids will require relieving the pressure and straining of constipation. Doctors will often recommend increasing fiber and fluids in the diet. Eating the right amount of fiber and drinking six to eight glasses of fluid (not alcohol) result in softer, bulkier stools. A softer stool makes emptying the bowels easier and lessens the pressure on hemorrhoids caused by straining. Eliminating straining also helps prevent the hemorrhoids from protruding.

Good sources of fiber are fruits, vegetables, and whole grains. In addition, doctors may suggest a bulk stool softener or a fiber supplement such as psyllium (Metamucil) or methylcellulose (Citrucel).

In some cases, hemorrhoids must be treated endoscopically or surgically. These methods are used to shrink and destroy the hemorrhoidal tissue. The doctor will perform the procedure during an office or hospital visit.

A number of methods may be used to remove or reduce the size of internal hemorrhoids. These techniques include:

- **Rubber band ligation.** A rubber band is placed around the base of the hemorrhoid inside the rectum. The band cuts off circulation, and the hemorrhoid withers away within a few days.

- **Sclerotherapy.** A chemical solution is injected around the blood vessel to shrink the hemorrhoid.

- **Infrared coagulation.** A special device is used to burn hemorrhoidal tissue.

- **Hemorrhoidectomy.** Occasionally, extensive or severe internal or external hemorrhoids may require removal by surgery known as hemorrhoidectomy.

How are hemorrhoids prevented?

The best way to prevent hemorrhoids is to keep stools soft so they pass easily, thus decreasing pressure and straining, and to empty bowels as soon as possible after the urge occurs. Exercise, including walking, and increased fiber in the diet help reduce constipation and straining by producing stools that are softer and easier to pass.

Chapter 29

Other Disorders of the Lower Gastrointestinal Tract

Chapter Contents

Section 29.1

Intestinal Adhesions

Reprinted from "Intestinal Adhesions,"
National Institute of Diabetes and Digestive and Kidney Diseases,
NIH Publication No. 04-5037, February 2004.

Intestinal adhesions are bands of fibrous tissue that can connect the loops of the intestines to each other, or the intestines to other abdominal organs, or the intestines to the abdominal wall. These bands can pull sections of the intestines out of place and may block passage of food. Adhesions are a major cause of intestinal obstruction.

Adhesions may be present at birth (congenital) or may form after abdominal surgery or inflammation. Most form after surgery. They are more common after procedures on the colon, appendix, or uterus than after surgery on the stomach, gall bladder, or pancreas. The risk of developing adhesions increases with the passage of time after the surgery.

Symptoms

Some adhesions will cause no symptoms. If the adhesions cause partial or complete obstruction of the intestines, the symptoms one would feel would depend on the degree and the location of the obstruction. They include crampy abdominal pain, vomiting, bloating, an inability to pass gas, and constipation.

Diagnosis

X-rays (computed tomography) or barium contrast studies may be used to locate the obstruction. Exploratory surgery can also locate the adhesions and the source of pain.

Treatment

Some adhesions will cause no symptoms and go away by themselves. For people whose intestines are only partially blocked, a diet low in fiber, called a low-residue diet, allows food to move more easily through the affected area. In some cases, surgery may be necessary to remove the adhesions, reposition the intestine, and relieve symptoms, but the risk of developing more adhesions increases with each additional surgery.

Prevention

Methods to prevent adhesions include using biodegradable membranes or gels to separate organs at the end of surgery or performing laparoscopic (keyhole) surgery, which reduces the size of the incision and the handling of the organs.

Section 29.2

Intestinal Pseudo-Obstruction

Reprinted from "Intestinal Pseudo-Obstruction,"
National Institute of Diabetes and Digestive and Kidney Diseases,
NIH Publication No. 03-4550, March 2003.

Intestinal pseudo-obstruction (false blockage) is a condition that causes symptoms like those of a bowel obstruction (blockage). Yet when the intestines are examined, no obstruction is found. A problem in how the muscles and nerves in the intestines work causes the symptoms.

Pseudo-obstruction symptoms include cramps, stomach pain, nausea, vomiting, bloating, fewer bowel movements than usual, and loose stools. Over time, pseudo-obstruction can cause bacterial infections, malnutrition, and muscle problems in other parts of the body. Some people also have bladder problems.

Diseases that affect muscles and nerves, such as lupus erythematosus, scleroderma, or Parkinson disease, can cause symptoms. When a disease causes the symptoms, the condition is called secondary intestinal pseudo-obstruction. Medications that affect muscles and nerves, such as opiates and antidepressants, might also cause secondary pseudo-obstruction.

To diagnose the condition, the doctor will take a complete medical history, do a physical exam, and take x-rays. The usual treatments are nutritional support (intravenous feeding) to prevent malnutrition and antibiotics to treat bacterial infections. Medication might also be given to treat intestinal muscle problems. In severe cases, surgery to remove part of the intestine might be necessary.

Section 29.3

Inguinal Hernia

Reprinted from "Inguinal Hernia,"
National Institute of Diabetes and Digestive and Kidney Diseases,
NIH Publication No. 02-4634, January 2002.

A hernia is a condition in which part of the intestine bulges through a weak area in muscles in the abdomen. An inguinal hernia occurs in the groin (the area between the abdomen and thigh). It is called "inguinal" because the intestines push through a weak spot in the inguinal canal, which is a triangle-shaped opening between layers of abdominal muscle near the groin. Obesity, pregnancy, heavy lifting, and straining to pass stool can cause the intestine to push against the inguinal canal.

Symptoms of inguinal hernia may include a lump in the groin near the thigh; pain in the groin; and, in severe cases, partial or complete blockage of the intestine. The doctor diagnoses hernia by doing a physical exam and by taking x-rays and blood tests to check for blockage in the intestine.

The main treatment for inguinal hernia is surgery to repair the opening in the muscle wall. This surgery is called herniorrhaphy. Sometimes the weak area is reinforced with steel mesh or wire. This operation is called hernioplasty. If the protruding intestine becomes twisted or traps stool, part of the intestine might need to be removed. This surgery is called bowel resection. (Bowel is another word for intestine.)

Section 29.4

Short Bowel Syndrome

Reprinted from "Short Bowel Syndrome,"
National Institute of Diabetes and Digestive and Kidney Diseases,
NIH Publication No. 02-4631, January 2002.

Short bowel syndrome is a group of problems affecting people who have had half or more of their small intestine removed. The most common reason for removing part of the small intestine is to treat Crohn disease.

Diarrhea is the main symptom of short bowel syndrome. Other symptoms include cramping, bloating, and heartburn. Many people with short bowel syndrome are malnourished because their remaining small intestine is unable to absorb enough water, vitamins, and other nutrients from food. They may also become dehydrated, which can be life threatening. Problems associated with dehydration and malnutrition include weakness, fatigue, depression, weight loss, bacterial infections, and food sensitivities.

Short bowel syndrome is treated through changes in diet, intravenous feeding, vitamin and mineral supplements, and medicine to relieve symptoms.

Part Five

Disorders of the Digestive System's Solid Organs: The Liver and Pancreas

Chapter 30

Pancreatitis

Pancreatitis is an inflammation of the pancreas. The pancreas is a large gland behind the stomach and close to the duodenum. The duodenum is the upper part of the small intestine. The pancreas secretes digestive enzymes into the small intestine through a tube called the pancreatic duct. These enzymes help digest fats, proteins, and carbohydrates in food. The pancreas also releases the hormones insulin and glucagon into the bloodstream. These hormones help the body use the glucose it takes from food for energy.

Normally, digestive enzymes do not become active until they reach the small intestine, where they begin digesting food, but if these enzymes

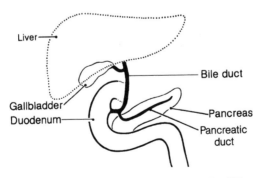

Figure 30.1. *The Pancreas and the Gastrointestinal Tract.*

Reprinted from "Pancreatitis," National Institute of Diabetes and Digestive and Kidney Diseases, NIH Publication No. 04-1596, February 2004.

become active inside the pancreas, they start "digesting" the pancreas itself.

Acute pancreatitis occurs suddenly, lasts for a short period of time, and usually resolves. Chronic pancreatitis does not resolve itself and results in a slow destruction of the pancreas. Either form can cause serious complications. In severe cases, bleeding, tissue damage, and infection may occur. Pseudocysts, accumulations of fluid and tissue debris, may also develop. Enzymes and toxins may enter the bloodstream, injuring the heart, lungs, and kidneys, or other organs.

Acute Pancreatitis

Some people have more than one attack and recover completely after each, but acute pancreatitis can be a severe, life-threatening illness with many complications. About eighty thousand cases occur in the United States each year; some 20 percent of them are severe. Acute pancreatitis occurs more often in men than women.

Acute pancreatitis is usually caused by gallstones or by drinking too much alcohol, but these aren't the only causes. If alcohol use and gallstones are ruled out, other possible causes of pancreatitis should be carefully examined so that appropriate treatment—if available—can begin.

Symptoms

Acute pancreatitis usually begins with pain in the upper abdomen that may last for a few days. The pain may be severe and may become constant—just in the abdomen—or it may reach to the back and other areas. It may be sudden and intense or begin as a mild pain that gets worse when food is eaten. Someone with acute pancreatitis often looks and feels very sick. Other symptoms may include the following:

- swollen and tender abdomen
- nausea
- vomiting
- fever
- rapid pulse

Severe cases may cause dehydration and low blood pressure. The heart, lungs, or kidneys may fail. If bleeding occurs in the pancreas, shock and sometimes even death follow.

Diagnosis

Besides asking about a person's medical history and doing a physical exam, a doctor will order a blood test to diagnose acute pancreatitis. During acute attacks, the blood contains at least three times more amylase and lipase than usual. Amylase and lipase are digestive enzymes formed in the pancreas. Changes may also occur in blood levels of glucose, calcium, magnesium, sodium, potassium, and bicarbonate. After the pancreas improves, these levels usually return to normal.

A doctor may also order an abdominal ultrasound to look for gallstones and a CAT (computerized axial tomography) scan to look for inflammation or destruction of the pancreas. CAT scans are also useful in locating pseudocysts.

Treatment

Treatment depends on the severity of the attack. If no kidney or lung complications occur, acute pancreatitis usually improves on its own. Treatment, in general, is designed to support vital bodily functions and prevent complications. A hospital stay will be necessary so that fluids can be replaced intravenously.

If pancreatic pseudocysts occur and are considered large enough to interfere with the pancreas's healing, your doctor may drain or surgically remove them.

Unless the pancreatic duct or bile duct is blocked by gallstones, an acute attack usually lasts only a few days. In severe cases, a person may require intravenous feeding for three to six weeks while the pancreas slowly heals. This process is called total parenteral nutrition. However, for mild cases of the disease, total parenteral nutrition offers no benefit.

Before leaving the hospital, a person will be advised not to drink alcohol and not to eat large meals. After all signs of acute pancreatitis are gone, the doctor will try to decide what caused it in order to prevent future attacks. In some people, the cause of the attack is clear, but in others, more tests are needed.

Complications

Acute pancreatitis can cause breathing problems. Many people develop hypoxia, which means that cells and tissues are not receiving enough oxygen. Doctors treat hypoxia by giving oxygen through a face mask. Despite receiving oxygen, some people still experience lung failure and require a ventilator.

Sometimes a person cannot stop vomiting and needs to have a tube placed in the stomach to remove fluid and air. In mild cases, a person may not eat for three or four days and instead may receive fluids and pain relievers through an intravenous line.

If an infection develops, the doctor may prescribe antibiotics. Surgery may be needed for extensive infections. Surgery may also be necessary to find the source of bleeding, to rule out problems that resemble pancreatitis, or to remove severely damaged pancreatic tissue.

Acute pancreatitis can sometimes cause kidney failure. If your kidneys fail, you will need dialysis to help your kidneys remove wastes from your blood.

Gallstones and Pancreatitis

Gallstones can cause pancreatitis and they usually require surgical removal. Ultrasound or a CAT scan can detect gallstones and can sometimes give an idea of the severity of the pancreatitis. When gallstone surgery can be scheduled depends on how severe the pancreatitis is. If the pancreatitis is mild, gallstone surgery may proceed within about a week. More severe cases may mean gallstone surgery is delayed for a month or more.

After the gallstones are removed and inflammation goes away, the pancreas usually returns to normal.

Chronic Pancreatitis

If injury to the pancreas continues, chronic pancreatitis may develop. Chronic pancreatitis occurs when digestive enzymes attack and destroy the pancreas and nearby tissues, causing scarring and pain. The usual cause of chronic pancreatitis is many years of alcohol abuse, but the chronic form may also be triggered by only one acute attack, especially if the pancreatic ducts are damaged. The damaged ducts cause the pancreas to become inflamed, tissue to be destroyed, and scar tissue to develop.

While common, alcoholism is not the only cause of chronic pancreatitis. The main causes of chronic pancreatitis are the following:

- alcoholism
- blocked or narrowed pancreatic duct because of trauma or pseudocysts have formed
- heredity
- unknown cause (idiopathic)

Damage from alcohol abuse may not appear for many years, and then a person may have a sudden attack of pancreatitis. In up to 70 percent of adult patients, chronic pancreatitis appears to be caused by alcoholism. This form is more common in men than in women and often develops between the ages of thirty and forty.

Hereditary pancreatitis usually begins in childhood but may not be diagnosed for several years. A person with hereditary pancreatitis usually has the typical symptoms that come and go over time. Episodes last from two days to two weeks. A determining factor in the diagnosis of hereditary pancreatitis is two or more family members with pancreatitis in more than one generation. Treatment for individual attacks is usually the same as it is for acute pancreatitis. Any pain or nutrition problems are treated just as they are for acute pancreatitis. Surgery can often ease pain and help manage complications.

There are other causes of chronic pancreatitis:

- congenital conditions such as pancreas divisum
- cystic fibrosis
- high levels of calcium in the blood (hypercalcemia)
- high levels of blood fats (hyperlipidemia or hypertriglyceridemia)
- some drugs
- certain autoimmune conditions

Symptoms

Most people with chronic pancreatitis have abdominal pain, although some people have no pain at all. The pain may get worse when eating or drinking, spread to the back, or become constant and disabling. In certain cases, abdominal pain goes away as the condition advances, probably because the pancreas is no longer making digestive enzymes. Other symptoms include nausea, vomiting, weight loss, and fatty stools.

People with chronic disease often lose weight, even when their appetite and eating habits are normal. The weight loss occurs because the body does not secrete enough pancreatic enzymes to break down food, so nutrients are not absorbed normally. Poor digestion leads to excretion of fat, protein, and sugar into the stool. If the insulin-producing cells of the pancreas (islet cells) have been damaged, diabetes may also develop at this stage.

Diagnosis

Diagnosis may be difficult, but new techniques can help. Pancreatic function tests help a doctor decide whether the pancreas is still making enough digestive enzymes. Using ultrasonic imaging, endoscopic retrograde cholangiopancreatography (ERCP), and CAT scans, a doctor can see problems indicating chronic pancreatitis. Such problems include calcification of the pancreas, in which tissue hardens from deposits of insoluble calcium salts. In more advanced stages of the disease, when diabetes and malabsorption occur, a doctor can use a number of blood, urine, and stool tests to help diagnose chronic pancreatitis and to monitor its progression.

Treatment

Relieving pain is the first step in treating chronic pancreatitis. The next step is to plan a diet that is high in carbohydrates and low in fat.

A doctor may prescribe pancreatic enzymes to take with meals if the pancreas does not secrete enough of its own. The enzymes should be taken with every meal to help the body digest food and regain some weight. Sometimes insulin or other drugs are needed to control blood glucose.

In some cases, surgery is needed to relieve pain. The surgery may involve draining an enlarged pancreatic duct or removing part of the pancreas.

For fewer and milder attacks, people with pancreatitis must stop drinking alcohol, stick to their prescribed diet, and take the proper medications.

Pancreatitis in Children

Chronic pancreatitis is rare in children. Trauma to the pancreas and hereditary pancreatitis are two known causes of childhood pancreatitis. Children with cystic fibrosis, a progressive, disabling, and incurable lung disease, may also have pancreatitis. But more often the cause is not known.

Points to Remember

- Pancreatitis begins when the digestive enzymes become active inside the pancreas and start "digesting" it.

- Pancreatitis has two forms: acute and chronic

344

- Common causes of pancreatitis are gallstones or alcohol abuse.

- Sometimes no cause for pancreatitis can be found.

- Symptoms of acute pancreatitis include pain in the abdomen, nausea, vomiting, fever, and a rapid pulse.

- Treatment for acute pancreatitis can include intravenous fluids, oxygen, antibiotics, or surgery.

- Acute pancreatitis becomes chronic when pancreatic tissue is destroyed and scarring develops.

- Treatment for chronic pancreatitis includes easing the pain; eating a high-carbohydrate, low-fat diet; and taking enzyme supplements. Surgery is sometimes needed as well.

Chapter 31

Hepatitis

Introduction

Hepatitis is a disorder in which viruses or other mechanisms produce inflammation in liver cells, resulting in their injury or destruction.

The esophagus, stomach, and large and small intestine, aided by the liver, gallbladder, and pancreas, convert the nutritive components of food into energy and break down the non-nutritive components into waste to be excreted.

Damage to the liver can impair these and many other processes. Hepatitis varies in severity from a self-limited condition with total recovery to a life-threatening or lifelong disease. It can occur from many different causes:

- In the most common hepatitis cases, specific viruses incite the immune system to fight off infections (called viral hepatitis). Specific immune factors become overproduced that cause injury.

- Hepatitis can also result from an autoimmune condition, in which abnormal immune factors attack the body's own liver cells.

- Inflammation of the liver can also occur from medical problems, drugs, alcoholism, chemicals, and environmental toxins.

No matter what the cause of hepatitis, it can take either an acute (short term) or chronic form (persistent). In some cases, acute hepatitis develops into a chronic condition, but chronic hepatitis can also occur on its own. Although chronic hepatitis is generally the more serious condition, patients having either condition can experience varying degrees of severity.

Acute Hepatitis

Acute hepatitis can begin suddenly or gradually, but it has a limited course and rarely lasts beyond one or two months. Usually there is only spotty liver cell damage and evidence of immune system activity, but on rare occasions, acute hepatitis can cause severe, even life-threatening, liver damage.

Chronic Hepatitis

The chronic forms of hepatitis persist for prolonged periods. Experts usually categorize chronic hepatitis by indications of severity as one of the following:

- *Chronic persistent hepatitis:* Chronic persistent hepatitis is usually mild and nonprogressive or slowly progressive, causing limited damage to the liver.

- *Chronic active hepatitis:* Chronic active hepatitis involves extensive liver damage and cell injury beyond the portal tract.

Viral Hepatitis

Most cases of hepatitis are caused by viruses that infect liver cells and begin replicating. They are defined by the letters A through G:

- Hepatitis A, B, and C are the most common viral forms of hepatitis. Investigators are still looking for additional viruses that may be implicated in hepatitis unexplained by the current known viruses.

- Other hepatitis viruses include hepatitis E and hepatitis G. Like hepatitis A, hepatitis E is caused by contact with contaminated food or water. It is not serious except in pregnant women, when it can be life threatening. Hepatitis G is always chronic with probably the same modes of transmission as hepatitis C, but to date it does not appear to have serious effects.

Autoimmune Chronic Hepatitis

Autoimmune chronic hepatitis accounts for about 20 percent of all chronic hepatitis cases. Like other autoimmune disorders, this condition develops because a genetically defective immune system attacks the body's own cells and organs (in this case the liver) after being triggered by an environmental agent, probably a virus. Suspects include the measles virus, a hepatitis virus, or the Epstein-Barr virus, which causes mononucleosis. It is also possible that a reaction to a drug or other toxin that affects the liver also triggers an autoimmune response in susceptible individuals. In about 30 percent of cases, autoimmune hepatitis is associated with other disorders that involve autoimmune attacks on other parts of the body.

Hepatitis Caused by Alcohol and Drugs

Alcohol. About 10 to 35 percent of heavy drinkers develop alcoholic hepatitis. In the body, alcohol breaks down into various chemicals, some of which are very toxic in the liver. After years of drinking, liver damage can be very severe, leading to cirrhosis in about 10 to 20 percent of cases. Although heavy drinking itself is the major risk factor for alcoholic hepatitis, genetic factors may play a role in increasing a person's risk for alcoholic hepatitis. Women who abuse alcohol are at higher risk for alcoholic hepatitis and cirrhosis than are men who drink heavily. High-fat diets may also increase the risk in heavy drinkers.

Drugs. Because the liver plays such a major role in metabolizing drugs, hundreds of medications can cause reactions that are similar to those of acute viral hepatitis. Symptoms can appear anywhere from two weeks to six months after starting drug treatment. In most cases, they disappear when the drug is withdrawn, but, in rare circumstances, they may progress to serious liver disease. Notably, very high doses of acetaminophen (Tylenol) have been known to cause severe liver damage and even death, particularly when used with alcohol.

Nonalcoholic Fatty Liver Disease (NAFLD)

Nonalcoholic fatty liver disease (NAFLD) affects between 10 and 24 percent of the population and covers a number of conditions, notably nonalcoholic steatohepatitis (NASH). NAFLD has features similar to alcohol-induced hepatitis, particularly a fatty liver, but it occurs in individuals who do not consume significant amounts of alcohol. Severe obesity and diabetes are the major risk factors and may pose a risk for more severe conditions. NAFLD may also occur in conjunction with small intestine surgery or other factors.

NAFLD is usually benign and very slowly progressive. In certain patients, however, it can lead to cirrhosis, liver failure, or liver cancer.

Weight reduction and management of any accompanying medical condition are the primary approaches to nonalcoholic fatty liver disease. To date, however, there is no effective treatment for NAFLD. Drugs, such as fibrates, used to lower triglycerides or those that increase insulin levels, such as metformin, may help protect against liver damage. Other drugs showing some promise include ursodiol and betaine. Vitamin E may help reduce liver injury.

Diagnosis

In people suspected of having or carrying viral hepatitis, physicians will measure certain substances in the blood.

- *Bilirubin:* Bilirubin is one of the most important factors indicative of hepatitis. It is a red-yellow pigment that is normally metabolized in the liver and then excreted in the urine. In patients with hepatitis, the liver cannot process bilirubin, and blood levels of this substance rise. (High levels of bilirubin cause the yellowish skin tone known as jaundice.)

- *Liver Enzymes (Aminotransferases):* Enzymes known as aminotransferases, including aspartate (AST) and alanine (ALT), are released when the liver is damaged. Measurements of these enzymes, particularly ALT, are the least expensive and least invasive tests for determining severity of the underlying liver disease and monitoring treatment effectiveness. Enzyme levels vary, however, and are not always an accurate indicator of disease activity.

General Tests to Determine Causes of Viral Hepatitis

Radioimmunoassays

To identify the particular virus causing hepatitis, blood tests called radioimmunoassays are performed. Typically, radioimmunoassays identify particular antibodies, which are molecules in the immune system that attack specific antigens.

Polymerase Chain Reaction

In some cases of hepatitis C, a polymerase chain reaction (PCR) may be performed. PCR is able to make multiple copies of the virus's genetic material to the point where it is detectable.

Liver Biopsies

A liver biopsy may be performed for acute viral hepatitis caught in a late stage or for severe cases of chronic hepatitis. No laboratory tests for enzyme or viral levels can truly determine the actual damage to the liver. A biopsy helps determine treatment possibilities, the extent of damage, and the long-term outlook.

Screening for Liver Cancer

Patients with cirrhosis are usually screened for liver cancer using tests for a substance called alpha-fetoprotein (AFP) and ultrasound. It is not known, however, if such screening has much impact on survival, since it is not very sensitive and has a high rate of false positives (suggesting the presence of cancer when it is not actually present). Screening is not necessary in patients without cirrhosis.

Hepatitis B and D

Hepatitis B and D were formerly called serum hepatitis. Hepatitis B is mainly transmitted through blood transfusions, contaminated needles, and sexual contact. Blood screening has reduced the risk from transfusions. It can also be passed from cuts, scrapes, and other breaks in the skin. Hepatitis D virus can replicate only by attaching to hepatitis B and therefore cannot exist without the B virus being present.

Risk Factors for Hepatitis B

About 1.2 million Americans are chronically infected with HBV and between 20 percent and 30 percent acquired the infection when they were children. Men are at higher risk than women. Fortunately, in the United States the number of new infections has declined dramatically—by 67 percent between 1990 and 2002. In 2002, 8,064 cases were reported compared to over 20,000 in 1990.

The following are some people at risk:

- Drug users who share needles

- Children of infected mothers

- People with multiple sex partners or other high-risk sexual behavior

- Hospital workers and others exposed to blood products

- Staff members of institutions for mentally impaired people

- Prisoners

- Emigrants from areas where the disease rate is high. (International travelers who spend long periods in such areas may also be at risk.)

People at highest risk for becoming chronic carriers of the virus are the following:

- Children infected before they are five, including newborns, most of whom become carriers

- Infected people with damaged immune systems, such as AIDS patients

Risk Factors for Hepatitis D

Hepatitis D occurs only in people with hepatitis B. Those who recover from hepatitis B are immune to further infection from both hepatitis B and D viruses.

Lifestyle Precautions for Preventing Hepatitis B and C Virus Transmission

The following are some precautions for preventing the transmission of HBV or HCV:

- All objects contaminated by blood from patients with hepatitis B or C must be handled with special care. (Restrictions on food preparation are not necessary for these hepatitis viruses.)

- Patients with viral hepatitis should abstain from sexual activity or take strict precautions if they cannot. Infected patients should use condoms and contraceptives that prevent passage of the virus, possibly even in relationships that last for years. Women partners or infected women should abstain from sexual activity during menstruation. Either partner with infections that cause bleeding in the genital or urinary areas should avoid sexual activity until the infection is no longer active.

- Couples with an infected partner or people sharing a household with an infected person should avoid sharing personal items, such as razors or toothbrushes.

There is no evidence that the viruses can be passed through casual contact, or other contact without exposure to blood, including kissing, hugging, sneezing, or coughing or by sharing eating utensils or drinking glasses. People infected with chronic hepatitis B or C should not be excluded from work, school, play, and childcare or any social or work settings on the basis of their infection.

Symptoms of Hepatitis B

Symptoms appear long after the initial infection, usually four to twenty-four weeks later. Many patients may not even experience them or they may be mild and flu-like. About 10 percent to 20 percent of patients have a fever and rash. Nausea is not common. Sometimes there is general aching in the joints. The pain can resemble arthritis, affecting specific joints and accompanied by redness and swelling.

Outlook for Patients with Hepatitis B

Acute Form

Acute hepatitis B is generally mild, but it can be lethal in about 1 percent of patients. Patients who are co-infected with hepatitis D or C are at risk for serious complications. In patients whose immune systems are severely compromised, such as in AIDS, there is risk of a rapidly progressive form of HBV called fibrosing cholestatic hepatitis. Even patients with mild symptoms can remain chronically infected with the virus.

Chronic Form

About 70 percent of patients infected with hepatitis B will eventually eliminate the virus without any treatment. The rest will progress to chronic hepatitis. Hepatitis B can also become chronic without an acute stage.

The great majority of people with hepatitis B have a good long-term outlook, especially children infected with the virus.

Specific Tests for Identifying Hepatitis B

A diagnosis of hepatitis B relies on measuring the liver enzymes aspartate (AST) and alanine (ALT), which are released when the liver is damaged, assays to identify the viral DNA, and a liver biopsy.

Physicians then must determine if the condition is chronic but inactive or whether it is more aggressive. This is suggested by identifying a specific antigen called HBsAg, which is a protein that is found in the blood in early stages of hepatitis B and suggests the presence of viral replication. About 5 percent to 10 percent of people do not clear the infection but become carriers of the antigen (called HBsAg-positive). Evidence of its persistence for more than six months suggests that the condition is chronic.

To diagnose hepatitis D using an antibody test, hepatitis B must already have been identified.

Vaccinations for Prevention of Hepatitis B

Several inactivated virus vaccines, including Recombivax HB, GenHevac B, Hepagene, and Engerix-B, can prevent hepatitis B (HBV) and are safe even for infants and children. A triple-antigen hepatitis B vaccine (Hepacare) is proving to be effective for people who do not respond to the standard vaccines. Vaccination programs are also proving to reduce the risk for liver cancer. A combination vaccine (Twinrix) that contains Engerix-B and Havrix, a hepatitis A vaccine, is now approved for people with risk factors for both hepatitis A and B.

Candidates for HBV Vaccinations

Experts now recommend that all infants and children not previously vaccinated be immunized by the time they reach the seventh grade.

Hepatitis B vaccine protection lasts at least eight to ten years. Booster shots after that may be recommended depending on continuing risk, such as sexual exposure. In fact, a 2002 study suggested that there is risk for infection in teenagers who were vaccinated in infancy, although protection against chronic hepatitis B may be maintained.

The following adults are at very high risk and should be vaccinated:

- Healthcare and public safety workers who may be exposed to blood products.

- People in the same household as HBV-infected individuals. (Unvaccinated people who have had intimate exposure to people with HBV may be protected with immune globulin, which is sometimes administered with the vaccine.)

- Travelers to developing countries.

- Patients who require transfusions and have not been infected with HBV. (Those with blood clotting disorders should have the vaccination administered under the skin, not injected in the muscle.)

- Sexually active homosexual or heterosexual individuals with multiple partners or who engage in high-risk sexual behavior.

- People with any sexually transmitted diseases.

Other people at risk who would benefit from vaccinations are the following:

- Patients and workers in mental institutions and morticians.

- Patients on hemodialysis. (People on hemodialysis may need larger doses or boosters; they also may need to be re-vaccinated if blood tests indicate they are losing immunity.)

- People who use injected drugs.

- Pregnant women at risk for the virus should be vaccinated; there is no evidence that the vaccine is dangerous to the fetus.

- People receiving treatments or who have conditions that suppress the immune system may need the vaccination, although its benefits for this group are unclear except for those at high risk, such as people with HIV or spleen abnormalities.

The regimen in adults is typically three doses given over six months. One study reported that older adults would benefit from a fourth dose without incurring serious side effects. People with alcoholism may need high doses.

Treatments for Chronic Hepatitis B

Interferon alpha and nucleoside analogues are the important treatments at this time for hepatitis B. At this time, interferon alpha-2b is the standard agent but experts expect the nucleoside analogue lamivudine to replace it as the primary agent. Lamivudine is not only effective, it is less expensive than the interferon. Most likely, the best approach in the future will be combinations of these and other agents to achieve the greatest possible viral reduction and to minimize the chances of drug resistance.

Interferon Alpha for Hepatitis B

Interferon alpha-2b (Intron) is the standard drug for hepatitis B. It has eliminated the virus and sustained significant remission in 25 percent to 40 percent of patients with chronic hepatitis B. The drug is usually taken by injection every day for sixteen weeks. (It does not appear to be effective for hepatitis D.) Unfortunately, even in hepatitis B, the virus recurs in almost all cases, although this recurring mutation may be weaker than the original strain.

Lamivudine and Other Nucleoside Analogues

Nucleoside analogues are drugs that can block viral replication, and they are important in hepatitis B. The primary agent used in hepatitis is lamivudine (Zeffix). It can be taken orally, has few severe side effects, and is less expensive than interferon. Experts expect it to become the first-line treatment for hepatitis B. Famciclovir is an alternative. Newer nucleoside analogues, adefovir (Hepsera) and entecavir, may prove to be even more effective than the older agents.

Lamivudine has reduced viral count in over half of hepatitis B patients who have taken it as sole therapy for about a year. It also appears to significantly reduce the risk for liver damage and cirrhosis, and appears to be effective and safe in patients with decompensated cirrhosis. The drug even suppresses hepatitis B viral replication in HIV-positive patients and liver transplant recipients. It appears to be effective for children as well as adults. It is not yet clear if it protects against liver cancer, particularly in patients who have harbored the virus since childhood.

A major problem with lamivudine is the development of mutated viral strains that become resistant to the drug, particularly in areas where the virus is common. The specific genetic hepatitis B strain may be an important marker for predicting resistance. Combinations with interferons may be able to help control viral breakthroughs from mutated viruses and help sustain its effectiveness. Other nucleosides, such as adefovir and entecavir, are proving to be effective in patients who become resistant to lamivudine.

Lamivudine causes muscle aches and chills but does not appear to have some of the distressing side effects of interferon, such as depression, hair loss, weight loss, or a drop in white blood cells (leukopenia).

Of some concern, however, is eventual resistance to the drug in many patients.

Investigative Therapies

A number of drugs are being studied that boost the body's own immune system to fight the virus.

- *Thymosin Alpha 1 (Zadaxin)*, also called thymalfasin, is a synthetic version of a peptide derived from the thymus gland (which is responsible for maturation of immune factors call T-cells). It is injected and has few side effects. It appears to be safe for hepatitis B patients when used alone or in combination. Combinations with interferon and nucleoside analogues are showing promise.

- *Vaccines as Treatments:* Some hepatitis B vaccines, including Hepagene, are being investigated for treating and preventing hepatitis B.

Some important research is targeting agents that inhibit RNA—the genetic molecules that serve as messengers for regulating cellular processes.

Liver Transplantation

If the disease progresses to the point where it becomes life-threatening, liver transplantation may be an option.

Hepatitis C

Each year about thirty thousand new cases of hepatitis C occur. It is the most common blood-borne infection in the country. Until blood screening began in 1990, the primary mode of known transmission was through transfusions. It is also transmitted through contaminated needles and possibly through sexual transmission. The cause of transmission is unknown in 40 percent of cases.

About 4 million Americans have had an initial HCV infection and an estimated 2.7 million are currently chronically infected. Hepatitis C also affects 170 million people worldwide. Most people with chronic HCV, however, are unaware that they have it, and experts believe that over the next twenty years there will be a fourfold increase in diagnosed cases in the United States. It is currently not possible to predict which patients will develop the chronic form of hepatitis C.

Ethnic Groups

In general, HCV occurs most commonly in non-Caucasian men between the ages of thirty and forty-nine years. Over 6 percent of African Americans are infected with HCV, which is about two to three times the risk for Caucasians.

Other High-Risk Groups

Some other specific groups are at higher than normal risk:

* Intravenous drug users
* People who had transfusions before 1992
* Homeless people and prison inmates
* Infants of infected mothers
* Organ transplant recipients
* Hospital workers
* Children who survive cancer
* Body piercing or tattoos

Symptoms of Hepatitis C

Most patients with hepatitis C do not experience symptoms. In some patients, itchy skin is the first symptom. Overall, fatigue is the most common symptom.

Some evidence suggests, however, that patients with chronic hepatitis C often experience an impaired quality of life, mostly from fatigue. The severity of the fatigue is not necessarily related to the degree of liver injury. Some patients develop pain in small joints in the body (such as the hand) that may be nearly indistinguishable from symptoms of rheumatoid arthritis, fibromyalgia, or carpal tunnel syndrome. Other nonspecific symptoms include abdominal discomfort, loss of appetite, depression, and difficulty in concentration.

Outlook for Patients with Hepatitis C

Acute Form

Acute hepatitis C is rarely recognized, since there are no symptoms in up to 80 percent of these patients. An estimated 15 percent to 30 percent of acute cases clear up without becoming chronic. Early treatment with interferons can significantly reduce the risk for progression to chronic hepatitis.

Chronic Form

About 60 percent to 85 percent of infected people develop chronic hepatitis. This poses a risk for cirrhosis, liver cancer, or both.

Specific Tests for Identifying Hepatitis C and Determining Its Severity

Tests for Liver Enzymes

Blood tests showing elevated liver enzymes, particularly alanine aminotransferase (ALT), plus symptoms of hepatitis (e.g., jaundice, fatigue) are often the first signs of acute hepatitis. In chronic hepatitis, however, liver enzymes may be normal or fluctuate. They also can be elevated even after the virus has cleared.

Tests to Identify the Virus

The standard first test for diagnosing hepatitis C is known as enzyme-linked immunosorbent assay (ELISA or EIA). The antibody for hepatitis C is used to identify the virus but it may not show up for six weeks to a year after the onset of the disease, so its absence is not necessarily an indication of a healthy liver. A test called an immunoblot assay (called RIBA) may also be used to confirm the presence of the virus. An accurate home test (Hepatitis C Check) is now available. It supplies a lancet for obtaining a drop of blood, which is sent to the laboratory for EIA and possibly RIBA analysis. Results take about a week.

Tests to Identify Genetic Types and Viral Load

Additional tests called HCV RNA assays may be used to confirm the diagnosis. They use a polymerase chain reaction (PCR) to detect the RNA (the genetic material) of the virus. Such tests may be performed if there is some doubt about a diagnosis but the physician still firmly believes the virus is present.

HCV RNA assays also determine virus levels (called viral load). Such levels do not reflect the severity of the condition or speed of progression, as they do for other viruses, such as HIV. However, high viral loads suggest a poorer response to treatment with interferons.

Such techniques may also be used to determine the genotype of the virus, which can be helpful in determining a treatment approach. There are six main genetic types of HCV and more than ninety subtypes. They do not appear to affect the rate of progression of the disease itself, but they can differ significantly in their effects on response to treatment. Genotype 1 is the most difficult to treat and is the cause of up to three-quarters of the cases in the United States. The other common genetic types are types 2 (15 percent) and 3 (7 percent), which are more responsive to treatment.

Liver Biopsy

Only a biopsy can determine the extent of injury in the liver. Some experts are now recommending biopsies for all chronic hepatitis C patients, regardless of severity, because of the risk for liver damage even in patients without symptoms. If a biopsy does not show any scarring and liver enzymes are normal, patients can be assured that the outlook is very favorable.

Prevention of Hepatitis C

No vaccines are available, but immune globulin helps protect against developing hepatitis C after transfusions. Periodic doses of immune globulin in sexual partners of infected people also appear to confer protection. In infected people, measures for preventing transmission are similar to those for hepatitis B.

Treatments for Hepatitis C

Interferons Alone and in Combination with Ribavirin for Hepatitis C

The current gold standard for treating chronic hepatitis C is a once-weekly injection of the interferon called pegylated interferon in combination with oral ribavirin (a nucleoside analogue). Patients are typically treated for twenty-four to forty-eight weeks depending on certain factors, such as the genotype. Interferons are also used for patients with acute hepatitis C to prevent the development of the chronic form.

Interferons are natural proteins that activate certain immune functions in the body and have anti-viral properties. Ribavirin is poor at inducing initial responses alone but it can double sustained response rates when combined with an interferon.

A number of natural and synthetic interferons are available:

- Natural interferons were the first used for HCV and include interferon alpha-2a (Intron) and interferon alpha-2b (Roferon). Rebetron is the combination of interferon alpha-2b and ribavirin.

- Pegylated interferons (PegINF) are long-acting formulations of interferon. They include alfa-2b (Peg-Intron) or alfa-2a (Pegasys). Both are now available in combination with ribavirin. (Rebetol is the alfa-2b combination.) The combination is now considered the gold standard for treating HCV. Response rates of up to 51 percent with genotype 1 and over 80 percent with genotypes 2 and 3 have been reported. PegINFs may even help patients with cirrhosis. Whether the combination treatment protects against future liver cancer is still unclear. (A higher total dose, rather than a longer duration of treatment, may be the critical factor for protection.)

- Alfacon-1 (Infergen), also called consensus interferon, is a genetically modified interferon. A combination of alfacon-1 with ribavirin is proving to help some patients who were nonresponsive to ribavirin with interferon.

Side Effects of the Combination Treatment

Significant side effects of the combination treatment include flu-like symptoms, blood disorders (e.g., hemolytic anemia and low white blood cell counts), and psychologic and neurologic symptoms (particularly depression). Side effects from the combination result in treatment discontinuation in 10 percent to 14 percent of patients. The most frequent reason cited in the United States is depression. Of note, combination of both drugs poses a very high risk for birth defects in children whose mothers used the drugs while pregnant.

Determining Treatment Success

Physicians gauge treatment success and approaches based on the patient's response to the treatments:

- *Early Response.* These are patients who respond to the drug right away. This means that their viral count drops very rapidly within the first few weeks of treatment and is still undetectable at twelve weeks. (One difficulty in deciding when to stop treatment even in responders is the inability to predict at twelve weeks which of these patients will relapse and which ones will have sustained response.)

- *Sustained Response.* Patients who are free of the virus longer than six months are considered to be sustained responders. The overall sustained response rates with the current standard combination of pegylated interferon and ribavirin is over 50 percent, with certain factors predicting higher or lower response rates.

- *Relapse.* In relapse, the virus comes back and requires retreatment. This occurs most likely because of the development of mutant strains that may be resistant to the drugs used or because the original dose was too low.

- *Nonresponse.* Patients are considered to be nonresponders if the virus is still detectable twelve weeks after interferon alone or twenty-four weeks after combination therapy. Retreating these patients has achieved only a 15 percent response. Those who achieved a response called breakthrough at some point in the initial treatment may be more likely to respond. (During a breakthrough there is a temporary reduction in liver enzymes or disappearance of the virus.) Alfacon-1 (Infergen) may be beneficial for some nonresponding patients. Patients should also ask their physician about any clinical trials that might be appropriate.

Investigative Drugs for Hepatitis C

The current drugs used for HCV still do not meet the needs of all patients. They are expensive, have significant side effects, do not work in half the patients who take them, and are unsuitable in many others. Investigation then is ongoing to find better solutions. Some showing promise include the following:

- IMPDH inhibitors
- Amantadine (Symmetrel)
- Thymosin Alpha 1 (Zadaxin), also called thymalfasin
- Protease inhibitors

Other agents under investigation include vaccines, genetic therapies known as antisense oligonucleotides or monoclonal antibodies, and drugs that will help prevent or reduce progression of liver scarring or progression to liver cancer. Even if successful, none of these agents would be available for some years.

Of interest are studies using phlebotomy (which is simply drawing blood) to reduce iron levels. In one study, maintenance therapy with this procedure reduced liver inflammation and possibly slowed progression of cirrhosis.

Liver Transplantation for Hepatitis C

If the disease progresses to the point where it becomes life-threatening, liver transplantation may be an option. In fact, nearly 40 percent of liver transplant patients are infected with hepatitis C. In any case, liver transplantation is not a cure for hepatitis C. The virus nearly always returns. One study of patients with hepatitis C reported five-year risks for viral recurrence of 80 percent and for cirrhosis of 10 percent. Retreatment with antiviral agents at this point is being investigated.

Disease Recurrence

In both hepatitis B and C, the disease often persists or returns despite treatment. The virus continually generates many "mutant viruses" that differ just slightly from the parent virus. These mutated viruses may be resistant to interferons and so, over time, the drugs become ineffective.

Hepatitis A

About one-third of the U.S. population has antibodies to hepatitis A, indicating previous infection by the virus. The hepatitis A virus infects up to 200,000 Americans every year and causes symptoms in about 134,000 of them. Almost 30 percent are children under age fifteen.

Hepatitis A (formerly called infectious hepatitis) is excreted in feces and transmitted by contaminated food and water. Eating shellfish taken from sewage-contaminated water is a common means of contracting hepatitis A. Infected people can transmit it to others if they do not take strict sanitary precautions. Hepatitis A is infectious for two to four weeks before symptoms develop and for a few days afterward.

Among the people at risk for passing the infection along or being infected are the following:

- International travelers
- Day care employees and children
- Sexually active homosexual men
- Intravenous drug users
- Health care, food industry, and sewage workers

Symptoms of Acute Hepatitis

Symptoms of acute viral hepatitis may begin suddenly or develop gradually. They may be so mild that patients mistake the disease for the flu. They include the following:

- Fatigue and mild fever.

- Gastrointestinal problems, including nausea, vomiting, a general feeling of discomfort in the abdomen, or a sharper pain that may occur in the upper right area of the abdomen.

- Loss of appetite, weight loss, and dehydration.

- Dark urine and jaundice (a yellowish color in the skin and whites of the eyes) develops in some, but not all, patients.

- Light-colored stools, muscle pain, drowsiness, irritability, and itching, usually mild.

- Diarrhea and joint aches.

- The liver may be tender and enlarged and most people have mild anemia.

- In about 10 percent of patients, the spleen is enlarged.

Vaccinations for Hepatitis A

Two vaccines (Havrix, Vaqta) are now available and both are very safe and effective for preventing hepatitis A (HAV). They can be given along with immune globulin and other vaccines. A combination vaccine (Twinrix) that contains both Havrix and Engerix-B (a hepatitis B vaccine) is now approved for people with risk factors for both hepatitis A and B.

Candidates for HAV Vaccinations

Vaccinations for hepatitis A are recommended for the following individuals:

- People in specific populations where outbreaks occur.

- Sexually active homosexual men.

- Patients with any form of chronic hepatitis.

- Health care workers exposed to the virus.

- Travelers to developing countries. (Travelers should also receive immune globulin if they are visiting high-risk areas within four weeks of the vaccination.)

- Experts now recommend routine vaccinations for children and adolescents in high-risk states. These states are Arizona, Alaska, California, Idaho, Nevada, New Mexico, Oklahoma, Oregon, South Dakota, Utah, Washington, Missouri, Texas, Colorado, Arkansas, Montana, and Wyoming.

- People who have had intimate exposure to patients with hepatitis A may be protected with immune globulin or possibly with the vaccine itself.

- People with chronic liver disease, including those with hepatitis C, should also be vaccinated, particularly if they have not been exposed to hepatitis A, since the infection can cause liver failure in these patients.

Side Effects

Although there are few side effects, allergic responses from the vaccination can occur. Hair loss has been reported in a very few people after a second administration. There may be pain at the injection site. (Havrix causes more pain at the injection site than Vaqta.)

Symptoms of Hepatitis A

Symptoms are usually mild, especially in children, and generally appear between two and six weeks after exposure to the virus. Adult patients are more likely to have fever, jaundice, and itching that can last one to several months.

General Outlook for People Infected with Hepatitis A

This is the least serious of the common hepatitis viruses. It does not directly kill liver cells and there is no risk for a chronic form. Fulminant hepatitis is the only major concern, but even if it develops, it is almost always less dangerous than with other viral types.

Specific Tests for Hepatitis A

Radioimmunoassays are generally used to identify IgM antibodies, first produced to fight hepatitis A. They appear early in the course of the disease and usually can be identified as soon as symptoms appear. IgM antibodies disappear during recovery, but those known as IgG antibodies persist, and their presence can be used to indicate a previous infection.

Treatments and Measures to Prevent Transmission of Hepatitis A

The primary goals for managing acute viral hepatitis are to provide adequate nutrition, to prevent additional damage to the liver, and to prevent transmission to others.

Precautions for Preventing Transmission of Hepatitis A

Because hepatitis A (and also hepatitis E) are usually passed through contaminated food, people with these viruses should not prepare food for others; unfortunately, these viruses are most contagious before symptoms appear.

- Using hot water when cleaning utensils or clothing is essential. Heating a contaminated article for a minute kills the virus. Simple household bleach is effective for disinfecting hard surfaces. Sterilizing is not necessary. Still, even with strong precautions, utensils used by the patient for eating and cooking should be kept separate from those used by others.

- Abstain from sexual activity or take strict precautions.

- Abstain from alcohol. Moderate drinking (one or two drinks per evening) after recovery is not harmful for most people.

Outlook

In most cases of acute viral hepatitis, recovery is complete and the liver returns to normal within two to eight weeks. In a small number of cases of hepatitis B or C, the condition can be prolonged and recovery may not occur for a year. People who have been infected with a hepatitis virus continue to produce antibodies to that specific virus. This means that they cannot be reinfected with the same hepatitis virus again. Unfortunately, they are not protected from other types.

Serious consequences of acute viral hepatitis are rare, but can be life threatening if they occur. Pregnant women with acute hepatitis B, C, or E are at higher risk for complications of acute hepatitis.

In very rare cases, within two months of onset of acute hepatitis, a very serious condition known as fulminant hepatitis can develop. In this event, the liver fails with catastrophic consequences.

No medications, including corticosteroids, have any effect against the condition itself. Liver transplantation is currently the only life-saving treatment for fulminant acute hepatitis and has survival rates of up to 60 percent. Without liver transplantation, the chance of survival is only 20 percent.

General Prognosis for Chronic Hepatitis

Chronic Persistent Hepatitis

Chronic persistent hepatitis is usually mild and nonprogressive or slowly progressive, causing limited damage to the liver. Cell injury in such cases is usually limited to the region of portal tracts, which contains vessels that carry blood to the liver from the digestive tract. In some cases, however, more extensive liver damage can occur over long periods of time and progress to chronic active hepatitis.

Chronic Active Hepatitis

If damage to the liver is extensive and cell injury occurs beyond the portal tract, chronic active hepatitis can develop. Significant liver damage has usually occurred by this time. Nearly every bodily process is affected by a damaged liver, including digestive, hormonal, and circulatory systems. Symptoms can significantly impair daily life.

Symptom Management

The primary goals for managing viral hepatitis are to provide adequate nutrition, to prevent additional damage to the liver, and to prevent transmission to others. For mild cases of acute viral hepatitis, no drug therapy or other treatment is either available or necessary. Hospitalization is needed only for people at high risk for complications, such as pregnant women, elderly people, patients with other serious conditions, or those who have severe nausea and vomiting and need to have fluids administered intravenously.

The following tips may be useful:

• In some cases, the physician may prescribe drugs that have minimal impact on the liver to alleviate the symptoms of hepatitis, such as nausea or severe itching.

- All patients should abstain from alcohol and sexual contact during the acute phase.

- Although most patients with hepatitis experience fatigue and require more rest than usual, they can be as physically active as they want without affecting recovery. In fact, patients should be encouraged to be as active as they can.

- Depression is common, particularly in people used to an active life. Patients should be reassured that in the great majority of hepatitis cases, recovery is complete.

- The liver processes many types of medications, so as soon as hepatitis is diagnosed, the patient should stop taking all drugs, including over-the-counter medications, except those a physician specifically prescribes or recommends. Of special note, ibuprofen (Advil, Motrin) apparently increases liver enzymes in hepatitis C patients and therefore should be avoided. Ibuprofen is one of the common painkillers known as nonsteroidal anti-inflammatory drugs (NSAIDs). Other NSAIDs include aspirin and naproxen. The usual alternative to an NSAID is acetaminophen (Tylenol). It should be noted that acetaminophen also can be toxic in the liver, particularly when drinking alcohol.

After the onset of acute hepatitis, periodic visits to the physician for repeat blood tests are necessary, the frequency of which depends on how well the patient feels. If symptoms still occur after three months and laboratory tests still indicate active presence of the virus, the patient should be evaluated every month. If symptoms persist beyond six months, a liver biopsy may be required to determine any liver damage.

Treatment for Chronic Hepatitis

Chronic Hepatitis B and C

Drug treatments for chronic hepatitis B and C are aimed at reducing or preventing liver damage and boosting or modifying the immune system to promote its attack on the viruses. The important agents for treating chronic hepatitis are interferons (particularly interferon alpha) and nucleoside analogues (ribavirin, lamivudine, famciclovir, and adefovir), which act directly against the virus. They are being used as sole therapy and in combinations. These drugs are used differently depending on the specific hepatitis. Other drugs with different mechanisms are also being tested. Smokers with hepatitis C should make every attempt to quit, as research now indicates that smoking is associated with increased severity of the infection.

Liver Transplantation

Liver transplantation may be indicated in the following patients:

- Those who have developed life-threatening cirrhosis and who have a life expectancy of more than twelve years.

- Patients with liver cancer that has not spread beyond the liver may also be candidates.

Autoimmune Hepatitis (AIH)

Autoimmune chronic hepatitis typically occurs in women between the ages of twenty and forty who have other autoimmune diseases, including systemic lupus erythematosus, rheumatoid arthritis, Sjögren syndrome, inflammatory bowel disease, glomerulonephritis, and hemolytic anemia. Some research indicates that the postmenopausal period may be another peak in incidence of AIH among women. About 30 percent of patients are men, however, and in both genders there is often no relationship to another autoimmune disease. In general, no major risk factors have been discovered for this condition.

Symptoms of Autoimmune Hepatitis

About 85 percent of people with chronic active autoimmune hepatitis do not have severe symptoms at all. When symptoms occur, they range from minimal to severe, and include fatigue, jaundice, fever, and weight loss. The liver and spleen are often enlarged. In addition, patients with this condition may experience skin disorders, including palmar erythema (red palms) and spider angioma (a blood-red spot, the size of a pinhead, from which tiny blood vessels radiate like spider legs). Itching is not common, however. The abdomen or legs may be swollen due to the accumulation of fluid.

Tests for Autoimmune Chronic Hepatitis

If a patient experiences symptoms of chronic active hepatitis for six months or more and a virus cannot be identified, then autoimmune hepatitis is usually suspected. There are other autoimmune liver diseases, however, that can confuse a diagnosis. To help confirm this condition, test results may show high levels of immune factors called serum globulins or certain antibodies to liver proteins. In some cases, a successful trial of steroid drugs may be the only way to diagnose autoimmune hepatitis.

Outlook for Autoimmune Hepatitis

Autoimmune hepatitis is usually benign and causes little trouble, although there is a very small risk that it can evolve into the active form. One study reported a ten-year survival rate of 95 percent, which was similar to that for the same age group in the general population. However, if the condition evolves into the chronic active form, five-year survival rate may be only 50 percent if the disease is not treated. (The survival rate can be higher in people with milder symptoms and less liver damage.)

Although very uncommon, severe autoimmune hepatitis can be life-threatening and require intensive therapy, including possibly liver transplantation. The risk for liver failure and bleeding in the stomach and esophagus is highest in the early years after disease onset. This risk diminishes over time but is replaced by an increase in liver cancer rates and bleeding in the stomach and intestines. The risk for liver cancer is not as high, however, as with chronic viral hepatitis.

Treatments for Autoimmune Hepatitis

Patients with autoimmune hepatitis who have mild symptoms and slight inflammation of the liver do not require any treatment except to alleviate symptoms. They should be monitored, however, for any signs of disease progression. Because of effective treatment options and in spite of a high rate of relapse, long-term survival rates in patients with autoimmune hepatitis are excellent. Drugs that block factors in the immune system and help reduce inflammation and symptoms of autoimmune hepatitis are most often used.

Corticosteroids

Corticosteroids, prednisone and prednisolone, are the standard agents used for autoimmune hepatitis. They produce remission of symptoms in about 80 percent of patients with autoimmune hepatitis. For most patients, steroids also reduce symptoms within three months, improve liver function within six months, and restore liver health within two years. Between 10 percent and 20 percent of patients continue to deteriorate despite steroid treatment, although higher doses may help some of these people.

Unfortunately, remission rarely lasts more than three years. About half of patients relapse within six months, and only about 20 percent of patients achieve remission (are disease-free) for more than five years. Re-administering prednisone therapy after relapse achieves another remission in 80 percent of patients.

Side effects can be very distressing and sometimes serious; they include weight gain, skin problems, moon-shaped face, high blood pressure, diabetes, cataracts, mental disturbances, infections, and osteoporosis.

Investigative Agents

In severe cases, drugs that block the immune system may be used:

- Azathioprine (Imuran) is often prescribed along with steroids to help reduce severe side effects caused by using steroids alone. Azathioprine also suppresses the immune system and helps prevent relapse, but the drug will not induce remission by itself. In one promising study, patients who continued to use azathioprine after prednisolone was withdrawn had no relapses for at least a year. Unfortunately, long-term use of azathioprine may increase the risk for cancer, although studies indicate that this risk is very low.

- Cyclosporine A (Neoral) is another immunosuppressant and may prove to be a safe and effective alternative to corticosteroids.

Some important research is targeting agents that inhibit RNA—the genetic molecules that serve as messengers for regulating cellular processes. In a 2003 animal study, an agent that targeted RNA specifically affecting cell receptors involved in liver injury protected against autoimmune hepatitis in mice.

Liver Transplantation and Autoimmune Hepatitis

If all therapies fail and the disease becomes life threatening, liver transplantation may be performed. Liver transplantation is problematic, however. In one study, half of patients who received a transplant required re-transplantation within a year. Autoimmune hepatitis recurred in 25 percent of patients studied.

Chapter 32

Cirrhosis of the Liver

The liver, the largest organ in the body, is essential in keeping the body functioning properly. It removes or neutralizes poisons from the blood, produces immune agents to control infection, and removes germs and bacteria from the blood. It makes proteins that regulate blood clotting and produces bile to help absorb fats and fat-soluble vitamins. You cannot live without a functioning liver.

In cirrhosis of the liver, scar tissue replaces normal, healthy tissue, blocking the flow of blood through the organ and preventing it from working as it should. Cirrhosis is the twelfth leading cause of death by disease, killing about twenty-six thousand people each year. Also, the cost of cirrhosis in terms of human suffering, hospital costs, and lost productivity is high.

Causes

Cirrhosis has many causes. In the United States, chronic alcoholism and hepatitis C are the most common ones.

Alcoholic Liver Disease: To many people, cirrhosis of the liver is synonymous with chronic alcoholism, but in fact, alcoholism is only one of the causes. Alcoholic cirrhosis usually develops after more than a decade of heavy drinking. The amount of alcohol that can injure the liver varies greatly from person to person. In women, as few as two

Reprinted from "Cirrhosis of the Liver," National Institute of Diabetes and Digestive and Kidney Diseases, NIH Publication No. 04-1134, December 2003.

to three drinks per day have been linked with cirrhosis and in men, as few as three to four drinks per day. Alcohol seems to injure the liver by blocking the normal metabolism of protein, fats, and carbohydrates.

Chronic Hepatitis C: The hepatitis C virus ranks with alcohol as a major cause of chronic liver disease and cirrhosis in the United States. Infection with this virus causes inflammation of and low-grade damage to the liver that over several decades can lead to cirrhosis.

Chronic Hepatitis B and D: The hepatitis B virus is probably the most common cause of cirrhosis worldwide, but it is less common in the United States and the Western world. Hepatitis B, like hepatitis C, causes liver inflammation and injury that over several decades can lead to cirrhosis. Hepatitis D is another virus that infects the liver, but only in people who already have hepatitis B.

Autoimmune Hepatitis: This disease appears to be caused by the immune system attacking the liver and causing inflammation, damage, and eventually scarring and cirrhosis.

Inherited Diseases: Alpha-1 antitrypsin deficiency, hemochromatosis, Wilson disease, galactosemia, and glycogen storage diseases are among the inherited diseases that interfere with the way the liver produces, processes, and stores enzymes, proteins, metals, and other substances the body needs to function properly.

Nonalcoholic Steatohepatitis (NASH): In NASH, fat builds up in the liver and eventually causes scar tissue. This type of hepatitis appears to be associated with diabetes, protein malnutrition, obesity, coronary artery disease, and treatment with corticosteroid medications.

Blocked Bile Ducts: When the ducts that carry bile out of the liver are blocked, bile backs up and damages liver tissue. In babies, blocked bile ducts are most commonly caused by biliary atresia, a disease in which the bile ducts are absent or injured. In adults, the most common cause is primary biliary cirrhosis, a disease in which the ducts become inflamed, blocked, and scarred. Secondary biliary cirrhosis can happen after gallbladder surgery if the ducts are inadvertently tied off or injured.

Drugs, Toxins, and Infections: Severe reactions to prescription drugs, prolonged exposure to environmental toxins, the parasitic infection schistosomiasis, and repeated bouts of heart failure with liver congestion can all lead to cirrhosis.

Symptoms

Many people with cirrhosis have no symptoms in the early stages of the disease. However, as scar tissue replaces healthy cells, liver function starts to fail and a person may experience the following symptoms:

- exhaustion
- fatigue
- loss of appetite
- nausea
- weakness
- weight loss
- abdominal pain
- spider-like blood vessels (spider angiomas) that develop on the skin

As the disease progresses, complications may develop. In some people, these may be the first signs of the disease.

Complications of Cirrhosis

Loss of liver function affects the body in many ways. Following are the common problems, or complications, caused by cirrhosis.

Edema and Ascites: When the liver loses its ability to make the protein albumin, water accumulates in the legs (edema) and abdomen (ascites).

Bruising and Bleeding: When the liver slows or stops production of the proteins needed for blood clotting, a person will bruise or bleed easily. The palms of the hands may be reddish and blotchy with palmar erythema.

Jaundice: Jaundice is a yellowing of the skin and eyes that occurs when the diseased liver does not absorb enough bilirubin.

Itching: Bile products deposited in the skin may cause intense itching.

Gallstones: If cirrhosis prevents bile from reaching the gallbladder, gallstones may develop.

Toxins in the Blood or Brain: A damaged liver cannot remove toxins from the blood, causing them to accumulate in the blood and eventually the brain. There, toxins can dull mental functioning and cause personality changes, coma, and even death. Signs of the buildup of toxins in the brain include neglect of personal appearance, unresponsiveness, forgetfulness, trouble concentrating, or changes in sleep habits.

Sensitivity to Medication: Cirrhosis slows the liver's ability to filter medications from the blood. Because the liver does not remove drugs from the blood at the usual rate, they act longer than expected and build up in the body. This causes a person to be more sensitive to medications and their side effects.

Portal Hypertension: Normally, blood from the intestines and spleen is carried to the liver through the portal vein. But cirrhosis slows the normal flow of blood through the portal vein, which increases the pressure inside it. This condition is called portal hypertension.

Varices: When blood flow through the portal vein slows, blood from the intestines and spleen backs up into blood vessels in the stomach and esophagus. These blood vessels may become enlarged because they are not meant to carry this much blood. The enlarged blood vessels, called varices, have thin walls and carry high pressure, and thus are more likely to burst. If they do burst, the result is a serious bleeding problem in the upper stomach or esophagus that requires immediate medical attention.

Insulin Resistance and Type 2 Diabetes: Cirrhosis causes resistance to insulin. This hormone, produced by the pancreas, enables blood glucose to be used as energy by the cells of the body. If you have insulin resistance, your muscle, fat, and liver cells do not use insulin properly. The pancreas tries to keep up with the demand for insulin by producing more. Eventually, the pancreas cannot keep up with the body's need for insulin, and type 2 diabetes develops as excess glucose builds up in the bloodstream.

Liver Cancer: Hepatocellular carcinoma, a type of liver cancer commonly caused by cirrhosis, starts in the liver tissue itself. It has a high mortality rate.

Problems in Other Organs: Cirrhosis can cause immune system dysfunction, leading to infection. Fluid in the abdomen (ascites) may become infected with bacteria normally present in the intestines. Cirrhosis can also lead to impotence, kidney dysfunction and failure, and osteoporosis.

Diagnosis

The doctor may diagnose cirrhosis on the basis of symptoms, laboratory tests, the medical history, and a physical examination. For example, during a physical examination, the doctor may notice that the liver feels harder or larger than usual and order blood tests that can show whether liver disease is present.

If looking at the liver is necessary to check for signs of disease, the doctor might order a computerized axial tomography (CAT) scan, ultrasound, magnetic resonance imaging (MRI), or a scan of the liver using a radioisotope (a harmless radioactive substance that highlights the liver). Or the doctor might look at the liver using a laparoscope, an instrument that is inserted through the abdomen and relays pictures back to a computer screen.

A liver biopsy will confirm the diagnosis. For a biopsy, the doctor uses a needle to take a tiny sample of liver tissue, then examines it under the microscope for scarring or other signs of disease.

Treatment

Liver damage from cirrhosis cannot be reversed, but treatment can stop or delay further progression and reduce complications. Treatment depends on the cause of cirrhosis and any complications a person is experiencing. For example, cirrhosis caused by alcohol abuse is treated by abstaining from alcohol. Treatment for hepatitis-related cirrhosis involves medications used to treat the different types of hepatitis, such as interferon for viral hepatitis and corticosteroids for autoimmune hepatitis. Cirrhosis caused by Wilson disease, in which copper builds up in organs, is treated with medications to remove the copper. These are just a few examples—treatment for cirrhosis resulting from other diseases depends on the underlying cause. In all cases, regardless of the cause, following a healthy diet and avoiding alcohol are essential because the body needs all the nutrients it can get, and alcohol will only lead to more liver damage. Light physical activity can help stop or delay cirrhosis as well.

Treatment will also include remedies for complications. For example, for ascites and edema, the doctor may recommend a low-sodium diet or the use of diuretics, which are drugs that remove fluid from the body. Antibiotics will be prescribed for infections, and various medications can help with itching. Protein causes toxins to form in the digestive tract, so eating less protein will help decrease the buildup of toxins in the blood and brain. The doctor may also prescribe laxatives to help absorb the toxins and remove them from the intestines.

For portal hypertension, the doctor may prescribe a blood pressure medication such as a beta-blocker. If varices bleed, the doctor may either inject them with a clotting agent or perform a so-called rubber-band ligation, which uses a special device to compress the varices and stop the bleeding.

When complications cannot be controlled or when the liver becomes so damaged from scarring that it completely stops functioning, a liver transplant is necessary. In liver transplantation surgery, a diseased liver is removed and replaced with a healthy one from an organ donor. About 80 to 90 percent of patients survive liver transplantation. Survival rates have improved over the past several years because of drugs such as cyclosporine and tacrolimus, which suppress the immune system and keep it from attacking and damaging the new liver.

Chapter 33

Primary Sclerosing Cholangitis

What is primary sclerosing cholangitis?

In primary sclerosing cholangitis (PSC), the bile ducts (a type of passageway) inside and outside the liver become narrowed due to inflammation and scarring. As the scarring increases, the ducts become blocked. The ducts are important because they carry bile out of the liver.

Bile is a liquid that removes toxins from the body and helps break down fat in food. If the ducts are blocked, toxins in bile remain in the liver and damage liver cells. In addition, fat and vitamins A, D, E, and K may not be well absorbed. Eventually, primary sclerosing cholangitis can cause liver failure.

Approximately three out of every one hundred thousand individuals in the world are diagnosed with sclerosing cholangitis.

What are the causes?

The causes of primary sclerosing cholangitis are not known, but many researchers think it might be an autoimmune disease. When the immune system is working correctly, it protects the body from infections caused by bacteria and viruses.

In the case of an autoimmune disease, the body does not recognize certain cells and body parts as part of itself. The body then goes to war against itself, damaging the body part it thinks is foreign.

In many cases, primary sclerosing cholangitis occurs along with a type of inflammatory bowel disease in which the colon becomes inflamed and develops ulcers, but it may also be associated with cystic fibrosis and disorders of the immune system.

What are the signs and symptoms?

Since primary sclerosing cholangitis progresses slowly, a person can have the disease for years before symptoms develop. Symptoms are caused by two things: the bile is not being drained properly through the bile ducts and the liver is damaged and not able to carry out its usual functions.

The main symptoms are:

- Itching (may occur when toxins in bile get into the bloodstream);

- Fatigue (when you feel tired all the time);

- Jaundice (causes yellowing of the eyes or skin; the color change is due to bile that gets in the blood and eventually in the skin and eyes);

- Fever, chills, and soreness in the upper part of the stomach (caused by infected bile ducts).

As the disease progresses, chronic fatigue, loss of appetite, weight loss, and continued jaundice may occur. In the advanced stages, swelling can occur in the stomach and feet. Liver failure may take many years to develop.

How is primary sclerosing cholangitis diagnosed?

Since people with primary sclerosing cholangitis may not have noticeable symptoms for many years, the disease often is suspected due to abnormal blood tests (taken for other reasons) that show a high level of liver enzymes (which indicate abnormal liver function). The disease also might be suspected due to a history of inflammatory bowel disease.

X-ray techniques can reveal whether bile ducts are blocked; however they may not be able to determine the cause or site of the possible obstruction.

Sclerosing cholangitis is diagnosed by injecting dye into the bile ducts and taking an x-ray. The test can determine the cause and site of the blockage. A lighted and flexible endoscope (instrument used to visually examine the inside of certain body parts) is inserted through the mouth, stomach, and then into the small intestine.

A thin tube is placed through the scope and into the pancreatic and bile ducts, and the dye is injected to show the bile ducts on the x-ray. If the x-ray shows the bile ducts are narrowed, the doctor diagnoses the problem as primary sclerosing cholangitis.

As the disease progresses, a liver biopsy usually is needed to determine how much liver damage has occurred.

How is primary sclerosing cholangitis treated?

Currently there is no cure for primary sclerosing cholangitis. Treatment is directed at managing symptoms and opening narrowed bile ducts. Symptoms of this disease can sometimes be managed by:

- Antibiotics to treat bile ducts that have become infected;

- Diets low in salt and medication to treat swelling of the stomach and feet caused by fluid retention;

- Vitamin supplements, since people with primary sclerosing cholangitis often do not have enough vitamins A, D, and K;

- Medications (such as Cholestyramine® and Ursodiol®) to control itching caused by too much bile in the bloodstream, and to improve bile flow.

Endoscopic or surgical procedures may be used to open major blockages in bile ducts. A catheter is a thin, flexible tube used to drain bile from the ducts and relieve the obstruction.

A prosthesis (artificial device in the form of a hollow tube) may be placed in the bile ducts after they have been opened in order to keep the ducts open. Some patients may undergo surgery in order to explore the bile ducts and open major blockages.

Liver transplantation may be an option if the liver begins to fail. Liver transplantation is very effective in the treatment of patients with advanced liver disease caused by primary sclerosing cholangitis.

If a transplant is the best treatment option, the care team will focus on preventing complications and treating symptoms while awaiting a donated liver.

If a liver transplant is the best treatment option, the doctor and the other members of the patient care team will focus on preventing complications and will treat symptoms while waiting for the donated liver.

What is the long-term prognosis?

Sclerosing cholangitis is a disease that continues to advance and tends to become more severe over time.

Medication does not have a major impact on slowing the progression of primary sclerosing cholangitis, but it has an important role in treating complications. For instance, Ursodiol® can help stop itching, but it does not help a patient survive longer, and it does not delay the time to referral for liver transplant.

Currently there are exciting studies being done to test the effectiveness of other drugs on the body's immune system, since that seems to be the underlying problem associated with primary sclerosing cholangitis.

Chapter 34

Other Liver Disorders

Chapter Contents

Section 34.1

Porphyria

Porphyrins are chemical compounds that are stepping stones along the pathway that leads to the formation of heme in humans, and to chlorophyll in plants. They are responsible for the fact that "blood is red, and grass is green." Heme is essential if the body is to work properly.

In porphyria, the cells do not convert porphyrins to heme in a normal manner. Because of this, porphyrins build up in the body and are excreted in the urine and stool in excessive amounts. When present in very high levels, they cause the urine to have a spectacular port wine color.

The symptoms of porphyria fall into two major groups. Some patients have attacks in which the nerves of the body do not function properly. Abdominal pain and weakness result. Other patients have problems with the parts of the skin that are exposed to the sun and this can cause pain and swelling of the skin or the formation of blisters. Treatment is available for both types of symptoms.

The disease can appear in childhood, but the onset most frequently occurs between the ages of twenty and forty. The disease affects men less often than women, in whom attacks are related to the menstrual cycle. Long latent periods may separate these attacks, which can be precipitated by drugs, infections, alcohol consumption, and dieting.

Proper diagnosis and treatment of porphyria depends on chemical studies of the blood, urine, and stool. Since certain types of porphyria are genetic diseases, studies should also be done on children and blood relatives of affected individuals.

Section 34.2

Type I Glycogen Storage Disease

Glycogen storage disease has been divided into at least ten different types based on the deficiency of a particular enzyme that controls blood sugar levels.

Type I glycogen storage disease is a deficiency of the enzyme glucose-6-phosphatase, which helps in maintaining a normal blood glucose (sugar concentration) during fasting. Patients with this particular disorder show a large number of abnormalities that exhibit themselves in growth failure, a greatly enlarged liver, and a distended (swollen) abdomen. The abnormal blood chemical condition is indicated by low blood sugar concentration and higher than normal levels of lipids and uric acid.

In the past, these patients have been treated by frequent feedings during the daytime and occasional feedings during the normal sleeping hours which required waking the patient. This was the accepted form of therapy until 1966 to 1967, but the patients continued to show various difficulties in physical development and blood chemistry.

Starting in 1967, surgeons began performing a surgical procedure, called a portacaval shunt, which bypassed the blood around the liver. In some patients this procedure resulted in improvement in observable physical condition and improved biochemical levels in the blood. In 1974 it was found that patients also did exceedingly well if the blood glucose level was maintained within the normal range by frequent daytime feedings and by continuous infusion of a solution high in glucose concentration into the stomach during the night. Maintenance of the blood glucose level either in total intravenous feedings or by continuous infusion of high glucose-containing foods into the stomach could reverse all of the physical and chemical signs of this disease.

A practical management technique for maintaining the blood glucose level has been devised in which a nasogastric tube is inserted into the stomach each evening and through this tube is infused a solution containing a high concentration of glucose so the blood sugar level remains between 75 and 120. In the daytime the tube is removed and the patient eats a high starch feeding approximately every 2½ to 3½ hours. Using this technique, most of the physical and biochemical abnormalities are completely reversed.

One study in which a total of fourteen patients were followed, nine for a period of greater than five years, has shown this to be an effective form of treatment. Although younger children will have to use the tube each evening, doctors feel that this may not be necessary past puberty.

Liver transplantation has been performed successfully in some cases, and greatly improves metabolic control. However, it does not correct all of the abnormalities seen in this disease, and its use is not routine at this point.

Section 34.3

Hemochromatosis

Hemochromatosis is an inherited condition that causes the body to absorb and store too much iron. It is the most common inherited disorder, affecting more than one million people in the United States who carry both copies of the abnormal gene. It is estimated that 10 percent of the population are carriers of one copy of the abnormal hemochromatosis gene. Many cases go undiagnosed because neither parents nor physicians have been alerted to the problem. The most vital factor in making an early diagnosis is enhanced recognition of the disease by doctors and patients. This is particularly important since early diagnosis and prompt treatment can prevent all of the long-term complications of the disease.

Who is most likely to get hemochromatosis?

The hemochromatosis gene, called *HFE*, was identified in 1996 and is inherited from both parents. It is most often diagnosed in people who exhibit symptoms and are between the ages of forty and sixty years old. Women who lose iron through menstruation, pregnancy, and breast-feeding often develop symptoms at a later age than men. Anyone who has a blood relative with hemochromatosis should be tested even if there are no symptoms.

What are the symptoms?

Many people have no symptoms, even in advanced cases. Others suffering from hemochromatosis frequently exhibit these symptoms:

- fatigue
- weakness
- abdominal pain
- pain in the joints
- slightly elevated liver enzymes
- bronze or greyish discoloration of the skin
- impotence

Are there special tests for iron overload?

Blood tests for serum iron and either total iron binding capacity (TIBC) or transferrin are good screening tests. The ratio of serum iron or transferrin or TIBC is normally about 0.30, or 30 percent. Figures above 50 percent (indicative of iron overload) or below 15 percent (iron deficiency) need more study. A good additional test is serum ferritin level, which is elevated in patients with hemochromatosis. If these tests are persistently high, a genetic test for the mutations in the HFE gene should be performed. A genetic test is commercially available and costs about $175. Depending on whether there is evidence of liver damage, a liver biopsy should be done to assess the damage to the liver. Excess iron is also frequently present in patients with alcoholic liver disease or chronic viral hepatitis. A liver biopsy is the only definitive way to determine if patients with these diseases also have iron overload.

How can hemochromatosis be treated?

Phlebotomy treatments (blood letting) are performed where one to two pints of blood (which contain iron in hemoglobin in red blood cells) are removed each week until iron stores go down to a normal level. It may take several months to several years to remove all excess iron. After the iron stores are reduced to normal, maintenance phlebotomy treatments should continue every two to four months for life to prevent re-accumulation of iron.

What is the outlook for patients?

Those who are treated early can look forward to a completely normal life. When the illness has advanced to the stage of cirrhosis, the situation is more serious. Liver cancer can occur in up to 30 percent of these patients. Damage to the pancreas by the excess iron can result in diabetes mellitus. Damage to other organs may cause arthritis, loss of body hair, heart problems, loss of sex drive (males), and impotence. In the latter stages of the disease, the patient may develop an enlarged liver (hepatomegaly), cirrhosis (scarring of the liver), and an enlargement of the spleen (splenomegaly).

Does having anemia rule out iron overload?

No. There are many forms of anemia, and a person can have both anemia and iron overload.

What effect does alcohol have on hemochromatosis?

Drinking alcoholic beverages should be avoided. Alcohol can accelerate liver damage in hemochromatosis.

Is there any relationship between diet and iron overload?

Hemochromatosis is unrelated to diet. It is rare for people to develop iron storage problems after taking large amounts of iron tonics and medications over a long period. However, no one should take iron supplements without a doctor's advice. Anyone with an iron overload problem should avoid tonics and medications containing iron.

Can diet help?

When hemochromatosis is diagnosed, a well-balanced diet low in iron-rich food is recommended. Consumption of iron-rich foods such as red meat should be limited to small quantities. Liver, a food high in iron content, should be avoided as it may enhance iron absorption from food. Read food labels carefully, as many foods, such as cereals, are fortified with iron.

Should damage appear in other organs, further dietary recommendations may be indicated:

- Damage to the pancreas will likely require a diabetic diet in which the main focus is avoidance of concentrated sweets. A high-fiber diet may be a benefit to help control blood sugar levels.

- Cardiac problems may require sodium restriction.

- Diabetes mellitus and cardiac problems related to obesity require a weight reduction, low-fat diet.

- Cirrhosis may require restriction of sodium.

Liver Transplantation and Hemochromatosis

Patients who under go liver transplantation for hemochromatosis generally have a one-year average survival rate of 50 percent, which is about 30 percent lower than those transplanted for other reasons. The lower rate is believed to be caused by infectious or cardiac complications. The survival rate is also lower for patients whose hemochromatosis is not diagnosed prior to liver transplantation for other reasons.

Section 34.4

Cystic Disease of the Liver

An important task of the liver is producing and excreting bile. This yellow-green, bitter-tasting fluid flows into the intestine through the bile ducts. The bile ducts in the liver are like the branches on a tree, and come together just below the stomach. A side branch leads to a sack for storing bile, called the gallbladder.

Gallbladder disease is a common type of illness involving the biliary tree. Less common, but significant, is cystic disease of the biliary tree. This can take several forms:

- cysts in the main trunk (choledochal cysts)

- cysts (or lakes) in the small branches within the liver (Caroli syndrome)

- cysts in the liver separate from the biliary tree (polycystic liver disease)

Choledochal Cyst

In this condition, the main trunk (the common bile duct) of the biliary tree is structurally abnormal. In some cases this is present from birth; in others, it appears to be acquired later on. Eventually (usually by age two or three but sometimes not until adolescence or adulthood) the bile accumulates in the duct. It forms a sack or cyst which then presses on the bile duct and prevents bile from reaching the intestine. Bile backs up into the liver and the patient becomes jaundiced (yellow). Occasionally this accumulation of bile becomes infected, causing abdominal pain and fever. In addition, some biliary cysts can become cancerous, although it remains somewhat unclear how large this risk is.

In some patients the cyst can be felt by the doctor examining the abdomen. In most patients the diagnosis can be confirmed by using sonic pictures (ultrasound) or by injecting a radioactive substance that gives an "image" of the abnormal duct (nuclear medicine). CT scanning and MRI can also be useful. Treatment is surgical. The abnormal bile duct is removed and a piece of intestine used to replace it. In most cases, surgery permanently corrects the disease, and decreases the risk of development of a bile duct cancer. Rarely, infection in the newly formed biliary tree recurs. If the condition is not correctly diagnosed the blockage of bile may result in scarring in the liver (cirrhosis).

Caroli Syndrome

Caroli syndrome (intrahepatic ductal ectasia) is another rare congenital (from birth) disease. In most cases, it appears to have autosomal recessive inheritance. Specific genes for the disease have not been identified, but it is suspected they are closely related to the genes that cause polycystic kidney disease. In Caroli syndrome, the small branches of the biliary tree in the liver are abnormal. Small lakes alternate with narrowed segments of bile ducts, instead of the normal smooth contour. These abnormalities may be present throughout the liver, or limited to only a small area. If the bile duct becomes infected, the patient develops fever, abdominal pain, and, rarely, jaundice. Patients with Caroli syndrome frequently also suffer from polycystic kidney disease, and initial symptoms may relate to the kidney disease rather than the liver disease. Complications may not occur until middle age or may first appear in childhood. This disease can be detected by ultrasound studies, MRI, or cholangiography. The latter procedure involves using radioisotopes to "image" the biliary tree and by injecting dye directly into the biliary tree. This may be done by inserting a needle through the skin into the liver (percutaneous transhepatic cholangiogram) or using a tube to pass dye through the intestine up into the bile duct (endoscopic retrograde cholangiography).

Congenital Hepatic Fibrosis

In patients with this condition, there is abnormal growth of fibrous tissue (scar) around the small branches of the bile ducts in the liver. As a result, the liver becomes enlarged and hard and blood can no longer flow freely through the liver. The spleen becomes enlarged and the blood must return to the heart through weak veins along the tube to the stomach (esophageal varices). These veins may burst and cause bleeding into the stomach and bowels. Patients with this condition are usually discovered in childhood, either because of the large liver or because of bleeding. The diagnosis is proven by liver biopsy and x-ray of blood vessels. There is no specific treatment for this condition but many patients require rerouting of blood from the intestines (shunt operation) to prevent more intestinal bleeding.

Polycystic Liver Disease

In some patients, large lakes (cysts) separate from the biliary tree form in the liver. In severe cases, the liver looks like a sponge. These cysts may cause pain, but do not affect liver function. In most patients, the kidneys are similarly affected with cysts, which may cause high blood pressure and kidney failure. The tendency to form cysts is probably present at birth in these patients, but usually the cysts do not enlarge and give problems until adulthood. This condition may be detected using ultrasound or CAT scan and x-rays of the kidney (intravenous pyelogram). Polycystic disease is inherited and once it has been detected in one member of a family, all the patient's relatives should be tested for it. There are two major categories of polycystic disease of the liver and kidney. In the more benign, the cysts are mostly in the liver and kidney function is near normal. These patients have a normal life expectancy. However those patients who have kidney damage need treatment for the equivalent of polycystic kidney disease.

All these conditions are rare and many people have never heard of them. They will probably be diagnosed with greater frequency in the future with the help of new tools such as ultrasonography. Several of these conditions are inherited. To help patients and their children, we need to know more about what causes these diseases and how to diagnose and treat them.

Section 34.5

Sarcoidosis

Sarcoidosis is a systemic disease of unknown cause. Nests of cells (noncaseating epithelioid cell granulomas) appear in many tissues, including the lung, lymph nodes, and liver. The disease is recognized in many parts of the world. Blacks are affected about fifteen times more often than whites in the United States, with the highest incidences in the southeastern states.

Pulmonary lymph node involvement is typical. Fibrosis or scarring may be widespread. Lung function may be abnormal. In addition to lung involvement, there may be enlargement of lymph nodes, facial nerve palsy, uveitis, erythema nodosum, subcutaneous nodules, lupus pernio, polyarthralgias, arthritis, cystic bone lesions, nephrocalcinosis, myocardial disease, and neurologic problems which may include peripheral nerve damage and diabetes.

Liver biopsy reveals hepatic granuloma in about 75 percent of patients. There is no specific treatment for sarcoidosis, however, symptoms are treated as needed.

Part Six

Cancers of the Gastrointestinal Tract

Chapter 35

Gastrointestinal Carcinoid Tumors

General Information about Gastrointestinal Carcinoid Tumors

A gastrointestinal carcinoid tumor is cancer that forms in the lining of the gastrointestinal tract.

The gastrointestinal tract includes the stomach, small intestine, and large intestine. These organs are part of the digestive system, which processes nutrients (vitamins, minerals, carbohydrates, fats, proteins, and water) in foods that are eaten and helps pass waste material out of the body. Gastrointestinal carcinoid tumors develop from a certain type of hormone-making cell in the lining of the gastrointestinal tract. These cells produce hormones that help regulate digestive juices and the muscles used in moving food through the stomach and intestines. A gastrointestinal carcinoid tumor may also produce hormones. Carcinoid tumors that start in the rectum (the last several inches of the large intestine) usually do not produce hormones.

Gastrointestinal carcinoid tumors grow slowly. Most of them occur in the appendix (an organ attached to the large intestine), small intestine, and rectum. It is common for more than one tumor to develop in the small intestine. Having a carcinoid tumor increases a person's chance of getting other cancers in the digestive system, either at the same time or later.

PDQ® Cancer Information Summary. National Cancer Institute; Bethesda, MD. Gastrointestinal Carcinoid Tumors (PDQ®): Treatment—Patient. Updated 5/2004. Available at: http://www.cancer.gov. Accessed February 10, 2005.

Risk Factors

Health history can affect the risk of developing gastrointestinal carcinoid tumors.

Risk factors include the following:

- Having a family history of multiple endocrine neoplasia type 1 (MEN1) syndrome

- Having certain conditions that affect the stomach's ability to produce stomach acid, such as atrophic gastritis, pernicious anemia, or Zollinger-Ellison syndrome

- Smoking tobacco

Symptoms

A gastrointestinal carcinoid tumor often has no signs in its early stages. Carcinoid syndrome may occur if the tumor spreads to the liver or other parts of the body.

The hormones produced by gastrointestinal carcinoid tumors are usually destroyed by blood and liver enzymes. If the tumor has spread to the liver, however, high amounts of these hormones may remain in the body and cause the following group of symptoms, called carcinoid syndrome:

- Redness or a feeling of warmth in the face and neck

- Diarrhea

- Shortness of breath, fast heartbeat, tiredness, or swelling of the feet and ankles

- Wheezing

- Pain or a feeling of fullness in the abdomen

These symptoms and others may be caused by gastrointestinal carcinoid tumors or by other conditions. A doctor should be consulted if any of these symptoms occur.

Diagnosis

Tests that examine the blood and urine are used to detect (find) and diagnose gastrointestinal carcinoid tumors.

The following tests and procedures may be used:

- **Complete blood count:** A procedure in which a sample of blood is drawn and checked for the following:

  - The number of red blood cells, white blood cells, and platelets.

  - The amount of hemoglobin (the protein that carries oxygen) in the red blood cells.

  - The portion of the sample made up of red blood cells.

- **Physical exam and history:** An exam of the body to check general signs of health, including checking for signs of disease, such as lumps or anything else that seems unusual. A history of the patient's health habits and past illnesses and treatments will also be taken.

- **Blood chemistry studies:** A procedure in which a blood sample is checked to measure the amounts of certain substances, such as hormones, released into the blood by organs and tissues in the body. An unusual (higher or lower than normal) amount of a substance can be a sign of disease in the organ or tissue that produces it. The blood sample is checked to see if it contains a hormone produced by carcinoid tumors. This test is used to help diagnose carcinoid syndrome.

- **Twenty-four-hour urine test:** A test in which a urine sample is checked to measure the amounts of certain substances, such as hormones. An unusual (higher or lower than normal) amount of a substance can be a sign of disease in the organ or tissue that produces it. The urine sample is checked to see if it contains a hormone produced by carcinoid tumors. This test is used to help diagnose carcinoid syndrome.

Prognosis

Certain factors affect prognosis (chance of recovery) and treatment options.

The prognosis (chance of recovery) and treatment options depend on the following:

- Whether the cancer can be completely removed by surgery.

- Whether the cancer has spread from the stomach and intestines to other parts of the body, such as the liver or lymph nodes.

- The size of the tumor.

- Where the tumor is in the gastrointestinal tract.
- Whether the cancer is newly diagnosed or has recurred.

Treatment options also depend on whether the cancer is causing symptoms. Most gastrointestinal carcinoid tumors are slow-growing and can be treated and often cured. Even when not cured, many patients may live for a long time.

Stages of Gastrointestinal Carcinoid Tumors

After a gastrointestinal carcinoid tumor has been diagnosed, tests are done to find out if cancer cells have spread within the stomach and intestines or to other parts of the body.

Staging is the process used to find out how far the cancer has spread. The information gathered from the staging process determines the stage of the disease. There are no standard stages for gastrointestinal carcinoid tumors. In order to plan treatment, it is important to know the extent of the disease and whether the tumor can be removed by surgery. The following tests and procedures may be used:

- **Gastrointestinal endoscopy:** A procedure to look inside the gastrointestinal tract for abnormal areas or cancer. An endoscope (a thin, lighted tube) is inserted through the mouth and esophagus into the stomach and first part of the small intestine. Also, a colonoscope (a thin, lighted tube) is inserted through the rectum into the colon (large intestine); this is called a colonoscopy.

- **CT scan (CAT scan):** A procedure that makes a series of detailed pictures of areas inside the body, taken from different angles. The pictures are made by a computer linked to an x-ray machine. A dye may be injected into a vein or swallowed to help the organs or tissues show up more clearly. This procedure is also called computed tomography, computerized tomography, or computerized axial tomography.

- **Somatostatin receptor scintigraphy (SRS):** A type of radionuclide scan used to find carcinoid tumors. In SRS, radioactive octreotide, a drug similar to somatostatin, is injected into a vein and travels through the bloodstream. The radioactive octreotide attaches to carcinoid tumor cells that have somatostatin receptors. A radiation-measuring device detects the radioactive material, showing where the carcinoid tumor cells are in the body. This procedure is also called an octreotide scan.

- **Biopsy:** The removal of cells or tissues so they can be viewed under a microscope to check for signs of cancer. Tissue samples may be taken during endoscopy and colonoscopy.

- **Angiogram:** A procedure to look at blood vessels and the flow of blood. A contrast dye is injected into the blood vessel. As the contrast dye moves through the blood vessel, x-rays are taken to see if there are any blockages.

- **PET scan (positron emission tomography scan):** A procedure to find malignant tumor cells in the body. A small amount of radionuclide glucose (sugar) is injected into a vein. The PET scanner rotates around the body and makes a picture of where glucose is being used in the body. Malignant tumor cells show up brighter in the picture because they are more active and take up more glucose than normal cells.

- **X-ray of the abdomen:** An x-ray of the organs and tissues inside the abdomen. An x-ray is a type of energy beam that can go through the body and onto film, making a picture of areas inside the body.

Gastrointestinal carcinoid tumors are grouped for treatment based on where they are in the body.

- **Localized:** Cancer is found in the appendix, colon, rectum, small intestine, or stomach only.

- **Regional:** Cancer has spread from the appendix, colon, rectum, stomach, or small intestine to nearby tissues or lymph nodes.

- **Metastatic:** Cancer has spread to other parts of the body.

Recurrent Gastrointestinal Carcinoid Tumors

A recurrent gastrointestinal carcinoid tumor is a tumor that has recurred (come back) after it has been treated. The tumor may come back in the stomach or intestines or in other parts of the body.

Treatment Option Overview

Different types of treatment are available for patients with gastrointestinal carcinoid tumors. Some treatments are standard (the currently used treatment), and some are being tested in clinical trials. Before starting treatment, patients may want to think about taking part in a clinical trial. A treatment clinical trial is a research study meant to help improve current treatments or obtain information on new treatments for patients with cancer. When clinical trials show that a new treatment is better than the standard treatment, the new treatment may become the standard treatment.

Clinical trials are taking place in many parts of the country. Choosing the most appropriate cancer treatment is a decision that ideally involves the patient, family, and health care team.

Seven types of standard treatment are used:

Surgery

Treatment of gastrointestinal carcinoid tumors usually includes surgery. One of the following surgical procedures may be used:

- **Appendectomy:** Removal of the appendix.

- **Fulguration:** Use of an electric current to burn away the tumor using a special tool.

- **Cryosurgery:** A treatment that uses an instrument to freeze and destroy abnormal tissue, such as carcinoma in situ. This type of treatment is also called cryotherapy. The doctor may use ultrasound to guide the instrument.

- **Resection:** Surgery to remove part or all of the organ that contains cancer. Resection of the tumor and a small amount of normal tissue around it is called a local excision.

- **Bowel resection and anastomosis:** Removal of the bowel tumor and a small section of healthy bowel on each side. The healthy parts of the bowel are then sewn together (anastomosis). Lymph nodes are removed and checked by a pathologist to see if they contain cancer.

- **Radiofrequency ablation:** The use of a special probe with tiny electrodes that release high-energy radio waves (similar to microwaves) that kill cancer cells. The probe may be inserted through the skin or through an incision (cut) in the abdomen.

- **Hepatic resection:** Surgery to remove part or all of the liver.

- **Hepatic artery ligation or embolization:** A procedure to ligate (tie off) or embolize (block) the hepatic artery, the main blood vessel that brings blood into the liver. Blocking the flow of blood to the liver helps kill cancer cells growing there.

Radiation Therapy

Radiation therapy is a cancer treatment that uses high-energy x-rays or other types of radiation to kill cancer cells. There are two types of radiation therapy. External radiation therapy uses a machine outside the body to send radiation toward the cancer. Internal radiation therapy uses a radioactive substance sealed in needles, seeds, wires, or catheters that are placed directly into or near the cancer. The way the radiation therapy is given depends on the type and stage of the cancer being treated.

Chemotherapy

Chemotherapy is a cancer treatment that uses drugs to stop the growth of cancer cells, either by killing the cells or by stopping the cells from dividing. When chemotherapy is taken by mouth or injected into a vein or muscle, the drugs enter the bloodstream and can reach cancer cells throughout the body (systemic chemotherapy). When chemotherapy is placed directly into the spinal column, an organ, or a body cavity such as the abdomen, the drugs mainly affect cancer cells in those areas (regional chemotherapy).

Chemoembolization of the hepatic artery is a type of regional chemotherapy that may be used to treat a gastrointestinal carcinoid tumor that has spread to the liver. The anticancer drug is injected into the hepatic artery through a catheter (thin tube). The drug is mixed with a substance that embolizes (blocks) the artery, cutting off blood flow to the tumor. Most of the anticancer drug is trapped near the tumor and only a small amount of the drug reaches other parts of the body. The blockage may be temporary or permanent, depending on the substance used to block the artery. The tumor is prevented from getting the oxygen and nutrients it needs to grow. The liver continues to receive blood from the hepatic portal vein, which carries blood from the stomach and intestine.

The way the chemotherapy is given depends on the type and stage of the cancer being treated.

Percutaneous Ethanol Injection

Percutaneous ethanol injection is a cancer treatment in which a small needle is used to inject ethanol (alcohol) directly into a tumor to kill cancer cells. This procedure is also called intratumoral ethanol injection.

Biologic Therapy

Biologic therapy is a treatment that uses the patient's immune system to fight cancer. Substances made by the body or made in a

laboratory are used to boost, direct, or restore the body's natural defenses against cancer. This type of cancer treatment is also called
biotherapy or immunotherapy.

Hormone Therapy

Hormone therapy is a cancer treatment that removes hormones
or blocks their action and stops cancer cells from growing. Hormones
are substances produced by glands in the body and circulated in the
bloodstream. The presence of some hormones can cause certain cancers to grow. If tests show that the cancer cells have places where
hormones can attach (receptors), drugs, surgery, or radiation therapy
are used to reduce the production of hormones or block them from
working.

Other Drug Therapy

MIBG (metaiodobenzylguanidine) is sometimes used, with or without radioactive iodine (I131), to lessen the symptoms of gastrointestinal carcinoid tumors.

Other types of treatment are being tested in clinical trials.

Treatments being studied in clinical trials for gastrointestinal carcinoid tumors include new combinations of chemotherapy.

Treatment Options for Gastrointestinal Carcinoid Tumors

Localized Gastrointestinal Carcinoid Tumors

Carcinoid Tumors in the Appendix: Treatment of localized
gastrointestinal carcinoid tumors in the appendix may include the
following:

- Appendectomy

- Appendectomy and local excision

- Appendectomy, bowel resection with anastomosis, and removal
  of lymph nodes

Rectal Carcinoid Tumors: Treatment of localized gastrointestinal carcinoid tumors in the rectum may include the following:

- Fulguration

- Local excision
- Resection

Surgery that saves the sphincter muscles (the muscles that open and close the anus) may be possible.

Small Bowel Carcinoid Tumors: Treatment of localized gastrointestinal carcinoid tumors in the small intestine may include the following:

- Local excision
- Resection with removal of nearby lymph nodes

Gastric, Colon, and Pancreatic Carcinoid Tumors: Treatment of localized gastrointestinal carcinoid tumors in the stomach, colon, or pancreas is usually resection.

Regional Gastrointestinal Carcinoid Tumors

Treatment is usually surgery to remove all the cancer that can be seen at the site of the original tumor, as well as nearby tissues and lymph nodes.

If the tumor cannot be completely removed by surgery, treatment is usually palliative therapy to relieve symptoms and improve the patient's quality of life. This may include the following:

- Resection, cryosurgery, or radiofrequency ablation to remove as much of the tumor as possible.
- Chemoembolization to shrink tumors in the liver.

Metastatic Gastrointestinal Carcinoid Tumors

Distant Metastases: If the metastatic gastrointestinal carcinoid tumor is not causing symptoms, there may be a period of watchful waiting before treatment is given. Treatment of distant metastases of gastrointestinal carcinoid tumors is usually palliative therapy that may include the following:

- Surgery to bypass or remove part of a tumor blocking the small intestine.
- Chemotherapy, which may include chemoembolization.

- Radiation therapy, sometimes with radioisotopes such as radio-active iodine (I131).

- MIBG (metaiodobenzylguanidine) therapy.

- Biologic therapy or hormone therapy.

- Clinical trials of new treatments.

Carcinoid Syndrome: Treatment of metastatic gastrointestinal carcinoid tumors that are causing carcinoid syndrome may include the following:

- Resection, cryosurgery, radiofrequency ablation, or percutaneous ethanol injection for tumors in the liver.

- Hepatic artery ligation or embolization, with or without regional or systemic chemotherapy.

- Hormone therapy.

- Biologic therapy with or without chemotherapy.

- Clinical trials of new combinations of chemotherapy.

A heart valve replacement may be done for some patients with carcinoid syndrome.

This summary section refers to specific treatments under study in clinical trials, but it may not mention every new treatment being studied.

Recurrent Gastrointestinal Carcinoid Tumors

Treatment of recurrent gastrointestinal carcinoid tumors may include the following:

- Surgery to remove part or all of the tumor.

- A clinical trial.

Chapter 36

Esophageal Cancer

General Information about Esophageal Cancer

Esophageal cancer is a disease in which malignant (cancer) cells form in the tissues of the esophagus.

The esophagus is the hollow, muscular tube that moves food and liquid from the throat to the stomach. The wall of the esophagus is made up of several layers of tissue, including mucous membrane, muscle, and connective tissue. Esophageal cancer starts at the inside lining of the esophagus and spreads outward through the other layers as it grows.

The two most common forms of esophageal cancer are named for the type of cells that become malignant (cancerous):

- **Squamous cell carcinoma:** Cancer that forms in squamous cells, the thin, flat cells lining the esophagus. This cancer is most often found in the upper and middle part of the esophagus, but can occur anywhere along the esophagus. This is also called epidermoid carcinoma.

- **Adenocarcinoma:** Cancer that begins in glandular (secretory) cells. Glandular cells in the lining of the esophagus produce and release fluids such as mucus. Adenocarcinomas usually form in the lower part of the esophagus, near the stomach.

PDQ® Cancer Information Summary. National Cancer Institute; Bethesda, MD. Esophageal Cancer (PDQ®): Treatment—Patient. Updated 11/2004. Available at: http://www.cancer.gov. Accessed February 10, 2005.

Risk Factors

Smoking, heavy alcohol use, and Barrett esophagus can affect the risk of developing esophageal cancer.

Risk factors include the following:

- Tobacco use

- Heavy alcohol use

- Barrett esophagus: A condition in which the cells lining the lower part of the esophagus have changed or been replaced with abnormal cells that could lead to cancer of the esophagus. Gastric reflux (the backing up of stomach contents into the lower section of the esophagus) may irritate the esophagus and, over time, cause Barrett esophagus.

- Older age

- Being male

- Being African-American

Symptoms

The most common signs of esophageal cancer are painful or difficult swallowing and weight loss.

These and other symptoms may be caused by esophageal cancer or by other conditions. A doctor should be consulted if any of the following problems occur:

- Painful or difficult swallowing

- Weight loss

- Pain behind the breastbone

- Hoarseness and cough

- Indigestion and heartburn

Diagnosis

Tests that examine the esophagus are used to detect (find) and diagnose esophageal cancer.

The following tests and procedures may be used:

- **Chest x-ray:** An x-ray of the organs and bones inside the chest. An x-ray is a type of energy beam that can go through the body and onto film, making a picture of areas inside the body.

- **Barium swallow:** A series of x-rays of the esophagus and stomach. The patient drinks a liquid that contains barium (a silver-white metallic compound). The liquid coats the esophagus and x-rays are taken. This procedure is also called an upper GI series.

- **Esophagoscopy:** A procedure to look inside the esophagus to check for abnormal areas. An esophagoscope (a thin, lighted tube) is inserted through the mouth or nose and down the throat into the esophagus. Tissue samples may be taken for biopsy.

- **Biopsy:** The removal of cells or tissues so they can be viewed under a microscope to check for signs of cancer. The biopsy is usually done during an esophagoscopy. Sometimes a biopsy shows changes in the esophagus that are not cancer but may lead to cancer.

Prognosis

Certain factors affect prognosis (chance of recovery) and treatment options.

The prognosis (chance of recovery) and treatment options depend on the following:

- The stage of the cancer (whether it affects part of the esophagus, involves the whole esophagus, or has spread to other places in the body)

- The size of the tumor

- The patient's general health

When esophageal cancer is found very early, there is a better chance of recovery. Esophageal cancer is often in an advanced stage when it is diagnosed. At later stages, esophageal cancer can be treated but rarely can be cured. Taking part in one of the clinical trials being done to improve treatment should be considered.

Stages of Esophageal Cancer

After esophageal cancer has been diagnosed, tests are done to find out if cancer cells have spread within the esophagus or to other parts of the body.

The process used to find out if cancer cells have spread within the esophagus or to other parts of the body is called staging. The information gathered from the staging process determines the stage of the disease. It is important to know the stage in order to plan treatment. The following tests and procedures may be used in the staging process:

- **Bronchoscopy:** A procedure to look inside the trachea and large airways in the lung for abnormal areas. A bronchoscope (a thin, lighted tube) is inserted through the nose or mouth into the trachea and lungs. Tissue samples may be taken for biopsy.

- **Chest x-ray:** An x-ray of the organs and bones inside the chest. An x-ray is a type of energy beam that can go through the body and onto film, making a picture of areas inside the body.

- **Laryngoscopy:** A procedure in which the doctor examines the larynx (voice box) with a mirror or with a laryngoscope (a thin, lighted tube).

- **CT scan (CAT scan):** A procedure that makes a series of detailed pictures of areas inside the body, taken from different angles. The pictures are made by a computer linked to an x-ray machine. A dye may be injected into a vein or swallowed to help the organs or tissues show up more clearly. This test is also called computed tomography, computerized tomography, or computerized axial tomography.

- **Endoscopic ultrasound (EUS):** A procedure in which an endoscope (a thin, lighted tube) is inserted into the body. The endoscope is used to bounce high-energy sound waves (ultrasound) off internal tissues or organs and make echoes. The echoes form a picture of body tissues called a sonogram. This procedure is also called endosonography.

- **Thoracoscopy:** A surgical procedure to look at the organs inside the chest to check for abnormal areas. An incision (cut) is made between two ribs and a thoracoscope (a thin, lighted tube) is inserted into the chest. Tissue samples and lymph nodes may be removed for biopsy. In some cases, this procedure may be used to remove portions of the esophagus or lung.

- **Laparoscopy:** A surgical procedure to look at the organs inside the abdomen to check for signs of disease. Small incisions (cuts) are made in the wall of the abdomen, and a laparoscope (a thin, lighted tube) is inserted into one of the incisions. Other instruments may be inserted through the same or other incisions to perform procedures such as removing organs or taking tissue samples for biopsy.

- **PET scan (positron emission tomography scan):** A procedure to find malignant tumor cells in the body. A small amount of radionuclide glucose (sugar) is injected into a vein. The PET scanner rotates around the body and makes a picture of where glucose is being used in the body. Malignant tumor cells show up brighter in the picture because they are more active and take up more glucose than normal cells. The use of PET for staging esophageal cancer is being studied in clinical trials.

The following stages are used for esophageal cancer:

Stage 0 (Carcinoma in Situ)

In stage 0, cancer is found only in the innermost layer of cells lining the esophagus. Stage 0 is also called carcinoma in situ.

Stage I

In stage I, cancer has spread beyond the innermost layer of cells to the next layer of tissue in the wall of the esophagus.

Stage II

Stage II esophageal cancer is divided into stage IIA and stage IIB, depending on where the cancer has spread.

- **Stage IIA:** Cancer has spread to the layer of esophageal muscle or to the outer wall of the esophagus.

- **Stage IIB:** Cancer may have spread to any of the first three layers of the esophagus and to nearby lymph nodes.

Stage III

In stage III, cancer has spread to the outer wall of the esophagus and may have spread to tissues or lymph nodes near the esophagus.

Stage IV

Stage IV esophageal cancer is divided into stage IVA and stage IVB, depending on where the cancer has spread.

- **Stage IVA:** Cancer has spread to nearby or distant lymph nodes.

- **Stage IVB:** Cancer has spread to distant lymph nodes or organs in other parts of the body.

411

Recurrent Esophageal Cancer

Recurrent esophageal cancer is cancer that has recurred (come back) after it has been treated. The cancer may come back in the esophagus or in other parts of the body.

Treatment Option Overview

Different types of treatment are available for patients with esophageal cancer. Some treatments are standard (the currently used treatment), and some are being tested in clinical trials. Before starting treatment, patients may want to think about taking part in a clinical trial. A treatment clinical trial is a research study meant to help improve current treatments or obtain information on new treatments for patients with cancer. When clinical trials show that a new treatment is better than the standard treatment, the new treatment may become the standard treatment.

Clinical trials are taking place in many parts of the country. Choosing the most appropriate cancer treatment is a decision that ideally involves the patient, family, and health care team.

Five types of standard treatment are used:

Surgery

Surgery is the most common treatment for cancer of the esophagus. Part of the esophagus may be removed in an operation called an esophagectomy. The doctor will connect the remaining healthy part of the esophagus to the stomach so the patient can still swallow. A plastic tube or part of the intestine may be used to make the connection. Lymph nodes near the esophagus may also be removed and viewed under a microscope to see if they contain cancer. If the esophagus is partly blocked by the tumor, an expandable metal stent (tube) may be placed inside the esophagus to help keep it open.

Radiation Therapy

Radiation therapy is a cancer treatment that uses high-energy x-rays or other types of radiation to kill cancer cells. There are two types of radiation therapy. External radiation therapy uses a machine outside the body to send radiation toward the cancer. Internal radiation therapy uses a radioactive substance sealed in needles, seeds, wires, or catheters that are placed directly into or near the cancer. The way the radiation therapy is given depends on the type and stage of the cancer being treated.

A plastic tube may be inserted into the esophagus to keep it open during radiation therapy. This is called intraluminal intubation and dilation.

Chemotherapy

Chemotherapy is a cancer treatment that uses drugs to stop the growth of cancer cells, either by killing the cells or by stopping the cells from dividing. When chemotherapy is taken by mouth or injected into a vein or muscle, the drugs enter the bloodstream and can reach cancer cells throughout the body (systemic chemotherapy). When chemotherapy is placed directly into the spinal column, an organ, or a body cavity such as the abdomen, the drugs mainly affect cancer cells in those areas (regional chemotherapy). The way the chemotherapy is given depends on the type and stage of the cancer being treated.

Laser Therapy

Laser therapy is a cancer treatment that uses a laser beam (a narrow beam of intense light) to kill cancer cells.

Electrocoagulation

Electrocoagulation is the use of an electric current to kill cancer cells.

Other types of treatment are being tested in clinical trials.

Patients have special nutritional needs during treatment for esophageal cancer.

Many people with esophageal cancer find it hard to eat because they have difficulty swallowing. The esophagus may be narrowed by the tumor or as a side effect of treatment. Some patients may receive nutrients directly into a vein. Others may need a feeding tube (a flexible plastic tube that is passed through the nose or mouth into the stomach) until they are able to eat on their own.

Treatment Options by Stage

Stage 0 Esophageal Cancer (Carcinoma in Situ)

Treatment of stage 0 esophageal cancer (carcinoma in situ) is usually surgery.

Stage I Esophageal Cancer

Treatment of stage I esophageal cancer may include the following:

- Surgery
- Clinical trials of chemotherapy plus radiation therapy, with or without surgery
- Clinical trials of new therapies used before or after surgery

Stage II Esophageal Cancer

Treatment of stage II esophageal cancer may include the following:

- Surgery
- Clinical trials of chemotherapy plus radiation therapy, with or without surgery
- Clinical trials of new therapies used before or after surgery

Stage III Esophageal Cancer

Treatment of stage III esophageal cancer may include the following:

- Surgery
- Clinical trials of chemotherapy plus radiation therapy, with or without surgery
- Clinical trials of new therapies used before or after surgery

Stage IV Esophageal Cancer

Treatment of stage IV esophageal cancer may include the following:

- External or internal radiation therapy as palliative therapy to relieve symptoms and improve quality of life
- Laser surgery or electrocoagulation as palliative therapy to relieve symptoms and improve quality of life
- Chemotherapy
- Clinical trials of chemotherapy

Treatment Options for Recurrent Esophageal Cancer

Treatment of recurrent esophageal cancer may include the following:

- Use of any standard treatments as palliative therapy to relieve symptoms and improve quality of life
- Clinical trials of new therapies used before or after surgery

This summary section refers to specific treatments under study in clinical trials, but it may not mention every new treatment being studied.

Chapter 37

Gastric Cancer

General Information about Gastric Cancer

Gastric cancer is a disease in which malignant (cancer) cells form in the lining of the stomach.

The stomach is a J-shaped organ in the upper abdomen. It is part of the digestive system, which processes nutrients (vitamins, minerals, carbohydrates, fats, proteins, and water) in foods that are eaten and helps pass waste material out of the body. Food moves from the throat to the stomach through a hollow, muscular tube called the esophagus. After leaving the stomach, partly digested food passes into the small intestine and then into the large intestine (the colon).

The wall of the stomach is made up of three layers of tissue: the mucosal (innermost) layer, the muscularis (middle) layer, and the serosal (outermost) layer. Gastric cancer begins in the cells lining the mucosal layer and spreads through the outer layers as it grows.

Stromal tumors of the stomach begin in supporting connective tissue and are treated differently from gastric cancer.

Risk Factors

Age, diet, and stomach disease can affect the risk of developing gastric cancer.

PDQ® Cancer Information Summary. National Cancer Institute; Bethesda, MD. Gastric Cancer (PDQ®): Treatment—Patient. Updated 4/2004. Available at http://www.cancer.gov. Accessed February 10, 2005.

Risk factors include the following:

- *Helicobacter pylori* infection of the stomach
- Chronic gastritis (inflammation of the stomach)
- Older age
- Being male
- A diet high in salted, smoked, or poorly preserved foods and low in fruits and vegetables
- Pernicious anemia
- Smoking cigarettes
- Intestinal metaplasia
- Familial adenomatous polyposis (FAP) or gastric polyps
- A mother, father, sister, or brother who has had stomach cancer

Symptoms

Possible signs of gastric cancer include indigestion and stomach discomfort or pain. These and other symptoms may be caused by gastric cancer or by other conditions.

In the early stages of gastric cancer, the following symptoms may occur:

- Indigestion and stomach discomfort
- A bloated feeling after eating
- Mild nausea
- Loss of appetite
- Heartburn

In more advanced stages of gastric cancer, the following symptoms may occur:

- Blood in the stool
- Vomiting
- Weight loss (unexplained)
- Stomach pain
- Jaundice (yellowing of eyes and skin)
- Ascites (buildup of fluid in the abdomen)
- Difficulty swallowing

A doctor should be consulted if any of these problems occur.

Diagnosis

Tests that examine the stomach and esophagus are used to detect (find) and diagnose gastric cancer.

The following tests and procedures may be used:

- **Physical exam and history:** An exam of the body to check general signs of health, including checking for signs of disease, such as lumps or anything else that seems unusual. A history of the patient's health habits and past illnesses and treatments will also be taken.

- **Blood chemistry studies:** A procedure in which a blood sample is checked to measure the amounts of certain substances released into the blood by organs and tissues in the body. An unusual (higher or lower than normal) amount of a substance can be a sign of disease in the organ or tissue that produces it.

- **Complete blood count:** A procedure in which a sample of blood is drawn and checked for the following:

  - The number of red blood cells, white blood cells, and platelets
  - The amount of hemoglobin (the protein that carries oxygen) in the red blood cells
  - The portion of the sample made up of red blood cells

- **Upper endoscopy:** A procedure to look inside the esophagus, stomach, and duodenum (first part of the small intestine) to check for abnormal areas. An endoscope (a thin, lighted tube) is passed through the mouth and down the throat into the esophagus.

- **Fecal occult blood test:** A test to check stool (solid waste) for blood that can only be seen with a microscope. Small samples of stool are placed on special cards and returned to the doctor or laboratory for testing.

- **Barium swallow:** A series of x-rays of the esophagus and stomach. The patient drinks a liquid that contains barium (a silver-white metallic compound). The liquid coats the esophagus and stomach and x-rays are taken. This procedure is also called an upper GI series.

- **Biopsy:** The removal of cells or tissues so they can be viewed under a microscope to check for signs of cancer. A biopsy of the stomach is usually done during the endoscopy.

- **CT scan (CAT scan):** A procedure that makes a series of detailed pictures of areas inside the body, taken from different angles. The pictures are made by a computer linked to an x-ray machine. A dye may be injected into a vein or swallowed to help the organs or tissues show up more clearly. This procedure is also called computed tomography, computerized tomography, or computerized axial tomography.

Prognosis

The prognosis (chance of recovery) and treatment options depend on the following:

- The stage and extent of the cancer (whether it is in the stomach only or has spread to lymph nodes or other places in the body)
- The patient's general health

When gastric cancer is found very early, there is a better chance of recovery. Gastric cancer is often in an advanced stage when it is diagnosed. At later stages, gastric cancer can be treated but rarely can be cured. Taking part in one of the clinical trials being done to improve treatment should be considered.

Stages of Gastric Cancer

After gastric cancer has been diagnosed, tests are done to find out if cancer cells have spread within the stomach or to other parts of the body.

The process used to find out if cancer has spread within the stomach or to other parts of the body is called staging. The information gathered from the staging process determines the stage of the disease. It is important to know the stage in order to plan treatment.

The following tests and procedures may be used in the staging process:

- **ß-hCG (beta-human chorionic gonadotropin), CA-125, and CEA (carcinoembryonic antigen) assays:** Tests that measure the levels of ß-hCG, CA-125, and CEA in the blood. These substances are released into the bloodstream from both cancer cells and normal cells. When found in higher than normal amounts, they can be a sign of gastric cancer or other conditions.

- **Chest x-ray:** An x-ray of the organs and bones inside the chest. An x-ray is a type of energy beam that can go through the body and onto film, making a picture of areas inside the body.

- **Endoscopic ultrasound (EUS):** A procedure in which an endoscope (a thin, lighted tube) is inserted into the body. The endoscope is used to bounce high-energy sound waves (ultrasound) off internal tissues or organs and make echoes. The echoes form a picture of body tissues called a sonogram. This procedure is also called endosonography.

- **CT scan (CAT scan):** A procedure that makes a series of detailed pictures of areas inside the body, taken from different angles. The pictures are made by a computer linked to an x-ray machine. A dye may be injected into a vein or swallowed to help the organs or tissues show up more clearly. This procedure is also called computed tomography, computerized tomography, or computerized axial tomography.

- **Laparoscopy:** A surgical procedure to look at the organs inside the abdomen to check for signs of disease. Small incisions (cuts) are made in the wall of the abdomen and a laparoscope (a thin, lighted tube) is inserted into one of the incisions. Other instruments may be inserted through the same or other incisions to remove lymph nodes or take tissue samples for biopsy.

- **PET scan (positron emission tomography scan):** A procedure to find malignant tumor cells in the body. A small amount of radionuclide glucose (sugar) is injected into a vein. The PET scanner rotates around the body and makes a picture of where glucose is being used in the body. Malignant tumor cells show up brighter in the picture because they are more active and take up more glucose than normal cells.

The following stages are used for gastric cancer:

Stage 0 (Carcinoma in Situ)

In stage 0, cancer is found only in the inside lining of the mucosal (innermost) layer of the stomach wall. Stage 0 is also called carcinoma in situ.

Stage I

Stage I gastric cancer is divided into stage IA and stage IB, depending on where the cancer has spread.

- **Stage IA:** Cancer has spread completely through the mucosal (innermost) layer of the stomach wall.

- **Stage IB:** Cancer has spread:
  - completely through the mucosal (innermost) layer of the stomach wall and is found in up to six lymph nodes near the tumor; or
  - to the muscularis (middle) layer of the stomach wall.

Stage II

In stage II gastric cancer, cancer has spread:

- completely through the mucosal (innermost) layer of the stomach wall and is found in seven to fifteen lymph nodes near the tumor; or
- to the muscularis (middle) layer of the stomach wall and is found in up to six lymph nodes near the tumor; or
- to the serosal (outermost) layer of the stomach wall but not to lymph nodes or other organs.

Stage III

Stage III gastric cancer is divided into stage IIIA and stage IIIB depending on where the cancer has spread.

- **Stage IIIA:** Cancer has spread to:
  - the muscularis (middle) layer of the stomach wall and is found in seven to fifteen lymph nodes near the tumor; or
  - the serosal (outermost) layer of the stomach wall and is found in one to six lymph nodes near the tumor; or
  - organs next to the stomach but not to lymph nodes or other parts of the body.
- **Stage IIIB:** Cancer has spread to the serosal (outermost) layer of the stomach wall and is found in seven to fifteen lymph nodes near the tumor.

Stage IV

In stage IV, cancer has spread to:

- organs next to the stomach and to at least one lymph node; or
- more than fifteen lymph nodes; or
- other parts of the body.

Recurrent Gastric Cancer

Recurrent gastric cancer is cancer that has recurred (come back) after it has been treated. The cancer may come back in the stomach or in other parts of the body such as the liver or lymph nodes.

Treatment Option Overview

Different types of treatments are available for patients with gastric cancer. Some treatments are standard (the currently used treatment), and some are being tested in clinical trials. Before starting treatment, patients may want to think about taking part in a clinical trial. A treatment clinical trial is a research study meant to help improve current treatments or obtain information on new treatments for patients with cancer. When clinical trials show that a new treatment is better than the "standard" treatment, the new treatment may become the standard treatment.

Clinical trials are taking place in many parts of the country. Choosing the most appropriate cancer treatment is a decision that ideally involves the patient, family, and health care team.

Standard Treatment

Four types of standard treatment are used:

Surgery: Surgery is a common treatment of all stages of gastric cancer. The following types of surgery may be used:

- *Subtotal gastrectomy:* Removal of the part of the stomach that contains cancer, nearby lymph nodes, and parts of other tissues and organs near the tumor. The spleen may be removed. The spleen is an organ in the upper abdomen that filters the blood and removes old blood cells.

- *Total gastrectomy:* Removal of the entire stomach, nearby lymph nodes, and parts of the esophagus, small intestine, and other tissues near the tumor. The spleen may be removed. The esophagus is connected to the small intestine so the patient can continue to eat and swallow.

If the tumor is blocking the opening to the stomach but the cancer cannot be completely removed by standard surgery, the following procedures may be used:

- *Endoluminal stent placement:* A procedure to insert a stent (a thin, expandable tube) in order to keep a passage (such as arteries or the esophagus) open. For tumors blocking the opening to the stomach, surgery may be done to place a stent from the esophagus to the stomach to allow the patient to eat normally.

- *Endoscopic laser surgery:* A procedure in which an endoscope (a thin, lighted tube) with a laser attached is inserted into the body. A laser is an intense beam of light that can be used as a knife.

- *Electrocautery:* A procedure that uses an electrical current to create heat. This is sometimes used to remove lesions or control bleeding.

Chemotherapy: Chemotherapy is a cancer treatment that uses drugs to stop the growth of cancer cells, either by killing the cells or by stopping the cells from dividing. When chemotherapy is taken by mouth or injected into a vein or muscle, the drugs enter the bloodstream and can reach cancer cells throughout the body (systemic chemotherapy). When chemotherapy is placed directly into the spinal column, an organ, or a body cavity such as the abdomen, the drugs mainly affect cancer cells in those areas. The way the chemotherapy is given depends on the type and stage of the cancer being treated.

Radiation Therapy: Radiation therapy is a cancer treatment that uses high-energy x-rays or other types of radiation to kill cancer cells. There are two types of radiation therapy. External radiation therapy uses a machine outside the body to send radiation toward the cancer. Internal radiation therapy uses a radioactive substance sealed in needles, seeds, wires, or catheters that are placed directly into or near the cancer. The way the radiation therapy is given depends on the type and stage of the cancer being treated.

Chemoradiation: Chemoradiation combines chemotherapy and radiation therapy to increase the effects of both. Chemoradiation treatment given after surgery to increase the chances of a cure is called adjuvant therapy. If it is given before surgery, it is called neoadjuvant therapy.

Clinical Trials

Other types of treatment are being tested in clinical trials. These include the following:

Biologic Therapy: Biologic therapy is a treatment that uses the patient's immune system to fight cancer. Substances made by the body or made in a laboratory are used to boost, direct, or restore the body's natural defenses against cancer. This type of cancer treatment is also called biotherapy or immunotherapy.

This summary section refers to specific treatments under study in clinical trials, but it may not mention every new treatment being studied.

Treatment Options by Stage

Stage 0 Gastric Cancer (Carcinoma in Situ)

Treatment of stage 0 gastric cancer is usually surgery (total or subtotal gastrectomy).

Stage I and Stage II Gastric Cancer

Treatment of stage I and stage II gastric cancer may include the following:

- Surgery (total or subtotal gastrectomy)
- Surgery (total or subtotal gastrectomy) followed by chemoradiation therapy
- A clinical trial of chemoradiation therapy given before surgery

Stage III Gastric Cancer

Treatment of stage III gastric cancer may include the following:

- Surgery (total gastrectomy)
- Surgery followed by chemoradiation therapy
- A clinical trial of chemoradiation therapy given before surgery

Stage IV Gastric Cancer

Treatment of stage IV gastric cancer that has not spread to distant organs may include the following:

- Surgery (total gastrectomy) followed by chemoradiation therapy
- A clinical trial of chemoradiation therapy given before surgery

Treatment of stage IV gastric cancer that has spread to distant organs may include the following:

- Chemotherapy as palliative therapy to relieve symptoms and improve the quality of life

- Endoscopic laser surgery or endoluminal stent placement as palliative therapy to relieve symptoms and improve the quality of life

- Radiation therapy as palliative therapy to stop bleeding, relieve pain, or shrink a tumor that is blocking the opening to the stomach

- Surgery as palliative therapy to stop bleeding or shrink a tumor that is blocking the opening to the stomach

Treatment Options for Recurrent Gastric Cancer

Treatment of recurrent gastric cancer may include the following:

- Chemotherapy as palliative therapy to relieve symptoms and improve the quality of life

- Endoscopic laser surgery or electrocautery as palliative therapy to relieve symptoms and improve the quality of life

- Radiation therapy as palliative therapy to stop bleeding, relieve pain, or shrink a tumor that is blocking the stomach

- A clinical trial of new anticancer drugs or biologic therapy

This summary section refers to specific treatments under study in clinical trials, but it may not mention every new treatment being studied.

Chapter 38

Small Intestine Cancer

General Information about Small Intestine Cancer

Small intestine cancer is a rare disease in which malignant (cancer) cells form in the tissues of the small intestine.

The small intestine is part of the body's digestive system, which also includes the esophagus, stomach, and large intestine. The digestive system removes and processes nutrients (vitamins, minerals, carbohydrates, fats, proteins, and water) from foods and helps pass waste material out of the body. The small intestine is a long tube that connects the stomach to the large intestine. It folds many times to fit inside the abdomen.

Types

There are five types of small intestine cancer.

The types of cancer found in the small intestine are adenocarcinoma, sarcoma, carcinoid tumors, gastrointestinal stromal tumors, and lymphoma. This summary discusses adenocarcinoma and leiomyosarcoma (a type of sarcoma).

Adenocarcinoma starts in glandular cells in the lining of the small intestine and is the most common type of small intestine cancer. Most of these tumors occur in the part of the small intestine near the stomach. They may grow and block the intestine.

PDQ® Cancer Information Summary. National Cancer Institute; Bethesda, MD. Small Intestine Cancer (PDQ®): Treatment—Patient. Updated 1/2005. Available at http://www.cancer.gov. Accessed February 11, 2005.

Leiomyosarcoma starts in the smooth muscle cells of the small intestine. Most of these tumors occur in the part of the small intestine near the large intestine.

Risk Factors

Diet and health history can affect the risk of developing small intestine cancer.

Risk factors include the following:

- Eating a high-fat diet
- Having Crohn disease
- Having celiac disease
- Having familial adenomatous polyposis (FAP)

Symptoms

Possible signs of small intestine cancer include abdominal pain and unexplained weight loss.

These and other symptoms may be caused by small intestine cancer or by other conditions. A doctor should be consulted if any of the following problems occur:

- Pain or cramps in the middle of the abdomen
- Weight loss with no known reason
- A lump in the abdomen
- Blood in the stool

Diagnosis

Tests that examine the small intestine are used to detect (find), diagnose, and stage small intestine cancer.

Procedures that create pictures of the small intestine and the area around it help diagnose small intestine cancer and show how far the cancer has spread. The process used to find out if cancer cells have spread within and around the small intestine is called staging.

In order to plan treatment, it is important to know the type of small intestine cancer and whether the tumor can be removed by surgery. Tests and procedures to detect, diagnose, and stage small intestine cancer are usually done at the same time. The following tests and procedures may be used:

- **Physical exam and history:** An exam of the body to check general signs of health, including checking for signs of disease, such as lumps or anything else that seems unusual. A history of the patient's health habits and past illnesses and treatments will also be taken.

- **Blood chemistry studies:** A procedure in which a blood sample is checked to measure the amounts of certain substances released into the blood by organs and tissues in the body. An unusual (higher or lower than normal) amount of a substance can be a sign of disease in the organ or tissue that produces it.

- **Liver function tests:** A procedure in which a blood sample is checked to measure the amounts of certain substances released into the blood by the liver. A higher than normal amount of a substance can be a sign of liver disease that may be caused by small intestine cancer.

- **Abdominal x-ray:** An x-ray of the organs in the abdomen. An x-ray is a type of energy beam that can go through the body onto film, making a picture of areas inside the body.

- **Barium enema:** A series of x-rays of the lower gastrointestinal (GI) tract. A liquid that contains barium (a silver-white metallic compound) is put into the rectum. The barium coats the lower gastrointestinal tract and x-rays are taken. This procedure is also called a lower GI series.

- **Fecal occult blood test:** A test to check stool (solid waste) for blood that can be seen only with a microscope. Small samples of stool are placed on special cards and returned to the doctor or laboratory for testing.

- **Upper endoscopy:** A procedure to look at the inside of the esophagus, stomach, and duodenum (first part of the small intestine, near the stomach). An endoscope (a thin, lighted tube) is inserted through the mouth and into the esophagus, stomach, and duodenum. Tissue samples may be taken for biopsy.

- **Upper GI series with small bowel follow-through:** A series of x-rays of the esophagus, stomach, and small bowel. The patient drinks a liquid that contains barium (a silver-white metallic compound). The liquid coats the esophagus, stomach, and small bowel. X-rays are taken at different times as the barium travels through the upper GI tract and small bowel.

- **Biopsy:** The removal of cells or tissues so they can be viewed under a microscope to check for signs of cancer. This may be done during the endoscopy. The sample is checked by a pathologist to see if it contains cancer cells.

- **CT scan (CAT scan):** A procedure that makes a series of detailed pictures of areas inside the body, taken from different angles. The pictures are made by a computer linked to an x-ray machine. A dye may be injected into a vein or swallowed to help the organs or tissues show up more clearly. This procedure is also called computed tomography, computerized tomography, or computerized axial tomography.

- **Lymph node biopsy:** The removal of all or part of a lymph node. A pathologist views the tissue under a microscope to look for cancer cells.

- **Laparotomy:** A surgical procedure in which an incision (cut) is made in the wall of the abdomen to check the inside of the abdomen for signs of disease. The size of the incision depends on the reason the laparotomy is being done. Sometimes organs are removed or tissue samples are taken for biopsy.

Prognosis

The prognosis (chance of recovery) and treatment options depend on the following:

- The type of small intestine cancer
- Whether the cancer has spread to other places in the body
- Whether the cancer can be completely removed by surgery
- Whether the cancer is newly diagnosed or has recurred

Stages of Small Intestine Cancer

Tests and procedures to stage small intestine cancer are usually done at the same time as diagnosis. Staging is used to find out how far the cancer has spread, but treatment decisions are not based on stage.

Small intestine cancer is grouped according to whether or not the tumor can be completely removed by surgery. Treatment depends on whether the tumor can be removed by surgery and if the cancer is being treated as a primary tumor or is metastatic cancer.

Recurrent Small Intestine Cancer

Recurrent small intestine cancer is cancer that has recurred (come back) after it has been treated. The cancer may come back in the small intestine or in other parts of the body.

Treatment Option Overview

Different types of treatments are available for patients with small intestine cancer. Some treatments are standard (the currently used treatment), and some are being tested in clinical trials. Before starting treatment, patients may want to think about taking part in a clinical trial. A treatment clinical trial is a research study meant to help improve current treatments or obtain information on new treatments for patients with cancer. When clinical trials show that a new treatment is better than the standard treatment, the new treatment may become the standard treatment.

Clinical trials are taking place in many parts of the country. Choosing the most appropriate cancer treatment is a decision that ideally involves the patient, family, and health care team.

Standard Treatment

Three types of standard treatment are used:

Surgery: Surgery is the most common treatment of small intestine cancer. One of the following types of surgery may be done:

- *Resection:* Surgery to remove part or all of an organ that contains cancer. The resection may include the small intestine and nearby organs (if the cancer has spread). The doctor may remove the section of the small intestine that contains cancer and perform an anastomosis (joining the cut ends of the intestine together). The doctor will usually remove lymph nodes near the small intestine and examine them under a microscope to see whether they contain cancer.

- *Bypass:* Surgery to allow food in the small intestine to go around (bypass) a tumor that is blocking the intestine but cannot be removed.

Even if the doctor removes all the cancer that can be seen at the time of the surgery, some patients may be given radiation therapy after surgery to kill any cancer cells that are left. Treatment given after the surgery, to increase the chances of a cure, is called adjuvant therapy.

Radiation Therapy: Radiation therapy is a cancer treatment that uses high-energy x-rays or other types of radiation to kill cancer cells. There are two types of radiation therapy. External radiation therapy uses a machine outside the body to send radiation toward the cancer. Internal radiation therapy uses a radioactive substance sealed in needles, seeds, wires, or catheters that are placed directly into or near the cancer. The way the radiation therapy is given depends on the type and stage of the cancer being treated.

Chemotherapy: Chemotherapy is a cancer treatment that uses drugs to stop the growth of cancer cells, either by killing the cells or by stopping the cells from dividing. When chemotherapy is taken by mouth or injected into a vein or muscle, the drugs enter the bloodstream and can reach cancer cells throughout the body (systemic chemotherapy). When chemotherapy is placed directly into the spinal column, an organ, or a body cavity such as the abdomen, the drugs mainly affect cancer cells in those areas (regional chemotherapy). The way the chemotherapy is given depends on the type and stage of the cancer being treated.

Clinical Trials

Other types of treatment are being tested in clinical trials. These include the following:

Biologic Therapy: Biologic therapy is a treatment that uses the patient's immune system to fight cancer. Substances made by the body or made in a laboratory are used to boost, direct, or restore the body's natural defenses against cancer. This type of cancer treatment is also called biotherapy or immunotherapy.

Radiation Therapy with Radiosensitizers: Radiosensitizers are drugs that make tumor cells more sensitive to radiation therapy. Combining radiation therapy with radiosensitizers may kill more tumor cells.

This summary section refers to specific treatments under study in clinical trials, but it may not mention every new treatment being studied.

Treatment Options for Small Intestine Cancer

Small Intestine Adenocarcinoma

When possible, treatment of small intestine adenocarcinoma will be surgery to remove the tumor and some of the normal tissue around it.

Treatment of small intestine adenocarcinoma that cannot be removed by surgery may include the following:

- Surgery to bypass the tumor

- Radiation therapy as palliative therapy to relieve symptoms and improve the patient's quality of life

- A clinical trial of radiation therapy with radiosensitizers, with or without chemotherapy

- A clinical trial of new anticancer drugs

- A clinical trial of biologic therapy

Small Intestine Leiomyosarcoma

When possible, treatment of small intestine leiomyosarcoma will be surgery to remove the tumor and some of the normal tissue around it.

Treatment of small intestine leiomyosarcoma that cannot be removed by surgery may include the following:

- Surgery (to bypass the tumor) and radiation therapy

- Surgery, radiation therapy, or chemotherapy as palliative therapy to relieve symptoms and improve the patient's quality of life

- A clinical trial of new anticancer drugs

- A clinical trial of biologic therapy

Recurrent Small Intestine Cancer

Treatment of recurrent small intestine cancer that has spread to other parts of the body is usually a clinical trial of new anticancer drugs or biologic therapy.

Treatment of locally recurrent small intestine cancer may include the following:

433

- Surgery

- Radiation therapy or chemotherapy as palliative therapy to relieve symptoms and improve the patient's quality of life

- A clinical trial of radiation therapy with radiosensitizers, with or without chemotherapy

This summary section refers to specific treatments under study in clinical trials, but it may not mention every new treatment being studied.

Chapter 39

Colon Cancer

General Information about Colon Cancer

Colon cancer is a disease in which malignant (cancer) cells form in the tissues of the colon.

The colon is part of the body's digestive system. The digestive system removes and processes nutrients (vitamins, minerals, carbohydrates, fats, proteins, and water) from foods and helps pass waste material out of the body. The digestive system is made up of the esophagus, stomach, and the small and large intestines. The first six feet of the large intestine are called the large bowel or colon. The last six inches are the rectum and the anal canal. The anal canal ends at the anus (the opening of the large intestine to the outside of the body).

Risk Factors

Age and health history can affect the risk of developing colon cancer.

Risk factors include the following:

- Age fifty or older

- A family history of cancer of the colon or rectum

PDQ® Cancer Information Summary. National Cancer Institute; Bethesda, MD. Colon Cancer (PDQ®): Treatment—Patient. Updated 1/2005. Available at http://www.cancer.gov. Accessed February 10, 2005.

- A personal history of cancer of the colon, rectum, ovary, endometrium, or breast

- A history of polyps in the colon

- A history of ulcerative colitis (ulcers in the lining of the large intestine) or Crohn disease

- Certain hereditary conditions, such as familial adenomatous polyposis and hereditary nonpolyposis colon cancer (HNPCC; Lynch syndrome)

Symptoms

Possible signs of colon cancer include a change in bowel habits or blood in the stool.

These and other symptoms may be caused by colon cancer or by other conditions. A doctor should be consulted if any of the following problems occur:

- A change in bowel habits

- Blood (either bright red or very dark) in the stool

- Diarrhea, constipation, or feeling that the bowel does not empty completely

- Stools that are narrower than usual

- General abdominal discomfort (frequent gas pains, bloating, fullness, or cramps)

- Weight loss with no known reason

- Constant tiredness

- Vomiting

Diagnosis

Tests that examine the rectum, rectal tissue, and blood are used to detect (find) and diagnose colon cancer.

The following tests and procedures may be used:

- **Physical exam and history:** An exam of the body to check general signs of health, including checking for signs of disease, such as lumps or anything else that seems unusual. A history of the patient's health habits and past illnesses and treatments will also be taken.

- **Fecal occult blood test:** A test to check stool (solid waste) for blood that can be seen only with a microscope. Small samples of stool are placed on special cards and returned to the doctor or laboratory for testing.

- **Digital rectal exam:** An exam of the rectum. The doctor or nurse inserts a lubricated, gloved finger into the rectum to feel for lumps or abnormal areas.

- **Barium enema:** A series of x-rays of the lower gastrointestinal tract. A liquid that contains barium (a silver-white metallic compound) is put into the rectum. The barium coats the lower gastrointestinal tract and x-rays are taken. This procedure is also called a lower GI series.

- **Sigmoidoscopy:** A procedure to look inside the rectum and sigmoid (lower) colon for polyps, abnormal areas, or cancer. A sigmoidoscope (a thin, lighted tube) is inserted through the rectum into the sigmoid colon. Polyps or tissue samples may be taken for biopsy.

- **Colonoscopy:** A procedure to look inside the rectum and colon for polyps, abnormal areas, or cancer. A colonoscope (a thin, lighted tube) is inserted through the rectum into the colon. Polyps or tissue samples may be taken for biopsy.

- **Biopsy:** The removal of cells or tissues so they can be viewed under a microscope to check for signs of cancer.

- **Virtual colonoscopy:** A procedure that uses a series of x-rays called computed tomography to make a series of pictures of the colon. A computer puts the pictures together to create detailed images that may show polyps and anything else that seems unusual on the inside surface of the colon. This test is also called colonography or CT colonography.

Prognosis

Certain factors affect prognosis (chance of recovery) and treatment options.

The prognosis (chance of recovery) depends on the following:

- The stage of the cancer (whether the cancer is in the inner lining of the colon only, involves the whole colon, or has spread to other places in the body)

- Whether the cancer has blocked or created a hole in the colon

- The blood levels of carcinoembryonic antigen (CEA; a substance in the blood that may be increased when cancer is present) before treatment begins
- Whether the cancer has recurred
- The patient's general health

Treatment options depend on the following:

- The stage of the cancer
- Whether the cancer has recurred
- The patient's general health

Stages of Colon Cancer

After colon cancer has been diagnosed, tests are done to find out if cancer cells have spread within the colon or to other parts of the body.

The process used to find out if cancer has spread within the colon or to other parts of the body is called staging. The information gathered from the staging process determines the stage of the disease. It is important to know the stage in order to plan treatment. The following tests and procedures may be used in the staging process:

- **CT scan (CAT scan):** A procedure that makes a series of detailed pictures of areas inside the body, taken from different angles. The pictures are made by a computer linked to an x-ray machine. A dye may be injected into a vein or swallowed to help the organs or tissues show up more clearly. This procedure is also called computed tomography, computerized tomography, or computerized axial tomography.

- **Lymph node biopsy:** The removal of all or part of a lymph node. A pathologist views the tissue under a microscope to look for cancer cells.

- **Complete blood count:** A procedure in which a sample of blood is drawn and checked for the following:
  - The number of red blood cells, white blood cells, and platelets
  - The amount of hemoglobin (the protein that carries oxygen) in the red blood cells
  - The portion of the sample made up of red blood cells

- **Carcinoembryonic antigen (CEA) assay:** A test that measures the level of CEA in the blood. CEA is released into the bloodstream from both cancer cells and normal cells. When found in higher than normal amounts, it can be a sign of colon cancer or other conditions.

- **MRI (magnetic resonance imaging):** A procedure that uses a magnet, radio waves, and a computer to make a series of detailed pictures of areas inside the colon. A substance called gadolinium is injected into the patient through a vein. The gadolinium collects around the cancer cells so they show up brighter in the picture. This procedure is also called nuclear magnetic resonance imaging (NMRI).

- **Chest x-ray:** An x-ray of the organs and bones inside the chest. An x-ray is a type of energy beam that can go through the body and onto film, making a picture of areas inside the body.

- **Surgery:** A procedure to remove the tumor and see how far it has spread through the colon.

The following stages are used for colon cancer:

Stage 0 (Carcinoma in Situ)

In stage 0, the cancer is found in the innermost lining of the colon only. Stage 0 cancer is also called carcinoma in situ.

Stage I

In stage I, the cancer has spread beyond the innermost tissue layer of the colon wall to the middle layers. Stage I colon cancer is sometimes called Dukes A colon cancer.

Stage II

Stage II colon cancer is divided into stage IIA and stage IIB.

- **Stage IIA:** Cancer has spread beyond the middle tissue layers of the colon wall or has spread to nearby tissues around the colon or rectum.

- **Stage IIB:** Cancer has spread beyond the colon wall into nearby organs or through the peritoneum.

Stage II colon cancer is sometimes called Dukes B colon cancer.

Stage III

Stage III colon cancer is divided into stage IIIA, stage IIIB, and stage IIIC.

- **Stage IIIA:** Cancer has spread from the innermost tissue layer of the colon wall to the middle layers and has spread to as many as three lymph nodes.

- **Stage IIIB:** Cancer has spread to as many as three nearby lymph nodes and has spread:

  - beyond the middle tissue layers of the colon wall; or

  - to nearby tissues around the colon or rectum; or

  - beyond the colon wall into nearby organs or through the peritoneum.

- **Stage IIIC:** Cancer has spread to four or more nearby lymph nodes and has spread:

  - to or beyond the middle tissue layers of the colon wall; or

  - to nearby tissues around the colon or rectum; or

  - to nearby organs or through the peritoneum.

Stage III colon cancer is sometimes called Dukes C colon cancer.

Stage IV

In stage IV, cancer may have spread to nearby lymph nodes and has spread to other parts of the body, such as the liver or lungs. Stage IV colon cancer is sometimes called Dukes D colon cancer.

Recurrent Colon Cancer

Recurrent colon cancer is cancer that has recurred (come back) after it has been treated. The cancer may come back in the colon or in other parts of the body, such as the liver, lungs, or both.

Treatment Option Overview

Different types of treatment are available for patients with colon cancer. Some treatments are standard (the currently used treatment), and some are being tested in clinical trials. Before starting treatment, patients may want to think about taking part in a clinical trial. A treatment clinical trial is a research study meant to help improve current treatments or obtain information on new treatments for patients with cancer. When clinical trials show that a new treatment is better than the "standard" treatment, the new treatment may become the standard treatment.

Clinical trials are taking place in many parts of the country. Choosing the most appropriate cancer treatment is a decision that ideally involves the patient, family, and health care team.

Standard Treatment

Three types of standard treatment are used. These include the following:

Surgery: Surgery (removing the cancer in an operation) is the most common treatment for all stages of colon cancer. A doctor may remove the cancer using one of the following types of surgery:

- *Local excision:* If the cancer is found at a very early stage, the doctor may remove it without cutting through the abdominal wall. Instead, the doctor may put a tube through the rectum into the colon and cut the cancer out. This is called a local excision. If the cancer is found in a polyp (a small bulging piece of tissue), the operation is called a polypectomy.

- *Resection:* If the cancer is larger, the doctor will perform a partial colectomy (removing the cancer and a small amount of healthy tissue around it). The doctor may then perform an anastomosis (sewing the healthy parts of the colon together). The doctor will also usually remove lymph nodes near the colon and examine them under a microscope to see whether they contain cancer.

- *Resection and colostomy:* If the doctor is not able to sew the two ends of the colon back together, a stoma (an opening) is made on the outside of the body for waste to pass through. This procedure is called a colostomy. Sometimes the colostomy is needed only until the lower colon has healed, and then it can be reversed. If the doctor needs to remove the entire lower colon, however, the colostomy may be permanent.

- *Radiofrequency ablation:* The use of a special probe with tiny electrodes that kill cancer cells. Sometimes the probe is inserted directly through the skin and only local anesthesia is needed. In other cases, the probe is inserted through an incision in the abdomen. This is done in the hospital with general anesthesia.

- *Cryosurgery:* A treatment that uses an instrument to freeze and destroy abnormal tissue, such as carcinoma in situ. This type of treatment is also called cryotherapy.

Even if the doctor removes all the cancer that can be seen at the time of the operation, some patients may be given chemotherapy or radiation therapy after surgery to kill any cancer cells that are left. Treatment given after the surgery, to increase the chances of a cure, is called adjuvant therapy.

Chemotherapy: Chemotherapy is a cancer treatment that uses drugs to stop the growth of cancer cells, either by killing the cells or by stopping the cells from dividing. When chemotherapy is taken by mouth or injected into a vein or muscle, the drugs enter the bloodstream and can reach cancer cells throughout the body (systemic chemotherapy). When chemotherapy is placed directly into the spinal column, an organ, or a body cavity such as the abdomen, the drugs mainly affect cancer cells in those areas.

Chemoembolization of the hepatic artery may be used to treat cancer that has spread to the liver. This involves blocking the hepatic artery (the main artery that supplies blood to the liver) and injecting anticancer drugs between the blockage and the liver. The liver's arteries then deliver the drugs throughout the liver. Only a small amount of the drug reaches other parts of the body. The blockage may be temporary or permanent, depending on what is used to block the artery. The liver continues to receive some blood from the hepatic portal vein, which carries blood from the stomach and intestine.

The way the chemotherapy is given depends on the type and stage of the cancer being treated.

Radiation Therapy: Radiation therapy is a cancer treatment that uses high-energy x-rays or other types of radiation to kill cancer cells. There are two types of radiation therapy. External radiation therapy uses a machine outside the body to send radiation toward the cancer. Internal radiation therapy uses a radioactive substance sealed in needles, seeds, wires, or catheters that are placed directly into or near the cancer. The way the radiation therapy is given depends on the type and stage of the cancer being treated.

Clinical Trials

Other types of treatment are being tested in clinical trials. These include the following:

Biologic Therapy: Biologic therapy is a treatment that uses the patient's immune system to fight cancer. Substances made by the body or made in a laboratory are used to boost, direct, or restore the body's natural defenses against cancer. This type of cancer treatment is also called biotherapy or immunotherapy.

This summary section refers to specific treatments under study in clinical trials, but it may not mention every new treatment being studied.

Follow-Up Exams

Follow-up exams may help find recurrent colon cancer earlier.

After treatment, a blood test to measure carcinoembryonic antigen (CEA; a substance in the blood that may be increased when colon cancer is present) may be done along with other tests to see if the cancer has come back.

Treatment Options for Colon Cancer

Stage 0 Colon Cancer (Carcinoma in Situ)

Treatment of stage 0 (carcinoma in situ) may include the following types of surgery:

- Local excision or simple polypectomy
- Resection/anastomosis. This is done when the cancerous tissue is too large to remove by local excision.

Stage I Colon Cancer

Treatment of stage I colon cancer is usually resection/anastomosis.

Stage II Colon Cancer

Treatment of stage II colon cancer may include the following:

- Resection/anastomosis
- Clinical trials of chemotherapy, radiation therapy, or biologic therapy after surgery

Stage III Colon Cancer

Treatment of stage III colon cancer may include the following:

- Resection/anastomosis with chemotherapy
- Clinical trials of chemotherapy, radiation therapy, or biologic therapy after surgery

Stage IV and Recurrent Colon Cancer

Treatment of stage IV and recurrent colon cancer may include the following:

- Resection/anastomosis (surgery to remove the cancer or bypass the tumor and join the cut ends of the colon)
- Surgery to remove parts of other organs, such as the liver, lungs, and ovaries, where the cancer may have recurred or spread
- Radiation therapy or chemotherapy may be offered to some patients as palliative therapy to relieve symptoms and improve quality of life.
- Clinical trials of chemotherapy or biologic therapy

Treatment of locally recurrent colon cancer may be local excision. Special treatments of cancer that has spread to or recurred in the liver may include the following:

- Radiofrequency ablation or cryosurgery
- Clinical trials of hepatic chemoembolization with radiation therapy

Patients whose colon cancer spreads or recurs after initial treatment with chemotherapy may be offered further chemotherapy with a different drug or combination of drugs.

This summary section refers to specific treatments under study in clinical trials, but it may not mention every new treatment being studied.

Chapter 40

Rectal Cancer

General Information about Rectal Cancer

Rectal cancer is a disease in which malignant (cancer) cells form in the tissues of the rectum.

The rectum is part of the body's digestive system. The digestive system removes and processes nutrients (vitamins, minerals, carbohydrates, fats, proteins, and water) from foods and helps pass waste material out of the body. The digestive system is made up of the esophagus, stomach, and the small and large intestines. The first six feet of the large intestine are called the large bowel or colon. The last six inches are the rectum and the anal canal. The anal canal ends at the anus (the opening of the large intestine to the outside of the body).

Risk Factors

Age and family history can affect the risk of developing rectal cancer.

The following are possible risk factors for rectal cancer:

- Age fifty years or older

PDQ® Cancer Information Summary. National Cancer Institute; Bethesda, MD. Rectal Cancer (PDQ®): Treatment—Patient. Updated 1/2005. Available at: http://www.cancer.gov. Accessed February 10, 2005.

- A family history of cancer of the colon or rectum

- A personal history of cancer of the colon, rectum, ovary, endometrium, or breast

- A history of ulcerative colitis (ulcers in the lining of the large intestine) or Crohn disease

- Certain hereditary conditions, such as familial adenomatous polyposis and hereditary nonpolyposis colon cancer (HNPCC; Lynch syndrome)

Symptoms

Possible signs of rectal cancer include a change in bowel habits or blood in the stool.

These and other symptoms may be caused by rectal cancer or other conditions. A doctor should be consulted if any of the following problems occur:

- A change in bowel habits

- Blood (either bright red or very dark) in the stool

- Diarrhea, constipation, or feeling that the bowel does not empty completely

- Stools that are narrower than usual

- General abdominal discomfort (frequent gas pains, bloating, fullness, or cramps)

- Weight loss with no known reason

- Constant tiredness

- Vomiting

Diagnosis

Tests that examine the rectum and colon are used to detect (find) and diagnose rectal cancer.

Tests used in diagnosing rectal cancer include the following:

- **Fecal occult blood test:** A test to check stool (solid waste) for blood that can be seen only with a microscope. Small samples of stool are placed on special cards and returned to the doctor or laboratory for testing.

- **Digital rectal exam:** An exam of the rectum. The doctor or nurse inserts a lubricated, gloved finger into the rectum to feel for lumps or abnormal areas.

- **Barium enema:** A series of x-rays of the lower gastrointestinal tract. A liquid that contains barium (a silver-white metallic compound) is put into the rectum. The barium coats the lower gastrointestinal tract and x-rays are taken. This procedure is also called a lower GI series.

- **Sigmoidoscopy:** A procedure to look inside the rectum and sigmoid (lower) colon for polyps, abnormal areas, or cancer. A sigmoidoscope (a thin, lighted tube) is inserted through the rectum into the sigmoid colon. Polyps or tissue samples may be taken for biopsy.

- **Colonoscopy:** A procedure to look inside the rectum and colon for polyps, abnormal areas, or cancer. A colonoscope (a thin, lighted tube) is inserted through the rectum into the colon. Polyps or tissue samples may be taken for biopsy.

- **Biopsy:** The removal of cells or tissues so they can be viewed under a microscope to check for signs of cancer.

Prognosis

The prognosis (chance of recovery) and treatment options depend on the following:

- The stage of the cancer (whether it affects the inner lining of the rectum only, involves the whole rectum, or has spread to other places in the body)

- The patient's general health

- Whether the cancer has just been diagnosed or has recurred (come back)

Stages of Rectal Cancer

After rectal cancer has been diagnosed, tests are done to find out if cancer cells have spread within the rectum or to other parts of the body.

The process used to find out whether cancer has spread within the rectum or to other parts of the body is called staging. The information gathered from the staging process determines the stage of the disease. It is important to know the stage in order to plan treatment. The following tests and procedures may be used in the staging process:

- **Digital rectal exam:** An exam of the rectum. The doctor or nurse inserts a lubricated, gloved finger into the rectum to feel for lumps or abnormal areas.

- **CT scan (CAT scan):** A procedure that makes a series of detailed pictures of areas inside the body, taken from different angles. The pictures are made by a computer linked to an x-ray machine. A dye may be injected into a vein or swallowed to help the organs or tissues show up more clearly. This procedure is also called computed tomography, computerized tomography, or computerized axial tomography.

- **MRI (magnetic resonance imaging):** A procedure that uses a magnet, radio waves, and a computer to make a series of detailed pictures of areas inside the body. This procedure is also called nuclear magnetic resonance imaging (NMRI).

- **Sigmoidoscopy or colonoscopy and biopsy:** A procedure to look inside the rectum and colon for polyps, abnormal areas, or cancer. A sigmoidoscope or colonoscope is inserted through the rectum into the colon. Polyps or tissue samples may be taken for biopsy.

- **Endoscopic ultrasound (EUS):** A procedure in which an endoscope (a thin, lighted tube) is inserted into the body. The endoscope is used to bounce high-energy sound waves (ultrasound) off internal tissues or organs and make echoes. The echoes form a picture of body tissues called a sonogram. This procedure is also called endosonography.

The following stages are used for rectal cancer:

Stage 0 (Carcinoma in Situ)

In stage 0, cancer is found in the innermost lining of the rectum only. Stage 0 cancer is also called carcinoma in situ.

Stage I

In stage I, cancer has spread beyond the innermost lining of the rectum to the second and third layers and involves the inside wall of the rectum, but it has not spread to the outer wall of the rectum or outside the rectum. Stage I rectal cancer is sometimes called Dukes A rectal cancer.

Stage II

In stage II, cancer has spread outside the rectum to nearby tissue, but it has not gone into the lymph nodes (small, bean-shaped structures found throughout the body that filter substances in a fluid called lymph and help fight infection and disease). Stage II rectal cancer is sometimes called Dukes B rectal cancer.

Stage III

In stage III, cancer has spread to nearby lymph nodes, but it has not spread to other parts of the body. Stage III rectal cancer is sometimes called Dukes C rectal cancer.

Stage IV

In stage IV, cancer has spread to other parts of the body, such as the liver, lungs, or ovaries. Stage IV rectal cancer is sometimes called Dukes D rectal cancer.

Recurrent Rectal Cancer

Recurrent rectal cancer is cancer that has recurred (come back) after it has been treated. The cancer may come back in the rectum or in other parts of the body, such as the colon, pelvis, liver, or lungs.

Treatment Option Overview

Different types of treatment are available for patients with rectal cancer. Some treatments are standard (the currently used treatment), and some are being tested in clinical trials. Before starting treatment, patients may want to think about taking part in a clinical trial. A treatment clinical trial is a research study meant to help improve current treatments or obtain information on new treatments for patients with cancer. When clinical trials show that a new treatment is better than the standard treatment, the new treatment may become the standard treatment

Clinical trials are taking place in many parts of the country. Choosing the most appropriate cancer treatment is a decision that ideally involves the patient, family, and health care team.

Standard Treatment

Three types of standard treatment are used:

Surgery: Surgery is the most common treatment for all stages of rectal cancer. A doctor may remove the cancer using one of the following types of surgery:

- *Local excision:* If the cancer is found at a very early stage, the doctor may remove it without cutting into the abdomen. If the cancer is found in a polyp (a growth that protrudes from the rectal mucous membrane), the operation is called a polypectomy.

- *Resection:* If the cancer is larger, the doctor will perform a resection of the rectum (removing the cancer and a small amount of healthy tissue around it). The doctor will then perform an anastomosis (sewing the healthy parts of the rectum together, sewing the remaining rectum to the colon, or sewing the colon to the anus). The doctor will also take out lymph nodes near the rectum and examine them under a microscope to see if they contain cancer.

- *Resection and colostomy:* If the doctor is not able to sew the rectum back together, a stoma (an opening) is made on the outside of the body for waste to pass through. This procedure is called a colostomy. Sometimes the colostomy is needed only until the rectum has healed, and then it can be reversed. If the doctor needs to remove the entire rectum, however, the colostomy may be permanent.

Even if the doctor removes all the cancer that can be seen at the time of the operation, some patients may be offered chemotherapy or radiation therapy after surgery to kill any cancer cells that are left. Treatment given after surgery to increase the chances of a cure is called adjuvant therapy.

Radiation Therapy: Radiation therapy is a cancer treatment that uses high-energy x-rays or other types of radiation to kill cancer cells. There are two types of radiation therapy. External radiation therapy uses a machine outside the body to send radiation toward the cancer. Internal radiation therapy uses a radioactive substance sealed in needles, seeds, wires, or catheters that are placed directly into or near the cancer. The way the radiation therapy is given depends on the type and stage of the cancer being treated.

Chemotherapy: Chemotherapy is a cancer treatment that uses drugs to stop the growth of cancer cells, either by killing the cells or by stopping the cells from dividing. When chemotherapy is taken by mouth or injected into a vein or muscle, the drugs enter the bloodstream and can reach cancer cells throughout the body (systemic chemotherapy). When chemotherapy is placed directly in the spinal column, an organ, or a body cavity such as the abdomen, the drugs mainly affect cancer cells in those areas (regional chemotherapy). The way the chemotherapy is given depends on the type and stage of the cancer being treated.

After treatment, a blood test to measure amounts of carcinoembryonic antigen (a substance in the blood that may be increased when cancer is present) may be done to see if the cancer has come back.

Clinical Trials

Other types of treatment are being tested in clinical trials. These include the following:

Chemotherapy and Biologic Therapy: Biologic therapy is a treatment that uses the patient's immune system to fight cancer. Substances made by the body or made in a laboratory are used to boost, direct, or restore the body's natural defenses against cancer. This type of cancer treatment is also called biotherapy or immunotherapy.

This summary section refers to specific treatments under study in clinical trials, but it may not mention every new treatment being studied.

Treatment Options by Stage

Stage 0 Rectal Cancer

Treatment of stage 0 (carcinoma in situ) rectal cancer may include the following:

- Local excision (surgery to remove the tumor without cutting into the abdomen) or simple polypectomy (surgery to remove a growth that protrudes from the rectal mucous membrane)

- Resection (surgery to remove the cancer). This is done when the cancerous tissue is too large to remove by local excision.

- Internal or external radiation therapy

Stage I Rectal Cancer

Treatment of stage I rectal cancer may include the following:

- Surgery to remove the tumor with or without anastomosis (joining the cut ends of the rectum)
- Surgery to remove the tumor with or without radiation therapy and chemotherapy
- Internal or external radiation therapy

Stage II Rectal Cancer

Treatment of stage II rectal cancer may include the following:

- Resection with or without anastomosis (joining the cut ends of the rectum and colon, or the colon and anus) followed by chemotherapy and radiation therapy
- Partial or total pelvic exenteration (surgery to remove the organs and nearby structures of the pelvis), depending on where the cancer has spread. Surgery is followed by radiation therapy and chemotherapy.
- Radiation therapy with or without chemotherapy followed by surgery and chemotherapy
- Radiation therapy during surgery followed by external-beam radiation therapy and chemotherapy
- A clinical trial evaluating new treatment options

Stage III Rectal Cancer

Treatment of stage III rectal cancer may include the following:

- Resection with or without anastomosis (joining the cut ends of the rectum and colon, or the colon and anus) followed by chemotherapy and radiation therapy
- Partial or total pelvic exenteration (surgery to remove the organs and nearby structures of the pelvis), depending on where the cancer has spread. Surgery is followed by radiation therapy and chemotherapy.
- Radiation therapy with or without chemotherapy followed by surgery and chemotherapy

- Radiation therapy during surgery followed by external-beam radiation therapy and chemotherapy
- Chemotherapy and radiation therapy to relieve symptoms caused by advanced cancer
- A clinical trial evaluating new treatment options

Stage IV Rectal Cancer

Treatment of stage IV rectal cancer may include the following:

- Resection/anastomosis (surgery to remove the cancer and join the cut ends of the rectum and colon, or colon and anus) to relieve symptoms caused by advanced cancer
- Surgery to remove parts of other organs, such as the liver, lung, and ovaries, where the cancer may have spread
- Chemotherapy and radiation therapy to relieve symptoms caused by advanced cancer
- Chemotherapy following surgery
- Clinical trials of chemotherapy and biological therapy

This summary section refers to specific treatments under study in clinical trials, but it may not mention every new treatment being studied.

Treatment Options for Recurrent Rectal Cancer

Treatment of recurrent rectal cancer may include the following:

- Surgery to remove the tumor or as palliative therapy to relieve symptoms caused by advanced cancer
- Surgery to remove parts of other organs, such as the liver, lungs, and ovaries, where the cancer may have spread
- Radiation therapy or chemotherapy as palliative therapy to reduce the size of the tumor and relieve symptoms caused by advanced cancer

Chapter 41

Gallbladder Cancer

General Information about Gallbladder Cancer

Gallbladder cancer is a rare disease in which malignant (cancer) cells are found in the tissues of the gallbladder. The gallbladder is a pear-shaped organ that lies just under the liver in the upper abdomen. The gallbladder stores bile, a fluid made by the liver to digest fat. When food is being broken down in the stomach and intestines, bile is released from the gallbladder through a tube called the common bile duct, which connects the gallbladder and liver to the first part of the small intestine.

The wall of the gallbladder has three main layers of tissue:

* Mucosal (innermost) layer
* Muscularis (middle, muscle) layer
* Serosal (outer) layer

Between these layers is supporting connective tissue. Primary gallbladder cancer starts in the innermost layer and spreads through the outer layers as it grows.

Risk Factors

Being female can affect the risk of developing gallbladder cancer.

PDQ® Cancer Information Summary. National Cancer Institute; Bethesda, MD. Gallbladder Cancer (PDQ®): Treatment—Patient. Updated 6/2005. Available at http://www.cancer.gov. Accessed August 17, 2005.

Symptoms

Possible signs of gallbladder cancer include jaundice, pain, and fever.

These and other symptoms may be caused by gallbladder cancer. Other conditions may cause the same symptoms. A doctor should be consulted if any of the following problems occur:

- Jaundice (yellowing of the skin and whites of the eyes)
- Pain above the stomach
- Fever
- Nausea and vomiting
- Bloating
- Lumps in the abdomen

Diagnosis

Gallbladder cancer is difficult to detect (find) and diagnose early. Gallbladder cancer is difficult to detect and diagnose for the following reasons:

- There aren't any noticeable signs or symptoms in the early stages of gallbladder cancer.
- The symptoms of gallbladder cancer, when present, are like the symptoms of many other illnesses.
- The gallbladder is hidden behind the liver.

Gallbladder cancer is sometimes found when the gallbladder is removed for other reasons. Patients with gallstones rarely develop gallbladder cancer.

Tests that examine the gallbladder and nearby organs are used to detect (find), diagnose, and stage gallbladder cancer.

Procedures that create pictures of the gallbladder and the area around it help diagnose gallbladder cancer and show how far the cancer has spread. The process used to find out if cancer cells have spread within and around the gallbladder is called staging.

In order to plan treatment, it is important to know if the gallbladder cancer can be removed by surgery. Tests and procedures to detect, diagnose, and stage gallbladder cancer are usually done at the same time. The following tests and procedures may be used:

- **Physical exam and history:** An exam of the body to check general signs of health, including checking for signs of disease, such as lumps or anything else that seems unusual. A history of the patient's health habits and past illnesses and treatments will also be taken.

- **Ultrasound exam:** A procedure in which high-energy sound waves (ultrasound) are bounced off internal tissues or organs and make echoes. The echoes form a picture of body tissues called a sonogram. An abdominal ultrasound is done to diagnose gallbladder cancer.

- **Liver function tests:** A procedure in which a blood sample is checked to measure the amounts of certain substances released into the blood by the liver. A higher than normal amount of a substance can be a sign of liver disease that may be caused by gallbladder cancer.

- **Carcinoembryonic antigen (CEA) assay:** A test that measures the level of CEA in the blood. CEA is released into the bloodstream from both cancer cells and normal cells. When found in higher than normal amounts, it can be a sign of gallbladder cancer or other conditions.

- **CA 19-9 assay:** A test that measures the level of CA 19-9 in the blood. CA 19-9 is released into the bloodstream from both cancer cells and normal cells. When found in higher than normal amounts, it can be a sign of gallbladder cancer or other conditions.

- **CT scan (CAT scan):** A procedure that makes a series of detailed pictures of areas inside the body, taken from different angles. The pictures are made by a computer linked to an x-ray machine. A dye may be injected into a vein or swallowed to help the organs or tissues show up more clearly. This procedure is also called computed tomography, computerized tomography, or computerized axial tomography.

- **Blood chemistry studies:** A procedure in which a blood sample is checked to measure the amounts of certain substances released into the blood by organs and tissues in the body. An unusual (higher or lower than normal) amount of a substance can be a sign of disease in the organ or tissue that produces it.

- **Chest x-ray:** An x-ray of the organs and bones inside the chest. An x-ray is a type of energy beam that can go through the body and onto film, making a picture of areas inside the body.

- **MRI (magnetic resonance imaging):** A procedure that uses a magnet, radio waves, and a computer to make a series of detailed pictures of areas inside the body. This procedure is also called nuclear magnetic resonance imaging (NMRI). A dye may be injected into the gallbladder area so the ducts (tubes) that carry bile from the liver to the gallbladder and from the gallbladder to the small intestine will show up better in the image. This procedure is called MRCP (magnetic resonance cholangiopancreatography). To create detailed pictures of blood vessels near the gallbladder, the dye is injected into a vein. This procedure is called MRA (magnetic resonance angiography).

- **ERCP (endoscopic retrograde cholangiopancreatography):** A procedure used to x-ray the ducts (tubes) that carry bile from the liver to the gallbladder and from the gallbladder to the small intestine. Sometimes gallbladder cancer causes these ducts to narrow and block or slow the flow of bile, causing jaundice. An endoscope (a thin, lighted tube) is passed through the mouth, esophagus, and stomach into the first part of the small intestine. A catheter (a smaller tube) is then inserted through the endoscope into the bile ducts. A dye is injected through the catheter into the ducts and an x-ray is taken. If the ducts are blocked by a tumor, a fine tube may be inserted into the duct to unblock it. This tube (or stent) may be left in place to keep the duct open. Tissue samples may also be taken.

- **Biopsy:** The removal of cells or tissues so they can be viewed under a microscope by a pathologist to check for signs of cancer. The biopsy may be done after surgery to remove the tumor. If the tumor clearly cannot be removed by surgery, the biopsy may be done using a fine needle to remove cells from the tumor.

- **Laparoscopy:** A surgical procedure to look at the organs inside the abdomen to check for signs of disease. Small incisions (cuts) are made in the wall of the abdomen and a laparoscope (a thin, lighted tube) is inserted into one of the incisions. Other instruments may be inserted through the same or other incisions to perform procedures such as removing organs or taking tissue samples for biopsy. The laparoscopy helps to determine if the cancer is within the gallbladder only or has spread to nearby tissues and if it can be removed by surgery.

- **PTC (percutaneous transhepatic cholangiography):** A procedure used to x-ray the liver and bile ducts. A thin needle is inserted through the skin below the ribs and into the liver. Dye is injected into the liver or bile ducts and an x-ray is taken. If a blockage is found, a thin, flexible tube called a stent is sometimes left in the liver to drain bile into the small intestine or a collection bag outside the body.

Prognosis

The prognosis (chance of recovery) and treatment options depend on the following:

- The stage of the cancer (whether the cancer has spread from the gallbladder to other places in the body)
- Whether the cancer can be completely removed by surgery
- The type of gallbladder cancer (how the cancer cell looks under a microscope)
- Whether the cancer has just been diagnosed or has recurred (come back)

Treatment may also depend on the age and general health of the patient and whether the cancer is causing symptoms.

Gallbladder cancer can be cured only if it is found before it has spread, when it can be removed by surgery. If the cancer has spread, palliative treatment can improve the patient's quality of life by controlling the symptoms and complications of this disease.

Taking part in one of the clinical trials being done to improve treatment should be considered.

Stages of Gallbladder Cancer

Tests and procedures to stage gallbladder cancer are usually done at the same time as diagnosis.

The following stages are used for gallbladder cancer:

Stage 0 (Carcinoma in Situ)

In stage 0, cancer is found only in the innermost (mucosal) layer of the gallbladder. Stage 0 cancer is also called carcinoma in situ.

Stage I

Stage I is divided into stage IA and stage IB.

459

- **Stage IA:** Cancer has spread beyond the innermost (mucosal) layer to the connective tissue or to the muscle (muscularis) layer.

- **Stage IB:** Cancer has spread beyond the muscle layer to the connective tissue around the muscle.

Stage II

Stage II is divided into stage IIA and stage IIB.

- **Stage IIA:** Cancer has spread beyond the visceral peritoneum (tissue that covers the gallbladder) or to the liver or one nearby organ (such as the stomach, small intestine, colon, pancreas, or bile ducts outside the liver).

- **Stage IIB:** Cancer has spread:
  - beyond the innermost layer to the connective tissue and to nearby lymph nodes; or
  - to the muscle layer and nearby lymph nodes; or
  - beyond the muscle layer to the connective tissue around the muscle and to nearby lymph nodes; or
  - through the visceral peritoneum (tissue that covers the gallbladder) or to the liver or to one nearby organ (such as the stomach, small intestine, colon, pancreas, or bile ducts outside the liver), and to nearby lymph nodes.

Stage III

In stage III, cancer has spread to a main blood vessel in the liver or to nearby organs and may have spread to nearby lymph nodes.

Stage IV

In stage IV, cancer has spread to nearby lymph nodes or to organs far away from the gallbladder.

For gallbladder cancer, stages are also grouped according to how the cancer may be treated. There are two treatment groups:

Localized (Stage I)

Cancer is found in the wall of the gallbladder and can be completely removed by surgery.

Unresectable (Stage II, Stage III, and Stage IV)

Cancer has spread through the wall of the gallbladder to surrounding tissues or organs or throughout the abdominal cavity. Except in patients whose cancer has spread only to lymph nodes, the cancer is unresectable (cannot be completely removed by surgery).

Recurrent Gallbladder Cancer

Recurrent gallbladder cancer is cancer that has recurred (come back) after it has been treated. The cancer may come back in the gallbladder or in other parts of the body.

Treatment Option Overview

Different types of treatments are available for patients with gallbladder cancer. Some treatments are standard (the currently used treatment), and some are being tested in clinical trials. Before starting treatment, patients may want to think about taking part in a clinical trial. A treatment clinical trial is a research study meant to help improve current treatments or obtain information on new treatments for patients with cancer. When clinical trials show that a new treatment is better than the standard treatment, the new treatment may become the standard treatment.

Clinical trials are taking place in many parts of the country. Choosing the most appropriate cancer treatment is a decision that ideally involves the patient, family, and health care team.

Standard Treatment

Three types of standard treatment are used:

Surgery: Gallbladder cancer may be treated with a cholecystectomy, surgery to remove the gallbladder and some of the tissues around it. Nearby lymph nodes may be removed. A laparoscope is sometimes used to guide gallbladder surgery. The laparoscope is attached to a video camera and inserted through an incision (port) in the abdomen. Surgical instruments are inserted through other ports to perform the surgery. Because there is a risk that gallbladder cancer cells may spread to these ports, tissue surrounding the port sites may also be removed.

If the cancer has spread and cannot be removed, the following types of palliative surgery may relieve symptoms:

- *Surgical biliary bypass:* If the tumor is blocking the small intestine and bile is building up in the gallbladder, a biliary bypass may be done. During this operation, the gallbladder or bile duct will be cut and sewn to the small intestine to create a new pathway around the blocked area.

- *Endoscopic stent placement:* If the tumor is blocking the bile duct, surgery may be done to put in a stent (a thin, flexible tube) to drain bile that has built up in the area. The stent may be placed through a catheter that drains to the outside of the body or the stent may go around the blocked area and drain the bile into the small intestine.

- *Percutaneous transhepatic biliary drainage:* A procedure done to drain bile when there is a blockage and endoscopic stent placement is not possible. An x-ray of the liver and bile ducts is done to locate the blockage. Images made by ultrasound are used to guide placement of a stent, which is left in the liver to drain bile into the small intestine or a collection bag outside the body. This procedure may be done to relieve jaundice before surgery.

Radiation therapy: Radiation therapy is a cancer treatment that uses high-energy x-rays or other types of radiation to kill cancer cells. There are two types of radiation therapy. External radiation therapy uses a machine outside the body to send radiation toward the cancer. Internal radiation therapy uses a radioactive substance sealed in needles, seeds, wires, or catheters that are placed directly into or near the cancer. The way the radiation therapy is given depends on the type and stage of the cancer being treated.

Chemotherapy: Chemotherapy is a cancer treatment that uses drugs to stop the growth of cancer cells, either by killing the cells or by stopping the cells from dividing. When chemotherapy is taken by mouth or injected into a vein or muscle, the drugs enter the bloodstream and can reach cancer cells throughout the body (systemic chemotherapy). When chemotherapy is placed directly into the spinal column, an organ, or a body cavity such as the abdomen, the drugs mainly affect cancer cells in those areas (regional chemotherapy). The way the chemotherapy is given depends on the type and stage of the cancer being treated.

Clinical Trials

New types of treatment are being tested in clinical trials. These include the following:

Radiosensitizers: Radiosensitizers are drugs that make tumor cells more sensitive to radiation therapy. Combining radiation therapy with radiosensitizers may kill more tumor cells.

This summary section refers to specific treatments under study in clinical trials, but it may not mention every new treatment being studied.

Treatment Options for Gallbladder Cancer

Localized Gallbladder Cancer

Treatment of localized gallbladder cancer may include the following:

- Surgery to remove the gallbladder and some of the tissue around it. The liver and nearby lymph nodes may also be removed. Radiation therapy with or without chemotherapy may follow surgery.

- Radiation therapy with or without chemotherapy

- A clinical trial of radiation therapy with radiosensitizers

Unresectable Gallbladder Cancer

Treatment of unresectable gallbladder cancer may include the following:

- Radiation therapy as palliative treatment, with or without surgery or the placement of stents, to relieve symptoms caused by blocked bile ducts

- Surgery as palliative treatment to relieve symptoms caused by blocked bile ducts

- Chemotherapy as palliative treatment to relieve symptoms caused by the cancer

- A clinical trial of internal radiation therapy or radiosensitizers

- A clinical trial of chemotherapy

This summary section refers to specific treatments under study in clinical trials, but it may not mention every new treatment being studied.

Recurrent Gallbladder Cancer

Treatment of recurrent gallbladder cancer is usually done in a clinical trial.

Chapter 42

Pancreatic Cancer

General Information about Pancreatic Cancer

Pancreatic cancer is a disease in which malignant (cancer) cells form in the tissues of the pancreas.

The pancreas is a gland about six inches long that is shaped like a thin pear lying on its side. The wider end of the pancreas is called the head, the middle section is called the body, and the narrow end is called the tail. The pancreas lies behind the stomach and in front of the spine.

The pancreas has two main jobs in the body:

- To produce juices that help digest (break down) food

- To produce hormones, such as insulin and glucagon, that help control blood sugar levels. Both of these hormones help the body use and store the energy it gets from food.

The digestive juices are produced by exocrine pancreas cells and the hormones are produced by endocrine pancreas cells. About 95 percent of pancreatic cancers begin in exocrine cells.

Risk Factors

Smoking and health history can affect the risk of developing pancreatic cancer.

PDQ® Cancer Information Summary. National Cancer Institute; Bethesda, MD. Pancreatic Cancer (PDQ®): Treatment—Patient. Updated 10/2004. Available at: http://www.cancer.gov. Accessed February 11, 2005.

The following are possible risk factors for pancreatic cancer:

- Smoking
- Long-standing diabetes
- Chronic pancreatitis
- Certain hereditary conditions, such as hereditary pancreatitis, multiple endocrine neoplasia type 1 syndrome, hereditary non-polyposis colon cancer (HNPCC; Lynch syndrome), von Hippel-Lindau syndrome, ataxia-telangiectasia, and the familial atypical multiple mole melanoma syndrome (FAMMM)

Symptoms

Possible signs of pancreatic cancer include jaundice, pain, and weight loss.

These symptoms can be caused by pancreatic cancer or other conditions. A doctor should be consulted if any of the following problems occur:

- Jaundice (yellowing of the skin and whites of the eyes)
- Pain in the upper or middle abdomen and back
- Unexplained weight loss
- Loss of appetite
- Fatigue

Diagnosis

Pancreatic cancer is difficult to detect and diagnose for the following reasons:

- There aren't any noticeable signs or symptoms in the early stages of pancreatic cancer
- The signs of pancreatic cancer, when present, are like the signs of many other illnesses
- The pancreas is hidden behind other organs such as the stomach, small intestine, liver, gallbladder, spleen, and bile ducts

Pancreatic cancer is usually diagnosed with tests and procedures that produce pictures of the pancreas and the area around it. The process used to find out if cancer cells have spread within and around the pancreas is called staging. Tests and procedures to detect, diagnose, and stage pancreatic cancer are usually done at the same time. In order to plan treatment, it is important to know the stage of the disease and whether or not the pancreatic cancer can be removed by surgery. The following tests and procedures may be used:

- **Chest x-ray:** An x-ray of the organs and bones inside the chest. An x-ray is a type of energy beam that can go through the body and onto film, making a picture of areas inside the body.

- **Physical exam and history:** An exam of the body to check general signs of health, including checking for signs of disease, such as lumps or anything else that seems unusual. A history of the patient's health habits and past illnesses and treatments will also be taken.

- **CT scan (CAT scan):** A procedure that makes a series of detailed pictures of areas inside the body, taken from different angles. The pictures are made by a computer linked to an x-ray machine. A dye may be injected into a vein or swallowed to help the organs or tissues show up more clearly. This procedure is also called computed tomography, computerized tomography, or computerized axial tomography. A spiral or helical CT scan makes a series of very detailed pictures of areas inside the body using an x-ray machine that scans the body in a spiral path.

- **MRI (magnetic resonance imaging):** A procedure that uses a magnet, radio waves, and a computer to make a series of detailed pictures of areas inside the body. This procedure is also called nuclear magnetic resonance imaging (NMRI).

- **PET scan (positron emission tomography scan):** A procedure to find malignant tumor cells in the body. A small amount of radionuclide glucose (sugar) is injected into a vein. The PET scanner rotates around the body and makes a picture of where glucose is being used in the body. Malignant tumor cells show up brighter in the picture because they are more active and take up more glucose than normal cells.

- **Endoscopic ultrasound (EUS):** A procedure in which an endoscope (a thin, lighted tube) is inserted into the body. The endoscope is used to bounce high-energy sound waves (ultrasound) off internal tissues or organs and make echoes. The echoes form a picture of body tissues called a sonogram. This procedure is also called endosonography.

- **Laparoscopy:** A surgical procedure to look at the organs inside the abdomen to check for signs of disease. Small incisions (cuts) are made in the wall of the abdomen and a laparoscope (a thin, lighted tube) is inserted into one of the incisions. Other instruments may be inserted through the same or other incisions to perform procedures such as removing organs or taking tissue samples for biopsy.

- **Endoscopic retrograde cholangiopancreatography (ERCP):** A procedure used to x-ray the ducts (tubes) that carry bile from the liver to the gallbladder and from the gallbladder to the small intestine. Sometimes pancreatic cancer causes these ducts to narrow and block or slow the flow of bile, causing jaundice. An endoscope (a thin, lighted tube) is passed through the mouth, esophagus, and stomach into the first part of the small intestine. A catheter (a smaller tube) is then inserted through the endoscope into the pancreatic ducts. A dye is injected through the catheter into the ducts and an x-ray is taken. If the ducts are blocked by a tumor, a fine tube may be inserted into the duct to unblock it. This tube (or stent) may be left in place to keep the duct open. Tissue samples may also be taken.

- **Percutaneous transhepatic cholangiography (PTC):** A procedure used to x-ray the liver and bile ducts. A thin needle is inserted through the skin below the ribs and into the liver. Dye is injected into the liver or bile ducts and an x-ray is taken. If a blockage is found, a thin, flexible tube called a stent is sometimes left in the liver to drain bile into the small intestine or a collection bag outside the body. This test is done only if ERCP cannot be done.

- **Biopsy:** The removal of cells or tissues so they can be viewed under a microscope to check for signs of cancer. There are several ways to do a biopsy for pancreatic cancer. A fine needle may be inserted into the pancreas during an x-ray or ultrasound to remove cells. Tissue may also be removed during a laparoscopy (a surgical incision made in the wall of the abdomen).

Prognosis

The prognosis (chance of recovery) and treatment options depend on the following:

- Whether or not the tumor can be removed by surgery

- The stage of the cancer (the size of the tumor and whether the cancer has spread outside the pancreas to nearby tissues or lymph nodes or to other places in the body)
- The patient's general health
- Whether the cancer has just been diagnosed or has recurred (come back)

Pancreatic cancer can be controlled only if it is found before it has spread, when it can be removed by surgery. If the cancer has spread, palliative treatment can improve the patient's quality of life by controlling the symptoms and complications of this disease.

Taking part in one of the clinical trials being done to improve treatment should be considered.

Stages of Pancreatic Cancer

Tests and procedures to stage pancreatic cancer are usually done at the same time as diagnosis.

The following stages are used for pancreatic cancer:

Stage I

In stage I, cancer is found in the pancreas only. Stage I is divided into stage IA and stage IB, based on the size of the tumor.

- **Stage IA:** The tumor is two centimeters or smaller.
- **Stage IB:** The tumor is larger than two centimeters.

Stage II

In stage II, cancer may have spread to nearby tissue and organs, and may have spread to lymph nodes near the pancreas. Stage II is divided into stage IIA and stage IIB, based on where the cancer has spread.

- **Stage IIA:** Cancer has spread to nearby tissue and organs but has not spread to nearby lymph nodes.
- **Stage IIB:** Cancer has spread to nearby lymph nodes and may have spread to nearby tissue and organs.

Stage III

In stage III, cancer has spread to the major blood vessels near the pancreas and may have spread to nearby lymph nodes.

Stage IV

In stage IV, cancer may be of any size and has spread to distant organs, such as the liver, lung, and peritoneal cavity. It may have also spread to organs and tissues near the pancreas or to lymph nodes.

Recurrent Pancreatic Cancer

Recurrent pancreatic cancer is cancer that has recurred (come back) after it has been treated. The cancer may come back in the pancreas or in other parts of the body.

Treatment Option Overview

Different types of treatment are available for patients with pancreatic cancer. Some treatments are standard (the currently used treatment), and some are being tested in clinical trials. Before starting treatment, patients may want to think about taking part in a clinical trial. A treatment clinical trial is a research study meant to help improve current treatments or obtain information on new treatments for patients with cancer. When clinical trials show that a new treatment is better than the standard treatment, the new treatment may become the standard treatment.

Clinical trials are taking place in many parts of the country. Choosing the most appropriate cancer treatment is a decision that ideally involves the patient, family, and health care team.

Standard Treatment

Three types of standard treatment are used:

Surgery: One of the following types of surgery may be used to take out the tumor:

- *Whipple procedure:* A surgical procedure in which the head of the pancreas, the gallbladder, part of the stomach, part of the small intestine, and the bile duct are removed. Enough of the pancreas is left to produce digestive juices and insulin.

- *Total pancreatectomy:* This operation removes the whole pancreas, part of the stomach, part of the small intestine, the common bile duct, the gallbladder, the spleen, and nearby lymph nodes.

- *Distal pancreatectomy:* The body and the tail of the pancreas and usually the spleen are removed.

If the cancer has spread and cannot be removed, the following types of palliative surgery may be done to relieve symptoms:

- *Surgical biliary bypass:* If cancer is blocking the small intestine and bile is building up in the gallbladder, a biliary bypass may be done. During this operation, the doctor will cut the gallbladder or bile duct and sew it to the small intestine to create a new pathway around the blocked area.

- *Endoscopic stent placement:* If the tumor is blocking the bile duct, surgery may be done to put in a stent (a thin tube) to drain bile that has built up in the area. The doctor may place the stent through a catheter that drains to the outside of the body or the stent may go around the blocked area and drain the bile into the small intestine.

- *Gastric bypass:* If the tumor is blocking the flow of food from the stomach, the stomach may be sewn directly to the small intestine so the patient can continue to eat normally.

Radiation Therapy: Radiation therapy is a cancer treatment that uses high-energy x-rays or other types of radiation to kill cancer cells. There are two types of radiation therapy. External radiation therapy uses a machine outside the body to send radiation toward the cancer. Internal radiation therapy uses a radioactive substance sealed in needles, seeds, wires, or catheters that are placed directly into or near the cancer. The way the radiation therapy is given depends on the type and stage of the cancer being treated.

Chemotherapy: Chemotherapy is a cancer treatment that uses drugs to stop the growth of cancer cells, either by killing the cells or by stopping the cells from dividing. When chemotherapy is taken by mouth or injected into a vein or muscle, the drugs enter the bloodstream and can reach cancer cells throughout the body (systemic chemotherapy). When chemotherapy is placed directly into the spinal column, an organ, or a body cavity such as the abdomen, the drugs mainly affect cancer cells in those areas (regional chemotherapy). The way the chemotherapy is given depends on the type and stage of the cancer being treated.

Clinical Trials

Other types of treatment are being tested in clinical trials. These include the following:

Biologic Therapy: Biologic therapy is a treatment that uses the patient's immune system to fight cancer. Substances made by the body or made in a laboratory are used to boost, direct, or restore the body's natural defenses against cancer. This type of cancer treatment is also called biotherapy or immunotherapy.

This summary section refers to specific treatments under study in clinical trials, but it may not mention every new treatment being studied.

Pain Treatment

Pain can occur when the tumor presses on nerves or other organs near the pancreas. When pain medicine is not enough, there are treatments that act on nerves in the abdomen to relieve the pain. The doctor may inject medicine into the area around affected nerves or may cut the nerves to block the feeling of pain. Radiation therapy with or without chemotherapy can also help relieve pain by shrinking the tumor.

Nutritional Issues

Surgery to remove the pancreas may interfere with the production of pancreatic enzymes that help to digest food. As a result, patients may have problems digesting food and absorbing nutrients into the body. To prevent malnutrition, the doctor may prescribe medicines that replace these enzymes.

Treatment Options by Stage

Stage I Pancreatic Cancer

Treatment of stage I pancreatic cancer may include the following:

- Surgery alone
- Surgery with chemotherapy and radiation therapy
- A clinical trial of surgery followed by radiation therapy with chemotherapy. Chemotherapy is given before, during, and after the radiation therapy.
- A clinical trial of surgery followed by chemotherapy

Stage IIA Pancreatic Cancer

Treatment of stage IIA pancreatic cancer may include the following:

- Surgery with or without chemotherapy and radiation therapy
- Radiation therapy with chemotherapy
- Palliative surgery to bypass blocked areas in ducts or the small intestine
- A clinical trial of surgery followed by radiation therapy with chemotherapy. Chemotherapy is given before, during, and after the radiation therapy.
- A clinical trial of surgery followed by chemotherapy
- A clinical trial of biologic therapy with radiation therapy or chemotherapy
- A clinical trial of radiation therapy combined with chemotherapy or radiosensitizers (drugs that make cancer cells more sensitive to radiation so more tumor cells are killed), followed by surgery
- A clinical trial of radiation therapy given during surgery or internal radiation therapy

Stage IIB Pancreatic Cancer

Treatment of stage IIB pancreatic cancer may include the following:

- Surgery with or without chemotherapy and radiation therapy
- Radiation therapy with chemotherapy
- Palliative surgery to bypass blocked areas in ducts or the small intestine
- A clinical trial of surgery followed by radiation therapy with chemotherapy. Chemotherapy is given before, during, and after the radiation therapy.
- A clinical trial of surgery followed by chemotherapy
- A clinical trial of biologic therapy with radiation therapy or chemotherapy
- A clinical trial of radiation therapy combined with chemotherapy or radiosensitizers, followed by surgery
- A clinical trial of radiation therapy given during surgery or internal radiation therapy

Stage III Pancreatic Cancer

Treatment of stage III pancreatic cancer may include the following:

- Surgery with or without chemotherapy and radiation therapy

- Radiation therapy with chemotherapy

- Palliative surgery or stent placement to bypass blocked areas in ducts or the small intestine

- A clinical trial of surgery followed by radiation therapy with chemotherapy. Chemotherapy is given before, during, and after the radiation therapy.

- A clinical trial of surgery followed by chemotherapy

- A clinical trial of biologic therapy with radiation therapy or chemotherapy

- A clinical trial of radiation therapy combined with chemotherapy or radiosensitizers, which may be followed by surgery

- A clinical trial of radiation therapy given during surgery or internal radiation therapy

Stage IV Pancreatic Cancer

Treatment of stage IV pancreatic cancer may include the following:

- Chemotherapy

- Palliative treatments for pain, such as nerve blocks, and other supportive care

- Palliative surgery or stent placement to bypass blocked areas in ducts or the small intestine

- Clinical trials of chemotherapy or biologic therapy

Treatment Options for Recurrent Pancreatic Cancer

Treatment of recurrent pancreatic cancer may include the following:

- Chemotherapy

- Palliative surgery or stent placement to bypass blocked areas in ducts or the small intestine

- Palliative radiation therapy

- Other palliative medical care to reduce symptoms, such as nerve blocks to relieve pain

- Clinical trials of chemotherapy or biologic therapy

This summary section refers to specific treatments under study in clinical trials, but it may not mention every new treatment being studied.

Chapter 43

Islet Cell Carcinoma

What Is Islet Cell Cancer?

Islet cell cancer, a rare cancer, is a disease in which cancer (malignant) cells are found in certain tissues of the pancreas. The pancreas is about six inches long and is shaped like a thin pear, wider at one end and narrower at the other. The pancreas lies behind the stomach, inside a loop formed by part of the small intestine. The broader right end of the pancreas is called the head, the middle section is called the body, and the narrow left end is the tail.

The pancreas has two basic jobs in the body. It produces digestive juices that help break down (digest) food, and hormones (such as insulin) that regulate how the body stores and uses food. The area of the pancreas that produces digestive juices is called the exocrine pancreas. About 95 percent of pancreatic cancers begin in the exocrine pancreas. The hormone-producing area of the pancreas has special cells called islet cells and is called the endocrine pancreas. Only about 5 percent of pancreatic cancers start here.

The islet cells in the pancreas make many hormones, including insulin, which help the body store and use sugars. When islet cells in the pancreas become cancerous, they may make too many hormones. Islet cell cancers that make too many hormones are called functioning

PDQ® Cancer Information Summary. National Cancer Institute; Bethesda, MD. Islet Cell Carcinoma (PDQ®): Treatment—Patient. Updated 6/2003. Available at: http://www.cancer.gov. Accessed March 13, 2005.

tumors. Other islet cell cancers may not make extra hormones and are called nonfunctioning tumors. Tumors that do not spread to other parts of the body can also be found in the islet cells. These are called benign tumors and are not cancer. A doctor will need to determine whether the tumor is cancer or a benign tumor.

A doctor should be seen if there is pain in the abdomen, diarrhea, stomach pain, a tired feeling all the time, fainting, or weight gain without eating too much.

If there are symptoms, the doctor will order blood and urine tests to see whether the amounts of hormones in the body are normal. Other tests, including x-rays and special scans, may also be done.

The chance of recovery (prognosis) depends on the type of islet cell cancer the patient has, how far the cancer has spread, and the patient's overall health.

Stages of Islet Cell Cancer

Once islet cell cancer is found, more tests will be done to find out if cancer cells have spread to other parts of the body. This is called staging. The staging system for islet cell cancer is still being developed. These tumors are most often divided into one of three groups:

- islet cell cancers occurring in one site within the pancreas,

- islet cell cancers occurring in several sites within the pancreas, or

- islet cell cancers that have spread to lymph nodes near the pancreas or to distant sites.

Types of Islet Cell Cancer

A doctor also needs to know the type of islet cell tumor to plan treatment. The following types of islet cell tumors are found:

- **Gastrinoma:** The tumor makes large amounts of a hormone called gastrin, which causes too much acid to be made in the stomach. Ulcers may develop as a result of too much stomach acid.

- **Insulinoma:** The tumor makes too much of the hormone insulin and causes the body to store sugar instead of burning the sugar for energy. This causes too little sugar in the blood, a condition called hypoglycemia.

- **Glucagonoma:** This tumor makes too much of the hormone glucagon and causes too much sugar in the blood, a condition called hyperglycemia.

- **Miscellaneous:** Other types of islet cell cancer can affect the pancreas or small intestine. Each type of tumor may affect different hormones in the body and cause different symptoms.

- **Recurrent:** Recurrent disease means that the cancer has come back (recurred) after it has been treated. It may come back in the pancreas or in another part of the body.

Treatment Option Overview

There are treatments for all patients with islet cell cancer. Three types of treatment are used:

- Surgery (taking out the cancer)
- Chemotherapy (using drugs to kill cancer cells)
- Hormone therapy (using hormones to stop cancer cells from growing)

Surgery is the most common treatment of islet cell cancer. The doctor may take out the cancer and most or part of the pancreas. Sometimes the stomach is taken out (gastrectomy) because of ulcers. Lymph nodes in the area may also be removed and looked at under a microscope to see if they contain cancer.

Chemotherapy uses drugs to kill cancer cells. Chemotherapy may be taken by pill, or it may be put into the body by a needle in the vein or muscle. Chemotherapy is called a systemic treatment because the drug enters the bloodstream, travels through the body, and can kill cancer cells throughout the body.

Hormone therapy uses hormones to stop the cancer cells from growing or to relieve symptoms caused by the tumor.

Hepatic arterial occlusion or embolization uses drugs or other agents to reduce or block the flow of blood to the liver in order to kill cancer cells growing in the liver.

Treatment by Type

Treatment of islet cell cancer depends on the type of tumor, the stage, and the patient's overall health.

479

Standard treatment may be considered because of its effectiveness in patients in past studies, or participation in a clinical trial may be considered. Not all patients are cured with standard therapy, and some standard treatments may have more side effects than are desired. For these reasons, clinical trials are designed to find better ways to treat cancer patients and are based on the most up-to-date information. Clinical trials are ongoing in many parts of the country for patients with islet cell cancer.

Gastrinoma

Treatment may be one of the following:

- Surgery to remove the cancer
- Surgery to remove the stomach (gastrectomy)
- Surgery to cut the nerve that stimulates the pancreas
- Chemotherapy
- Hormone therapy
- Hepatic arterial occlusion or embolization to kill cancer cells growing in the liver

Insulinoma

Treatment may be one of the following:

- Surgery to remove the cancer
- Chemotherapy
- Hormone therapy
- Drugs to relieve symptoms
- Hepatic arterial occlusion or embolization to kill cancer cells growing in the liver

Glucagonoma

Treatment may be one of the following:

- Surgery to remove the cancer
- Chemotherapy
- Hormone therapy
- Hepatic arterial occlusion or embolization to kill cancer cells growing in the liver

Miscellaneous Islet Cell Cancer

Treatment may be one of the following:

* Surgery to remove the cancer
* Chemotherapy
* Hormone therapy
* Hepatic arterial occlusion or embolization to kill cancer cells growing in the liver

Recurrent Islet Cell Carcinoma

Treatment depends on many factors, including what treatment the patient had before and where the cancer has come back. Treatment may be chemotherapy, or patients may want to consider taking part in a clinical trial.

Chapter 44

Liver Cancer

General Information about Adult Primary Liver Cancer

Adult primary liver cancer is a disease in which malignant (cancer) cells form in the tissues of the liver.

The liver is one of the largest organs in the body, filling the upper right side of the abdomen inside the rib cage. It has two parts, a right lobe and a smaller left lobe. The liver has many important functions, including:

- Filtering harmful substances from the blood so they can be passed from the body in stools and urine
- Making bile to help digest fats from food
- Storing glycogen (sugar), which the body uses for energy

Risk Factors

The following are possible risk factors for adult primary liver cancer:

- Having hepatitis B or hepatitis C
- Having a close relative with both hepatitis and liver cancer
- Having cirrhosis

PDQ® Cancer Information Summary. National Cancer Institute; Bethesda, MD. Adult Primary Liver Cancer (PDQ®): Treatment—Patient. Updated 1/2005. Available at: http://www.cancer.gov. Accessed February 11, 2005.

- Eating foods tainted with aflatoxin (poison from a fungus that can grow on foods, such as grains and nuts, that have not been stored properly)

Symptoms

Possible signs of adult primary liver cancer include a lump or pain on the right side.

These symptoms may be caused by swelling of the liver. These and other symptoms may be caused by adult primary liver cancer or by other conditions. A doctor should be consulted if any of the following problems occur:

- A hard lump on the right side just below the rib cage
- Discomfort in the upper abdomen on the right side
- Pain around the right shoulder blade
- Unexplained weight loss
- Jaundice (yellowing of the skin and whites of the eyes)
- Unusual tiredness
- Nausea
- Loss of appetite

Diagnosis

Tests that examine the liver and the blood are used to detect (find) and diagnose adult primary liver cancer.

The following tests and procedures may be used:

- **Physical exam and history:** An exam of the body to check general signs of health, including checking for signs of disease, such as lumps or anything else that seems unusual. A history of the patient's health habits and past illnesses and treatments will also be taken.

- **Serum tumor marker test:** A procedure in which a sample of blood is examined to measure the amounts of certain substances released into the blood by organs, tissues, or tumor cells in the body. Certain substances are linked to specific types of cancer when found in increased levels in the blood. These are called tumor markers. An increased level of alpha-fetoprotein (AFP) in the blood may be a sign of liver cancer. Other cancers and certain noncancerous conditions, including cirrhosis and hepatitis, may also increase AFP levels.

- **Complete blood count (CBC):** A procedure in which a sample of blood is drawn and checked for the following:

  - The number of red blood cells, white blood cells, and platelets

  - The amount of hemoglobin (the protein that carries oxygen) in the red blood cells

  - The portion of the blood sample made up of red blood cells

- **Laparoscopy:** A surgical procedure to look at the organs inside the abdomen to check for signs of disease. Small incisions (cuts) are made in the wall of the abdomen and a laparoscope (a thin, lighted tube) is inserted into one of the incisions. Other instruments may be inserted through the same or other incisions to perform procedures such as removing organs or taking tissue samples for biopsy.

- **Biopsy:** The removal of cells or tissues so they can be viewed under a microscope by a pathologist to check for signs of cancer. The sample may be taken using a fine needle inserted into the liver during an x-ray or ultrasound. This is called needle biopsy or fine-needle aspiration. The biopsy may be done during a laparoscopy.

- **CT scan (CAT scan):** A procedure that makes a series of detailed pictures of areas inside the body, taken from different angles. The pictures are made by a computer linked to an x-ray machine. A dye may be injected into a vein or swallowed to help the organs or tissues show up more clearly. This procedure is also called computed tomography, computerized tomography, or computerized axial tomography.

- **MRI (magnetic resonance imaging):** A procedure that uses a magnet, radio waves, and a computer to make a series of detailed pictures of areas inside the body. This procedure is also called nuclear magnetic resonance imaging (NMRI).

- **Ultrasound:** A procedure in which high-energy sound waves (ultrasound) are bounced off internal tissues or organs and make echoes. The echoes form a picture of body tissues called a sonogram.

Prognosis

The prognosis (chance of recovery) and treatment options depend on the following:

- The stage of the cancer (the size of the tumor, whether it affects part or all of the liver, or has spread to other places in the body)

- How well the liver is working

- The patient's general health, including whether there is cirrhosis of the liver

Prognosis is also affected by alpha-fetoprotein (AFP) levels.

Stages of Adult Primary Liver Cancer

After adult primary liver cancer has been diagnosed, tests are done to find out if cancer cells have spread within the liver or to other parts of the body.

The process used to find out if cancer has spread within the liver or to other parts of the body is called staging. The information gathered from the staging process determines the stage of the disease. It is important to know the stage in order to plan treatment. The following tests and procedures may be used in the staging process:

- **Chest x-ray:** An x-ray of the organs and bones inside the chest. An x-ray is a type of energy beam that can go through the body and onto film, making a picture of areas inside the body.

- **CT scan (CAT scan):** A procedure that makes a series of detailed pictures of areas inside the body, taken from different angles. The pictures are made by a computer linked to an x-ray machine. A dye may be injected into a vein or swallowed to help the organs or tissues show up more clearly. This procedure is also called computed tomography, computerized tomography, or computerized axial tomography.

- **MRI (magnetic resonance imaging):** A procedure that uses a magnet, radio waves, and a computer to make a series of detailed pictures of areas inside the body. This procedure is also called nuclear magnetic resonance imaging (NMRI).

- **Bone scan:** A procedure to check if there are rapidly dividing cells, such as cancer cells, in the bone. A very small amount of radioactive material is injected into a vein and travels through the bloodstream. The radioactive material collects in the bones and is detected by a scanner.

- **Doppler ultrasound:** A type of ultrasound that uses differences in the ultrasound echoes to measure the speed and direction of blood flow.

The following stages are used for adult primary liver cancer:

Stage I

In stage I, there is one tumor and it has not spread to nearby blood vessels.

Stage II

In stage II, one of the following is found:

- one tumor that has spread to nearby blood vessels; or
- more than one tumor, none of which is larger than five centimeters.

Stage III

Stage III is divided into stage IIIA, IIIB, and IIIC.

- In stage IIIA, one of the following is found:
  - more than one tumor larger than five centimeters; or
  - one tumor that has spread to a major branch of blood vessels near the liver.
- In stage IIIB, there are one or more tumors of any size that have either:
  - spread to nearby organs other than the gallbladder; or
  - broken through the lining of the peritoneal cavity.
- In stage IIIC, the cancer has spread to nearby lymph nodes.

Stage IV

In stage IV, cancer has spread beyond the liver to other places in the body, such as the bones or lungs. The tumors may be of any size and may also have spread to nearby blood vessels or lymph nodes.

For adult primary liver cancer, stages are also grouped according to how the cancer may be treated. There are three treatment groups:

Localized Resectable

The cancer is found in the liver only, has not spread, and can be completely removed by surgery.

Localized and Locally Advanced Unresectable

The cancer is found in the liver only and has not spread, but cannot be completely removed by surgery.

Advanced

Cancer has spread throughout the liver or has spread to other parts of the body, such as the lungs and bone.

Recurrent Adult Primary Liver Cancer

Recurrent adult primary liver cancer is cancer that has recurred (come back) after it has been treated. The cancer may come back in the liver or in other parts of the body.

Treatment Option Overview

Different types of treatments are available for patients with adult primary liver cancer. Some treatments are standard (the currently used treatment), and some are being tested in clinical trials. Before starting treatment, patients may want to think about taking part in a clinical trial. A treatment clinical trial is a research study meant to help improve current treatments or obtain information on new treatments for patients with cancer. When clinical trials show that a new treatment is better than the standard treatment, the new treatment may become the standard treatment.

Clinical trials are taking place in many parts of the country. Choosing the most appropriate cancer treatment is a decision that ideally involves the patient, family, and health care team.

Standard Treatment

Four types of standard treatment are used:

Surgery: The following types of surgery may be used to treat liver cancer:

- *Cryosurgery:* A treatment that uses an instrument to freeze and destroy abnormal tissue, such as carcinoma in situ (cancer that involves only the cells in which it began and that has not spread to nearby tissues). This type of treatment is also called cryotherapy. The doctor may use ultrasound to guide the instrument.

- *Partial hepatectomy:* Removal of the part of the liver where cancer is found. The part removed may be a wedge of tissue, an entire lobe, or a larger portion of the liver, along with some of the healthy tissue around it. The remaining liver tissue takes over the functions of the liver.

- *Total hepatectomy and liver transplant:* Removal of the entire liver and replacement with a healthy donated liver. A liver transplant may be done when the disease is in the liver only and a donated liver can be found. If the patient has to wait for a donated liver, other treatment is given as needed.

- *Radiofrequency ablation:* The use of a special probe with tiny electrodes that kill cancer cells. Sometimes the probe is inserted directly through the skin and only local anesthesia is needed. In other cases, the probe is inserted through an incision in the abdomen. This is done in the hospital with general anesthesia.

Radiation Therapy: Radiation therapy is a cancer treatment that uses high-energy x-rays or other types of radiation to kill cancer cells. Radiation therapy is given in different ways:

- External radiation therapy uses a machine outside the body to send radiation toward the cancer.

- Internal radiation therapy uses a radioactive substance sealed in needles, seeds, wires, or catheters that are placed directly into or near the cancer.

- Drugs called radiosensitizers may be given with the radiation therapy to make the cancer cells more sensitive to radiation therapy.

- Radiation may be delivered to the tumor using radiolabeled antibodies. Radioactive substances are attached to antibodies made in the laboratory. These antibodies, which target tumor cells, are injected into the body and the tumor cells are killed by the radioactive substance.

The way the radiation therapy is given depends on the type and stage of the cancer being treated.

Chemotherapy: Chemotherapy is a cancer treatment that uses drugs to stop the growth of cancer cells, either by killing the cells or by stopping the cells from dividing. When chemotherapy is taken by mouth or injected into a vein or muscle, the drugs enter the bloodstream and can reach cancer cells throughout the body (systemic chemotherapy). When chemotherapy is placed directly into the spinal column, an organ, or a body cavity such as the abdomen, the drugs mainly affect cancer cells in those areas (regional chemotherapy).

Regional chemotherapy is usually used to treat liver cancer. A small pump containing anticancer drugs may be placed in the body. The pump puts the drugs directly into the blood vessels that go to the tumor.

Another type of regional chemotherapy is chemoembolization of the hepatic artery. The anticancer drug is injected into the hepatic artery through a catheter (thin tube). The drug is mixed with a substance that blocks the artery, cutting off blood flow to the tumor. Most of the anticancer drug is trapped near the tumor and only a small amount of the drug reaches other parts of the body. The blockage may be temporary or permanent, depending on the substance used to block the artery. The tumor is prevented from getting the oxygen and nutrients it needs to grow. The liver continues to receive blood from the hepatic portal vein, which carries blood from the stomach and intestine.

The way the chemotherapy is given depends on the type and stage of the cancer being treated.

Percutaneous Ethanol Injection: Percutaneous ethanol injection is a cancer treatment in which a small needle is used to inject ethanol (alcohol) directly into a tumor to kill cancer cells. The procedure may be done once or twice a week. Usually local anesthesia is used, but if the patient has many tumors in the liver, general anesthesia may be needed.

Clinical Trials

Other types of treatment are being tested in clinical trials. These include the following:

Hyperthermia Therapy: Hyperthermia therapy is a type of treatment in which body tissue is exposed to high temperatures to damage and kill cancer cells or to make cancer cells more sensitive to the effects of radiation and certain anticancer drugs. Because some cancer cells are more sensitive to heat than normal cells are, the cancer cells die and the tumor shrinks.

Biologic Therapy: Biologic therapy is a treatment that uses the patient's immune system to fight cancer. Substances made by the body or made in a laboratory are used to boost, direct, or restore the body's natural defenses against cancer. This type of cancer treatment is also called biotherapy or immunotherapy.

This summary section refers to specific treatments under study in clinical trials, but it may not mention every new treatment being studied.

Treatment Options for Adult Primary Liver Cancer

Localized Resectable Adult Primary Liver Cancer

Treatment of localized resectable adult primary liver cancer may include the following:

* Surgery (partial hepatectomy)
* Surgery (total hepatectomy) and liver transplant
* A clinical trial of regional or systemic chemotherapy or biologic therapy following surgery

Localized and Locally Advanced Unresectable Adult Primary Liver Cancer

Treatment of localized and locally advanced unresectable adult primary liver cancer may include the following:

* Surgery (cryosurgery or radiofrequency ablation)
* Chemotherapy (chemoembolization, regional chemotherapy, or systemic chemotherapy)
* Percutaneous ethanol injection
* Surgery (total hepatectomy) and liver transplant
* Radiation therapy with radiosensitizers
* A clinical trial of a combination of surgery, chemotherapy, and radiation therapy. Hyperthermia therapy may also be used. Chemotherapy and radiation therapy may be used to shrink the tumor before surgery.

Advanced Adult Primary Liver Cancer

There is no standard treatment for advanced adult primary liver cancer. Patients may consider taking part in a clinical trial. Treatment may be a clinical trial of biologic therapy, chemotherapy, or radiation therapy with or without radiosensitizers. These treatments may be given as palliative therapy to help relieve symptoms and improve the quality of life.

This summary section refers to specific treatments under study in clinical trials, but it may not mention every new treatment being studied.

Recurrent Adult Primary Liver Cancer

Treatment of recurrent adult primary liver cancer may include the following:

- Surgery (partial hepatectomy)
- Surgery (total hepatectomy) and liver transplant
- Chemotherapy (chemoembolization or systemic chemotherapy)
- Percutaneous ethanol injection
- A clinical trial of a new therapy

Chapter 45

Anal Cancer

General Information about Anal Cancer

Anal cancer is a disease in which malignant (cancer) cells form in the tissues of the anus.

The anus is the end of the large intestine, below the rectum, through which stool (solid waste) leaves the body. The anus is formed partly from the outer, skin layers of the body and partly from the intestine. Two ring-like muscles, called sphincter muscles, open and close the anal opening to let stool pass out of the body. The anal canal, the part of the anus between the rectum and the anal opening, is about one and a half inches long.

The skin around the outside of the anus is called the perianal area. Tumors in this area are skin tumors, not anal cancer.

Risk Factors

Being infected with the human papillomavirus (HPV) can affect the risk of developing anal cancer.

Risk factors include the following:

- Being over fifty years old
- Being infected with human papillomavirus (HPV)
- Having many sexual partners

PDQ® Cancer Information Summary. National Cancer Institute; Bethesda, MD. Anal Cancer (PDQ®): Treatment—Patient. Updated 1/2005. Available at: http://www.cancer.gov. Accessed February 10, 2005.

- Having receptive anal intercourse (anal sex)
- Frequent anal redness, swelling, and soreness
- Having anal fistulas (abnormal openings)
- Smoking cigarettes

Symptoms

Possible signs of anal cancer include bleeding from the anus or rectum or a lump near the anus.

These and other symptoms may be caused by anal cancer or by other conditions. A doctor should be consulted if any of the following problems occur:

- Bleeding from the anus or rectum
- Pain or pressure in the area around the anus
- Itching or discharge from the anus
- A lump near the anus
- A change in bowel habits

Diagnosis

Tests that examine the rectum and anus are used to detect (find) and diagnose anal cancer.

The following tests and procedures may be used:

- **Physical exam and history:** An exam of the body to check general signs of health, including checking for signs of disease, such as lumps or anything else that seems unusual. A history of the patient's health habits and past illnesses and treatments will also be taken.

- **Digital rectal examination (DRE):** An exam of the anus and rectum. The doctor or nurse inserts a lubricated, gloved finger into the rectum to feel for lumps or anything else that seems unusual.

- **Anoscopy:** An exam of the anus and lower rectum using a short, lighted tube called an anoscope.

- **Proctoscopy:** An exam of the rectum using a short, lighted tube called a proctoscope.

- **Endo-anal or endorectal ultrasound:** A procedure in which an ultrasound transducer (probe) is inserted into the anus or rectum and used to bounce high-energy sound waves (ultrasound) off internal tissues or organs and make echoes. The echoes form a picture of body tissues called a sonogram.

- **Biopsy:** The removal of cells or tissues so they can be viewed under a microscope to check for signs of cancer. If an abnormal area is seen during the anoscopy, a biopsy may be done at that time.

Prognosis

Certain factors affect the prognosis (chance of recovery) and treatment options.

The prognosis (chance of recovery) depends on the following:

- The size of the tumor
- Where the tumor is in the anus
- Whether the cancer has spread to the lymph nodes

The treatment options depend on the following:

- The stage of the cancer
- Where the tumor is in the anus
- Whether the patient has human immunodeficiency virus (HIV)
- Whether cancer remains after initial treatment or has recurred

Stages of Anal Cancer

After anal cancer has been diagnosed, tests are done to find out if cancer cells have spread within the anus or to other parts of the body.

The process used to find out if cancer has spread within the anus or to other parts of the body is called staging. The information gathered from the staging process determines the stage of the disease. It is important to know the stage in order to plan treatment. The following tests may be used in the staging process:

- **CT scan (CAT scan):** A procedure that makes a series of detailed pictures of areas inside the body, taken from different angles. The pictures are made by a computer linked to an x-ray machine. A dye may be injected into a vein or swallowed to help the organs or tissues show up more clearly. This procedure is also called computed tomography, computerized tomography, or computerized axial tomography. For anal cancer, a CT scan of the pelvis and abdomen may be done.

- **Chest x-ray:** An x-ray of the organs and bones inside the chest. An x-ray is a type of energy beam that can go through the body and onto film, making a picture of areas inside the body.

- **Endo-anal or endorectal ultrasound:** A procedure in which an ultrasound transducer (probe) is inserted into the anus or rectum and used to bounce high-energy sound waves (ultrasound) off internal tissues or organs and make echoes. The echoes form a picture of body tissues called a sonogram.

The following stages are used for anal cancer:

Stage 0 (Carcinoma in Situ)

In stage 0, cancer is found in the innermost lining of the anus only. Stage 0 cancer is also called carcinoma in situ.

Stage I

In stage I, the tumor is no larger than two centimeters.

Stage II

In stage II, the tumor is larger than two centimeters.

Stage IIIA

In stage IIIA, the tumor may be any size and has spread to either:

- lymph nodes near the rectum; or
- nearby organs, such as the vagina, urethra, and bladder.

Stage IIIB

In stage IIIB, the tumor may be any size and has spread:

- to nearby organs and to lymph nodes near the rectum; or
- to lymph nodes on one side of the pelvis or groin; or
- to lymph nodes near the rectum and in the groin, or to lymph nodes on both sides of the pelvis or groin.

Stage IV

In stage IV, the tumor may be any size and cancer may have spread to lymph nodes and has spread to distant parts of the body.

Recurrent Anal Cancer

Recurrent anal cancer is cancer that has recurred (come back) after it has been treated. The cancer may come back in the anus or in other parts of the body.

Treatment Option Overview

Different types of treatments are available for patients with anal cancer. Some treatments are standard (the currently used treatment), and some are being tested in clinical trials. Before starting treatment, patients may want to think about taking part in a clinical trial. A treatment clinical trial is a research study meant to help improve current treatments or obtain information on new treatments for patients with cancer. When clinical trials show that a new treatment is better than the standard treatment, the new treatment may become the standard treatment.

Clinical trials are taking place in many parts of the country. Choosing the most appropriate cancer treatment is a decision that ideally involves the patient, family, and health care team.

Standard Treatments

Three types of standard treatment are used:

Radiation Therapy: Radiation therapy is a cancer treatment that uses high-energy x-rays or other types of radiation to kill cancer cells. There are two types of radiation therapy. External radiation therapy uses a machine outside the body to send radiation toward the cancer. Internal radiation therapy uses a radioactive substance sealed in needles, seeds, wires, or catheters that are placed directly into or near the cancer. The way the radiation therapy is given depends on the type and stage of the cancer being treated.

Chemotherapy: Chemotherapy is a cancer treatment that uses drugs to stop the growth of cancer cells, either by killing the cells or by stopping the cells from dividing. When chemotherapy is taken by mouth or injected into a vein or muscle, the drugs enter the bloodstream and can reach cancer cells throughout the body (systemic chemotherapy). When chemotherapy is placed directly into the spinal column, an organ, or a body cavity such as the abdomen, the drugs mainly affect cancer cells in those areas (regional chemotherapy). The way the chemotherapy is given depends on the type and stage of the cancer being treated.

Surgery:

- *Local resection:* A surgical procedure in which the tumor is cut from the anus along with some of the healthy tissue around it. Local resection may be used if the cancer is small and has not spread. This procedure may save the sphincter muscles so the patient can still control bowel movements. Tumors that develop in the lower part of the anus can often be removed with local resection.

- *Abdominoperineal resection:* A surgical procedure in which the anus, the rectum, and part of the sigmoid colon are removed through an incision made in the abdomen. The doctor sews the end of the intestine to an opening, called a stoma, made in the surface of the abdomen so body waste can be collected in a disposable bag outside of the body. This is called a colostomy. Lymph nodes that contain cancer may also be removed during this operation.

Cancer therapy can further damage the already weakened immune systems of patients who have the human immunodeficiency virus (HIV). For this reason, patients who have anal cancer and HIV are usually treated with lower doses of anticancer drugs and radiation than patients who do not have HIV.

Clinical Trials

Other types of treatment are being tested in clinical trials. These include the following:

Radiosensitizers: Radiosensitizers are drugs that make tumor cells more sensitive to radiation therapy. Combining radiation therapy with radiosensitizers may kill more tumor cells.

This summary section refers to specific treatments under study in clinical trials, but it may not mention every new treatment being studied.

Treatment Options by Stage

Stage 0 Anal Cancer (Carcinoma in Situ)

Treatment of stage 0 anal cancer is usually local resection.

Stage I Anal Cancer

Treatment of stage I anal cancer may include the following:

- Local resection

- External-beam radiation therapy with or without chemotherapy. If cancer remains after treatment, additional chemotherapy and radiation therapy may be given to avoid the need for a permanent colostomy.

- Internal radiation therapy

- Abdominoperineal resection, if cancer remains or comes back after treatment with radiation therapy and chemotherapy

- Internal radiation therapy for cancer that remains after treatment with external-beam radiation therapy

Patients who have had treatment that saves the sphincter muscles may receive follow-up exams every three months for the first two years, including rectal exams with endoscopy and biopsy, as needed.

Stage II Anal Cancer

Treatment of stage II anal cancer may include the following:

- Local resection

- External-beam radiation therapy with chemotherapy. If cancer remains after treatment, additional chemotherapy and radiation therapy may be given to avoid the need for a permanent colostomy.

- Internal radiation therapy

- Abdominoperineal resection, if cancer remains or comes back after treatment with radiation therapy and chemotherapy

- A clinical trial of new treatment options

Patients who have had treatment that saves the sphincter muscles may receive follow-up exams every three months for the first two years, including rectal exams with endoscopy and biopsy, as needed.

Stage IIIA Anal Cancer

Treatment of stage IIIA anal cancer may include the following:

- External-beam radiation therapy with chemotherapy. If cancer remains after treatment, additional chemotherapy and radiation therapy may be given to avoid the need for a permanent colostomy.

- Internal beam radiation
- Abdominoperineal resection, if cancer remains or comes back after treatment with chemotherapy and radiation therapy
- A clinical trial of new treatment options

Stage IIIB Anal Cancer

Treatment of stage IIIB anal cancer may include the following:

- External-beam radiation therapy with chemotherapy
- Local resection or abdominoperineal resection, if cancer remains or comes back after treatment with chemotherapy and radiation therapy. Lymph nodes may also be removed.
- A clinical trial of new treatment options

Stage IV Anal Cancer

Treatment of stage IV anal cancer may include the following:

- Surgery as palliative therapy to relieve symptoms and improve the quality of life
- Radiation therapy as palliative therapy
- Chemotherapy with radiation therapy as palliative therapy
- A clinical trial of new treatment options

Treatment Options for Recurrent Anal Cancer

Treatment of recurrent anal cancer may include the following:

- Radiation therapy and chemotherapy, for recurrence after surgery
- Surgery, for recurrence after radiation therapy or chemotherapy
- A clinical trial of radiation therapy with chemotherapy or radiosensitizers

This summary section refers to specific treatments under study in clinical trials, but it may not mention every new treatment being studied.

Part Seven

Food Intolerances and Infectious Disorders of the Gastrointestinal Tract

Chapter 46

Lactose Intolerance

What is lactose intolerance?

Lactose intolerance is the inability to digest significant amounts of lactose, the predominant sugar of milk. This inability results from a shortage of the enzyme lactase, which is normally produced by the cells that line the small intestine. Lactase breaks down milk sugar into simpler forms that can then be absorbed into the bloodstream. When there is not enough lactase to digest the amount of lactose consumed, the results, although not usually dangerous, may be very distressing. While not all persons deficient in lactase have symptoms, those who do are considered to be lactose intolerant.

Common symptoms include nausea, cramps, bloating, gas, and diarrhea, which begin about thirty minutes to two hours after eating or drinking foods containing lactose. The severity of symptoms varies depending on the amount of lactose each individual can tolerate.

Some causes of lactose intolerance are well known. For instance, certain digestive diseases and injuries to the small intestine can reduce the amount of enzymes produced. In rare cases, children are born without the ability to produce lactase. For most people, though, lactase deficiency is a condition that develops naturally over time. After about the age of two years, the body begins to produce less lactase. However, many people may not experience symptoms until they are much older.

Reprinted from "Lactose Intolerance," National Institute of Diabetes and Digestive and Kidney Diseases, NIH Publication No. 03-2751, March 2003.

Between thirty and fifty million Americans are lactose intolerant. Certain ethnic and racial populations are more widely affected than others. As many as 75 percent of all African Americans and American Indians and 90 percent of Asian Americans are lactose intolerant. The condition is least common among persons of northern European descent.

Researchers have identified a genetic variation associated with lactose intolerance; this discovery may be useful in developing a diagnostic test to identify people with this condition.

How is lactose intolerance diagnosed?

The most common tests used to measure the absorption of lactose in the digestive system are the lactose tolerance test, the hydrogen breath test, and the stool acidity test. These tests are performed on an outpatient basis at a hospital, clinic, or doctor's office.

The lactose tolerance test begins with the individual fasting (not eating) before the test and then drinking a liquid that contains lactose. Several blood samples are taken over a two-hour period to measure the person's blood glucose (blood sugar) level, which indicates how well the body is able to digest lactose.

Normally, when lactose reaches the digestive system, the lactase enzyme breaks it down into glucose and galactose. The liver then changes the galactose into glucose, which enters the bloodstream and raises the person's blood glucose level. If lactose is incompletely broken down, the blood glucose level does not rise and a diagnosis of lactose intolerance is confirmed.

The hydrogen breath test measures the amount of hydrogen in a person's breath. Normally, very little hydrogen is detectable. However, undigested lactose in the colon is fermented by bacteria, and various gases, including hydrogen, are produced. The hydrogen is absorbed from the intestines, carried through the bloodstream to the lungs, and exhaled. In the test, the patient drinks a lactose-loaded beverage, and the breath is analyzed at regular intervals. Raised levels of hydrogen in the breath indicate improper digestion of lactose. Certain foods, medications, and cigarettes can affect the accuracy of the test and should be avoided before taking it. This test is available for children and adults.

The lactose tolerance and hydrogen breath tests are not given to infants and very young children who are suspected of having lactose intolerance. A large lactose load may be dangerous for the very young because they are more prone to the dehydration that can result from diarrhea caused by the lactose. If a baby or young child is experiencing symptoms of lactose intolerance, many pediatricians simply recommend changing from cow's milk to soy formula and waiting for symptoms to abate.

If necessary, a stool acidity test, which measures the amount of acid in the stool, may be given to infants and young children. Undigested lactose fermented by bacteria in the colon creates lactic acid and other short-chain fatty acids that can be detected in a stool sample. In addition, glucose may be present in the sample as a result of unabsorbed lactose in the colon.

How is lactose intolerance treated?

Fortunately, lactose intolerance is relatively easy to treat. No treatment can improve the body's ability to produce lactase, but symptoms can be controlled through diet.

Young children with lactase deficiency should not eat any foods containing lactose. Most older children and adults need not avoid lactose completely, but people differ in the amounts and types of foods they can handle. For example, one person may have symptoms after drinking a small glass of milk, while another can drink one glass but not two. Others may be able to manage ice cream and aged cheeses, such as cheddar and Swiss, but not other dairy products. Dietary control of lactose intolerance depends on people learning through trial and error how much lactose they can handle.

For those who react to very small amounts of lactose or have trouble limiting their intake of foods that contain it, lactase enzymes are available without a prescription to help people digest foods that contain lactose. The tablets are taken with the first bite of dairy food. Lactase enzyme is also available as a liquid. Adding a few drops of the enzyme will convert the lactose in milk or cream, making it more digestible for people with lactose intolerance.

Lactose-reduced milk and other products are available at most supermarkets. The milk contains all of the nutrients found in regular milk and remains fresh for about the same length of time, or longer if it is super-pasteurized.

How is nutrition balanced?

Milk and other dairy products are a major source of nutrients in the American diet. The most important of these nutrients is calcium. Calcium is essential for the growth and repair of bones throughout life. In the middle and later years, a shortage of calcium may lead to thin, fragile bones that break easily, a condition called osteoporosis. A concern, then, for both children and adults with lactose intolerance, is getting enough calcium in a diet that includes little or no milk.

In 1997, the Institute of Medicine released a report recommending new requirements for daily calcium intake. How much calcium a person needs to maintain good health varies by age group. Recommendations from the report are shown in Table 46.1.

Table 46.1. Recommended Daily Calcium Intake

Age Group	Amount of Calcium to Consume Daily (mg)
0–6 months	210 mg
7–12 months	270 mg
1–3 years	500 mg
4–8 years	800 mg
9–18 years	1,300 mg
19–50 years	1,000 mg
51–70+ years	1,200 mg

Pregnant and nursing women under nineteen need 1,300 mg daily, while pregnant and nursing women over nineteen need 1,000 mg.

In planning meals, making sure that each day's diet includes enough calcium is important, even if the diet does not contain dairy products. Many nondairy foods are high in calcium. Green vegetables, such as broccoli and kale, and fish with soft, edible bones, such as salmon and sardines, are excellent sources of calcium.

Recent research shows that yogurt with active cultures may be a good source of calcium for many people with lactose intolerance, even though it is fairly high in lactose. Evidence shows that the bacterial cultures used to make yogurt produce some of the lactase enzyme required for proper digestion.

Clearly, many foods can provide the calcium and other nutrients the body needs, even when intake of milk and dairy products is limited. However, factors other than calcium and lactose content should be kept in mind when planning a diet. Some vegetables that are high in calcium (Swiss chard, spinach, and rhubarb, for instance) are not good sources of calcium because the body cannot use the calcium they contain. They also contain substances called oxalates, which stop calcium absorption. Calcium is absorbed and used only when there is enough vitamin D in the body. A balanced diet should provide an adequate supply of vitamin D. Sources of vitamin D include eggs and liver. However, sunlight helps the body naturally absorb or synthesize vitamin D, and with enough exposure to the sun, food sources may not be necessary.

Some people with lactose intolerance may think they are not getting enough calcium and vitamin D in their diet. Consultation with a doctor or dietitian may be helpful in deciding whether any dietary supplements are needed. Taking vitamins or minerals of the wrong kind or in the wrong amounts can be harmful. A dietitian can help in planning meals that will provide the most nutrients with the least chance of causing discomfort.

What is hidden lactose?

Although milk and foods made from milk are the only natural sources, lactose is often added to prepared foods. People with very low tolerance for lactose should know about the many food products that may contain even small amounts of lactose. The following are some examples:

- bread and other baked goods
- processed breakfast cereals
- instant potatoes, soups, and breakfast drinks
- margarine
- lunch meats (other than kosher)
- salad dressings
- candies and other snacks
- mixes for pancakes, biscuits, and cookies
- powdered meal-replacement supplements

Some products labeled nondairy, such as powdered coffee creamer and whipped toppings, may also include ingredients that are derived from milk and therefore contain lactose.

Smart shoppers learn to read food labels with care, looking not only for milk and lactose among the contents, but also for such words as whey, curds, milk by-products, dry milk solids, and nonfat dry milk powder. If any of these are listed on a label, the product contains lactose.

In addition, lactose is used as the base for more than 20 percent of prescription drugs and about 6 percent of over-the-counter medicines. Many types of birth control pills, for example, contain lactose, as do some tablets for stomach acid and gas. However, these products typically affect only people with severe lactose intolerance.

Summary

Even though lactose intolerance is widespread, it need not pose a serious threat to good health. People who have trouble digesting lactose can learn which dairy products and other foods they can eat without discomfort and which ones they should avoid. Many will be able to enjoy milk, ice cream, and other such products if they take them in small amounts or eat other food at the same time. Others can use lactase liquid or tablets to help digest the lactose. Even older women at risk for osteoporosis and growing children who must avoid milk and foods made with milk can meet most of their special dietary needs by eating greens, fish, and other calcium-rich foods that are free of lactose. A carefully chosen diet, with calcium supplements if the doctor or dietitian recommends them, is the key to reducing symptoms and protecting future health.

Chapter 47

Celiac Disease

What is celiac disease?

Celiac disease is a digestive disease that damages the small intestine and interferes with absorption of nutrients from food. People who have celiac disease cannot tolerate a protein called gluten, which is found in wheat, rye, and barley. When people with celiac disease eat foods containing gluten, their immune system responds by damaging the small intestine. Specifically, tiny finger-like protrusions, called villi, on the lining of the small intestine are lost. Nutrients from food are absorbed into the bloodstream through these villi. Without villi, a person becomes malnourished—regardless of the quantity of food eaten.

Because the body's own immune system causes the damage, celiac disease is considered an autoimmune disorder. However, it is also classified as a disease of malabsorption because nutrients are not absorbed. Celiac disease is also known as celiac sprue, nontropical sprue, and gluten-sensitive enteropathy.

Celiac disease is a genetic disease, meaning that it runs in families. Sometimes the disease is triggered—or becomes active for the first time—after surgery, pregnancy, childbirth, viral infection, or severe emotional stress.

Reprinted from "Celiac Disease," National Institute of Diabetes and Digestive and Kidney Diseases, NIH Publication No. 04-4269, February 2004.

What are the symptoms?

Celiac disease affects people differently. Some people develop symptoms as children, others as adults. One factor thought to play a role in when and how celiac appears is whether and how long a person was breastfed—the longer one was breastfed, the later symptoms of celiac disease appear and the more atypical the symptoms. Other factors include the age at which one began eating foods containing gluten and how much gluten is eaten.

Symptoms may or may not occur in the digestive system. For example, one person might have diarrhea and abdominal pain, while another person has irritability or depression. In fact, irritability is one of the most common symptoms in children.

Symptoms of celiac disease may include one or more of the following:

- recurring abdominal bloating and pain
- chronic diarrhea
- weight loss
- pale, foul-smelling stool
- unexplained anemia (low count of red blood cells)
- gas
- bone pain
- behavior changes
- muscle cramps
- fatigue
- delayed growth
- failure to thrive in infants
- pain in the joints
- seizures
- tingling numbness in the legs (from nerve damage)
- pale sores inside the mouth, called aphthous ulcers
- painful skin rash, called dermatitis herpetiformis
- tooth discoloration or loss of enamel
- missed menstrual periods (often because of excessive weight loss)

Anemia, delayed growth, and weight loss are signs of malnutrition—not getting enough nutrients. Malnutrition is a serious problem for anyone, but particularly for children because they need adequate nutrition to develop properly.

Some people with celiac disease may not have symptoms. The undamaged part of their small intestine is able to absorb enough nutrients to prevent symptoms. However, people without symptoms are still at risk for the complications of celiac disease.

How is celiac disease diagnosed?

Diagnosing celiac disease can be difficult because some of its symptoms are similar to those of other diseases, including irritable bowel syndrome, Crohn disease, ulcerative colitis, diverticulosis, intestinal infections, chronic fatigue syndrome, and depression.

Recently, researchers discovered that people with celiac disease have higher than normal levels of certain antibodies in their blood. Antibodies are produced by the immune system in response to substances that the body perceives to be threatening. To diagnose celiac disease, physicians test blood to measure levels of antibodies to endomysium and tissue transglutaminase.

If the tests and symptoms suggest celiac disease, the physician may remove a tiny piece of tissue from the small intestine to check for damage to the villi. This is done in a procedure called a biopsy: the physician eases a long, thin tube called an endoscope through the mouth and stomach into the small intestine, and then takes a sample of tissue using instruments passed through the endoscope. Biopsy of the small intestine is the best way to diagnose celiac disease.

Screening: Screening for celiac disease involves testing asymptomatic people for the antibodies. Americans are not routinely screened for celiac disease. However, because celiac disease is hereditary, family members—particularly first-degree relatives—of people who have been diagnosed may need to be tested for the disease. About 10 percent of an affected person's first-degree relatives (parents, siblings, or children) will also have the disease. The longer a person goes undiagnosed and untreated, the greater the chance of developing malnutrition and other complications.

What is the treatment?

The only treatment for celiac disease is to follow a gluten-free diet—that is, to avoid all foods that contain gluten. For most people, following this diet will stop symptoms, heal existing intestinal damage, and prevent further damage. Improvements begin within days of starting the diet, and the small intestine is usually completely healed—meaning the villi are intact and working—in three to six months. (It may take up to two years for older adults.)

The gluten-free diet is a lifetime requirement. Eating any gluten, no matter how small an amount, can damage the intestine. This is true for anyone with the disease, including people who do not have noticeable symptoms. Depending on a person's age at diagnosis, some problems, such as delayed growth and tooth discoloration, may not improve.

A small percentage of people with celiac disease do not improve on the gluten-free diet. These people often have severely damaged intestines that cannot heal even after they eliminate gluten from their diet. Because their intestines are not absorbing enough nutrients, they may need to receive intravenous nutrition supplements. Drug treatments are being evaluated for unresponsive celiac disease. These patients may need to be evaluated for complications of the disease.

The Gluten-Free Diet: A gluten-free diet means avoiding all foods that contain wheat (including spelt, triticale, and kamut), rye, and barley—in other words, most grain, pasta, cereal, and many processed foods. Despite these restrictions, people with celiac disease can eat a well-balanced diet with a variety of foods, including bread and pasta. For example, instead of wheat flour, people can use potato, rice, soy, or bean flour. Or, they can buy gluten-free bread, pasta, and other products from special food companies.

Whether people with celiac disease should avoid oats is controversial because some people have been able to eat oats without having a reaction. Scientists are doing studies to find out whether people with celiac disease can tolerate oats. Until the studies are complete, people with celiac disease should follow their physician or dietitian's advice about eating oats. A dietitian is a health care professional who specializes in food and nutrition.

Plain meat, fish, rice, fruits, and vegetables do not contain gluten, so people with celiac disease can eat as much of these foods as they like. Examples of foods that are safe to eat and those that are not are provided in the following.

The gluten-free diet is complicated. It requires a completely new approach to eating that affects a person's entire life. People with celiac disease have to be extremely careful about what they buy for lunch at school or work, eat at cocktail parties, or grab from the refrigerator for a midnight snack. Eating out can be a challenge as the person with celiac disease learns to scrutinize the menu for foods with gluten and question the waiter or chef about possible hidden sources of gluten. Hidden sources of gluten include additives, preservatives, and stabilizers found in processed food, medicines, and mouthwash. If ingredients are not itemized, you may want to check with the manufacturer of the product. With practice, screening for gluten becomes second nature.

A dietitian can help people learn about their new diet. Also, support groups are particularly helpful for newly diagnosed people and their families as they learn to adjust to a new way of life.

Tables 47.1 and 47.2 provide examples of foods that are allowed and those that should be questioned when eating gluten-free. Please note that these are not a complete lists. People are encouraged to discuss gluten-free food choices with a physician or dietitian who specializes in celiac disease. Also, it is important to read all food ingredient lists carefully to make sure that the food does not contain gluten.

What are the complications of celiac disease?

Damage to the small intestine and the resulting problems with nutrient absorption put a person with celiac disease at risk for several diseases and health problems.

- Lymphoma and adenocarcinoma are types of cancer that can develop in the intestine.

- Osteoporosis is a condition in which the bones become weak, brittle, and prone to breaking. Poor calcium absorption is a contributing factor to osteoporosis.

- Miscarriage and congenital malformation of the baby, such as neural tube defects, are risks for untreated pregnant women with celiac disease because of malabsorption of nutrients.

- Short stature results when childhood celiac disease prevents nutrient absorption during the years when nutrition is critical to a child's normal growth and development. Children who are diagnosed and treated before their growth stops may have a catch-up period.

- Seizures, or convulsions, result from inadequate absorption of folic acid. Lack of folic acid causes calcium deposits, called calcifications, to form in the brain, which in turn cause seizures.

How common is celiac disease?

Celiac disease is the most common genetic disease in Europe. In Italy about 1 in 250 people and in Ireland about 1 in 300 people have celiac disease. Recent studies have shown that it may be more common in Africa, South America, and Asia than previously believed.

Until recently, celiac disease was thought to be uncommon in the United States. However, studies have shown that celiac disease occurs in an estimated 1 in 133 Americans. Among people who have a first-degree relative diagnosed with celiac, as many as 1 in 22 people may have the disease. A recent study in which random blood samples from the Red Cross were tested for celiac disease suggests that as many as 1 in every 250 Americans may have it. Celiac disease could be under-diagnosed in the United States for a number of reasons:

- Celiac symptoms can be attributed to other problems.
- Many doctors are not knowledgeable about the disease.
- Only a handful of U.S. laboratories are experienced and skilled in testing for celiac disease.

More research is needed to find out the true prevalence of celiac disease among Americans.

What diseases are linked to celiac disease?

People with celiac disease tend to have other autoimmune diseases as well, including the following:

- dermatitis herpetiformis
- thyroid disease
- systemic lupus erythematosus
- type 1 diabetes
- liver disease
- collagen vascular disease
- rheumatoid arthritis
- Sjögren syndrome

The connection between celiac and these diseases may be genetic.

Dermatitis Herpetiformis: Dermatitis herpetiformis (DH) is a severe itchy, blistering skin disease caused by gluten intolerance. DH is related to celiac disease because both are autoimmune disorders caused by gluten intolerance, but they are separate diseases. The rash usually occurs on the elbows, knees, and buttocks.

Although people with DH do not usually have digestive symptoms, they often have the same intestinal damage as people with celiac disease.

DH is diagnosed by a skin biopsy, which involves removing a tiny piece of skin near the rash and testing it for the IgA antibody. DH is

Table 47.1. Flours, cereal, and starches allowed on a gluten-free diet.

Arrowroot

Amaranth

Buckwheat

Corn

Flax

Indian ricegrass (Montina™)

Legume flours (bean, chickpea/garbanzo, lentil, pea)

Millet

Nut flours (almond, hazelnut, pecan)

Potato flour

Potato starch

Quinoa

Rice (black, brown, glutinous/sweet, white, wild)

Rice bran

Rice polish

Sago

Sorghum

Soy

Sweet potato flour

Tapioca (cassava/manioc)

Teff

Source: From "Celiac Disease and the Gluten-free Diet: An Overview," by Marion Zarkadas, MSc, RD and Shelley Case, BSc, RD. Topics in Clinical Nutrition 2005 April—June; 20 (2):127–38.© 2005 Lippincott Williams and Willkins. Reprinted by permission.

Table 47.2. Examples of foods that are allowed on a gluten-free diet and foods to question

Foods allowed on a gluten-free diet		Foods to question
Grain products	Breads and baked goods, cereals, and pastas made with allowed cereals, flours, and starches	Rice and corn cereals (often have barley or malt added), buckwheat pasta
Fruits and vegetables	All fresh, frozen, and canned, with no gluten-containing sauces	Fruit pie fillings, dried fruits, French fries in restaurants
Meat and alternates	Meats: plain fresh, frozen, canned (no gluten fillers or thickened gravy) Eggs: fresh or frozen Legumes: lentils, chick peas, beans, peas, fresh, canned, and dried (no gluten-containing sauces) Seeds and nuts—plain	Processed meats, for example, ham, luncheon meats such as bologna, salami, meat loaf, meat patties, sausages, pate, wieners, imitation fish Dry roasted nuts Baked beans
Milk and milk products	Plain milk products, including milk, cream, yogurt, buttermilk, cheese, most ice creams, processed and plain cheeses	Milk drinks, flavored yogurt, frozen yogurt, sour cream, cheese sauces and spreads
Miscellaneous	Fats and oils: all fats and oils and some salad dressings Soups: all made with allowed ingredients Desserts: gelatin, sherbet, custard, some rice pudding, whipped toppings, baked goods, all made with allowed ingredients Beverages: regular tea, coffee, cocoa, soft drinks, distilled alcoholic beverages Sweets: honey, jam, jelly, marmalade, maple syrup, sugar, candy made with allowed ingredients Condiments: plain pickles, relish, olives, ketchup, plain mustard, spices, vinegar (except malt vinegar), gluten-free soy sauce Snacks: plain popcorn, nuts, and soy nuts	Salad dressings (may contain wheat flour or modified food starch) Canned soup, soup mixes, bases, bouillon cubes Milk puddings, custard powder, pudding mixes Flavored, herbal, and instant tea, coffee substitutes, chocolate drinks and mixes Chocolate bars Seasoning mixes Flavored potato chips, corn and taco chips

Source: From "Celiac Disease and the Gluten-free Diet: An Overview," by Marion Zarkadas, MSc, RD and Shelley Case, BSc, RD. Topics in Clinical Nutrition 2005 April—June; 20 (2):127–38.© 2005 Lippincott Williams and Willkins. Reprinted by permission.

treated with a gluten-free diet and medication to control the rash, such as dapsone or sulfapyridine. Drug treatment may last several years.

Points to Remember

- People with celiac disease cannot tolerate gluten, a protein in wheat, rye, barley, and possibly oats.
- Celiac disease damages the small intestine and interferes with nutrient absorption.
- Treatment is important because people with celiac disease could develop complications like cancer, osteoporosis, anemia, and seizures.
- A person with celiac disease may or may not have symptoms.
- Diagnosis involves blood tests and biopsy.
- Because celiac disease is hereditary, family members of a person with celiac disease may need to be tested.
- Celiac disease is treated by eliminating all gluten from the diet. The gluten-free diet is a lifetime requirement.

Chapter 48

Food- and
Water-Borne Diseases

Chapter Contents

Section 48.1

Foodborne Illnesses: An Overview

Excerpted from "Foodborne Illness,"
Centers for Disease Control and Prevention, January 2005.

What is foodborne disease?

Foodborne disease is caused by consuming contaminated foods or beverages. Many different disease-causing microbes, or pathogens, can contaminate foods, so there are many different foodborne infections. In addition, poisonous chemicals, or other harmful substances, can cause foodborne diseases if they are present in food.

More than 250 different foodborne diseases have been described. Most of these diseases are infections, caused by a variety of bacteria, viruses, and parasites that can be foodborne. Other diseases are poisonings, caused by harmful toxins or chemicals that have contaminated the food, for example, poisonous mushrooms. These different diseases have many different symptoms, so there is no one "syndrome" that is foodborne illness. However, the microbe or toxin enters the body through the gastrointestinal tract, and often causes the first symptoms there, so nausea, vomiting, abdominal cramps, and diarrhea are common symptoms in many foodborne diseases.

Many microbes can spread in more than one way, so we cannot always know that a disease is foodborne. The distinction matters, because public health authorities need to know how a particular disease is spreading to take the appropriate steps to stop it. For example, *Escherichia coli O157:H7* infections can spread through contaminated food, contaminated drinking water, contaminated swimming water, and from toddler to toddler at a daycare center. Depending on which means of spread caused a case, the measures to stop other cases from occurring could range from removing contaminated food from stores, to chlorinating a swimming pool, or to closing a child daycare center.

What are the most common foodborne diseases?

The most commonly recognized foodborne infections are those caused by the bacteria *Campylobacter*, *Salmonella*, and *E. coli O157:H7*, and by a group of viruses called calicivirus, also known as the Norwalk and Norwalk-like viruses.

Campylobacter is a bacterial pathogen that causes fever, diarrhea, and abdominal cramps. It is the most commonly identified bacterial cause of diarrheal illness in the world. These bacteria live in the intestines of healthy birds, and most raw poultry meat has *Campylobacter* on it. Eating undercooked chicken, or other food that has been contaminated with juices dripping from raw chicken, is the most frequent source of this infection.

Salmonella is also a bacterium that is widespread in the intestines of birds, reptiles, and mammals. It can spread to humans via a variety of different foods of animal origin. The illness it causes, salmonellosis, typically includes fever, diarrhea, and abdominal cramps. In persons with poor underlying health or weakened immune systems, it can invade the bloodstream and cause life-threatening infections.

E. coli O157:H7 is a bacterial pathogen that has a reservoir in cattle and other similar animals. Human illness typically follows consumption of food or water that has been contaminated with microscopic amounts of cow feces. The illness it causes is often a severe and bloody diarrhea and painful abdominal cramps, without much fever. In 3 percent to 5 percent of cases, a complication called hemolytic uremic syndrome (HUS) can occur several weeks after the initial symptoms. This severe complication includes temporary anemia, profuse bleeding, and kidney failure.

Calicivirus, or Norwalk-like virus, is an extremely common cause of foodborne illness, though it is rarely diagnosed, because the laboratory test is not widely available. It causes an acute gastrointestinal illness, usually with more vomiting than diarrhea, that resolves within two days. Unlike many foodborne pathogens that have animal reservoirs, it is believed that Norwalk-like viruses spread primarily from one infected person to another. Infected kitchen workers can contaminate a salad or sandwich as they prepare it, if they have the virus on their hands. Infected fishermen have contaminated oysters as they harvested them.

Some common diseases are occasionally foodborne, even though they are usually transmitted by other routes. These include infections caused by *Shigella*, hepatitis A, and the parasites *Giardia lamblia* and *Cryptosporidia*. Even strep throats have been transmitted occasionally through food.

In addition to disease caused by direct infection, some foodborne diseases are caused by the presence of a toxin in the food that was produced by a microbe in the food. For example, the bacterium *Staphylococcus aureus* can grow in some foods and produce a toxin that causes intense vomiting. The rare but deadly disease botulism occurs when the bacterium *Clostridium botulinum* grows and produces a powerful paralytic toxin in foods. These toxins can produce illness even if the microbes that produced them are no longer there.

Other toxins and poisonous chemicals can cause foodborne illness. People can become ill if a pesticide is inadvertently added to a food, or if naturally poisonous substances are used to prepare a meal. Every year, people become ill after mistaking poisonous mushrooms for safe species, or after eating poisonous reef fishes.

Are the types of foodborne diseases changing?

The spectrum of foodborne diseases is constantly changing. A century ago, typhoid fever, tuberculosis, and cholera were common foodborne diseases. Improvements in food safety, such as pasteurization of milk, safe canning, and disinfection of water supplies have conquered those diseases. Today other foodborne infections have taken their place, including some that have only recently been discovered. For example, in 1996, the parasite *Cyclospora* suddenly appeared as a cause of diarrheal illness related to Guatemalan raspberries. These berries had just started to be grown commercially in Guatemala, and somehow became contaminated in the field there with this unusual parasite. In 1998, a new strain of the bacterium *Vibrio parahaemolyticus* contaminated oyster beds in Galveston Bay and caused an epidemic of diarrheal illness in persons eating the oysters raw. The affected oyster beds were near the shipping lanes, which suggested that the bacterium arrived in the ballast water of freighters and tankers coming into the harbor from distant ports. Newly recognized microbes emerge as public health problems for several reasons: microbes can easily spread around the world, new microbes can evolve, the environment and ecology are changing, food production practices and consumption habits change, and because better laboratory tests can now identify microbes that were previously unrecognized.

In the last fifteen years, several important diseases of unknown cause have turned out to be complications of foodborne infections. For example, we now know that the Guillain-Barré syndrome can be caused by *Campylobacter* infection, and that the most common cause of acute kidney failure in children, hemolytic uremic syndrome, is caused by infection with *E. coli O157:H7* and related bacteria. In the future, other diseases whose origins are currently unknown may turn out be related to foodborne infections.

What happens in the body after the microbes that produce illness are swallowed?

After they are swallowed, there is a delay, called the incubation period, before the symptoms of illness begin. This delay may range from hours to days, depending on the organism, and on how many of them were swallowed. During the incubation period, the microbes pass through the stomach into the intestine, attach to the cells lining the intestinal walls, and begin to multiply there. Some types of microbes stay in the intestine, some produce a toxin that is absorbed into the bloodstream, and some can directly invade the deeper body tissues. The symptoms produced depend greatly on the type of microbe. Numerous organisms cause similar symptoms, especially diarrhea, abdominal cramps, and nausea. There is so much overlap that it is rarely possible to say which microbe is likely to be causing a given illness unless laboratory tests are done to identify the microbe, or unless the illness is part of a recognized outbreak.

How are foodborne diseases diagnosed?

The infection is usually diagnosed by specific laboratory tests that identify the causative organism. Bacteria such as *Campylobacter*, *Salmonella*, or *E. coli O157* are found by culturing stool samples in the laboratory and identifying the bacteria that grow on the agar or other culture medium. Parasites can be identified by examining stools under the microscope. Viruses are more difficult to identify, as they are too small to see under a light microscope and are difficult to culture. Viruses are usually identified by testing stool samples for genetic markers that indicate a specific virus is present.

Many foodborne infections are not identified by routine laboratory procedures and require specialized, experimental, or expensive tests that are not generally available. If the diagnosis is to be made, the patient has to seek medical attention, the physician must decide to order diagnostic tests, and the laboratory must use the appropriate procedures. Because many ill persons to not seek attention, and of those that do, many are not tested, many cases of foodborne illness go undiagnosed. For example, CDC estimates that thirty-eight cases of salmonellosis actually occur for every case that is actually diagnosed and reported to public health authorities.

How are foodborne diseases treated?

There are many different kinds of foodborne diseases and they may require different treatments, depending on the symptoms they cause. Illnesses that are primarily diarrhea or vomiting can lead to dehydration if the person loses more body fluids and salts (electrolytes) than he or she takes in. Replacing the lost fluids and electrolytes and keeping up with fluid intake are important. If diarrhea is severe, an oral rehydration solution, such as CeraLyte, Pedialyte, or Oralyte, should be drunk to replace the fluid losses and prevent dehydration. Sports drinks such as Gatorade do not replace the losses correctly and should not be used for the treatment of diarrheal illness. Preparations of bismuth subsalicylate (e.g., Pepto-Bismol) can reduce the duration and severity of simple diarrhea. If diarrhea and cramps occur, without bloody stools or fever, taking an antidiarrheal medication may provide symptomatic relief, but these medications should be avoided if there is high fever or blood in the stools because they may make the illness worse.

When should I consult my doctor about a diarrheal illness?

A health care provider should be consulted for a diarrheal illness is accompanied by the following symptoms:

- high fever (temperature over 101.5 F, measured orally)
- blood in the stools
- prolonged vomiting that prevents keeping liquids down (which can lead to dehydration)
- signs of dehydration, including a decrease in urination, a dry mouth and throat, and feeling dizzy when standing up
- diarrheal illness that lasts more than three days

Do not be surprised if your doctor does not prescribe an antibiotic. Many diarrheal illnesses are caused by viruses and will improve in two or three days without antibiotic therapy. In fact, antibiotics have no effect on viruses, and using an antibiotic to treat a viral infection could cause more harm than good. It is often not necessary to take an antibiotic even in the case of a mild bacterial infection. Other treatments can help the symptoms, and careful hand washing can prevent the spread of infection to other people. Overuse of antibiotics is the principal reason many bacteria are becoming resistant. Resistant bacteria are no longer killed by the antibiotic. This means that it is important to use antibiotics only when they are really needed. Partial treatment can also cause bacteria to become resistant. If an antibiotic is prescribed, it is important to take all of the medication as prescribed, and not stop early just because the symptoms seem to be improving.

How many cases of foodborne disease are there in the United States?

An estimated seventy-six million cases of foodborne disease occur each year in the United States. The great majority of these cases are mild and cause symptoms for only a day or two. Some cases are more serious, and CDC estimates that there are 325,000 hospitalizations and 5,000 deaths related to foodborne diseases each year. The most severe cases tend to occur in the very old, the very young, those who have an illness already that reduces their immune system function, and in healthy people exposed to a very high dose of an organism.

How does food become contaminated?

We live in a microbial world, and there are many opportunities for food to become contaminated as it is produced and prepared. Many foodborne microbes are present in healthy animals (usually in their intestines) raised for food. Meat and poultry carcasses can become contaminated during slaughter by contact with small amounts of intestinal contents. Similarly, fresh fruits and vegetables can be contaminated if they are washed or irrigated with water that is contaminated with animal manure or human sewage. Some types of *Salmonella* can infect a hen's ovary so that the internal contents of a normal-looking egg can be contaminated with *Salmonella* even before the shell is formed. Oysters and other filter feeding shellfish can concentrate *Vibrio* bacteria that are naturally present in seawater, or other microbes that are present in human sewage dumped into the sea.

Later in food processing, other foodborne microbes can be introduced from infected humans who handle the food, or by cross-contamination from some other raw agricultural product. For example, *Shigella* bacteria, hepatitis A virus, and Norwalk virus can be introduced by the unwashed hands of food handlers who are themselves infected. In the kitchen, microbes can be transferred from one food to another food by using the same knife, cutting board, or other utensil to prepare both without washing the surface or utensil in between. A food that is fully cooked can become recontaminated if it touches other raw foods or drippings from raw foods that contain pathogens.

The way that food is handled after it is contaminated can also make a difference in whether or not an outbreak occurs. Many bacterial microbes need to multiply to a larger number before enough are present in food to cause disease. Given warm, moist conditions and an ample supply of nutrients, one bacterium that reproduces by dividing itself every half hour can produce seventeen million progeny in twelve hours. As a result, lightly contaminated food left out overnight can be highly infectious by the next day. If the food were refrigerated promptly, the bacteria would not multiply at all. In general, refrigeration or freezing prevents virtually all bacteria from growing but generally preserves them in a state of suspended animation. This general rule has a few surprising exceptions. Two foodborne bacteria, *Listeria monocytogenes* and *Yersinia enterocolitica*, can actually grow at refrigerator temperatures. High salt, high sugar, or high acid levels keep bacteria from growing, which is why salted meats, jam, and pickled vegetables are traditional preserved foods.

Microbes are killed by heat. If food is heated to an internal temperature above 160°F, or 78°C, for even a few seconds this is sufficient to kill parasites, viruses or bacteria, except for the *Clostridium* bacteria, which produce a heat-resistant form called a spore. *Clostridium* spores are killed only at temperatures above boiling. This is why canned foods must be cooked to a high temperature under pressure as part of the canning process.

The toxins produced by bacteria vary in their sensitivity to heat. The staphylococcal toxin which causes vomiting is not inactivated even if it is boiled. Fortunately, the potent toxin that causes botulism is completely inactivated by boiling.

What foods are most associated with foodborne illness?

Raw foods of animal origin are the most likely to be contaminated; that is, raw meat and poultry, raw eggs, unpasteurized milk, and raw shellfish. Because filter-feeding shellfish strain microbes from the sea over many months, they are particularly likely to be contaminated if there are any pathogens in the seawater. Foods that mingle the products of many individual animals, such as bulk raw milk, pooled raw eggs, or ground beef, are particularly hazardous because a pathogen present in any one of the animals may contaminate the whole batch. A single hamburger may contain meat from hundreds of animals. A single restaurant omelet may contain eggs from hundreds of chickens.

A glass of raw milk may contain milk from hundreds of cows. A broiler chicken carcass can be exposed to the drippings and juices of many thousands of other birds that went through the same cold water tank after slaughter.

Fruits and vegetables consumed raw are a particular concern. Washing can decrease but not eliminate contamination, so consumers can do little to protect themselves. Recently, a number of outbreaks have been traced to fresh fruits and vegetables that were processed under less than sanitary conditions. These outbreaks show that the quality of the water used for washing and chilling the produce after it is harvested is critical. Using water that is not clean can contaminate many boxes of produce. Fresh manure used to fertilize vegetables can also contaminate them. Alfalfa sprouts and other raw sprouts pose a particular challenge, as the conditions under which they are sprouted are ideal for growing microbes as well as sprouts, and because they are eaten without further cooking. That means that a few bacteria present on the seeds can grow to high numbers of pathogens on the sprouts. Unpasteurized fruit juice can also be contaminated if there are pathogens in or on the fruit that is used to make it.

What can consumers do to protect themselves from foodborne illness?

A few simple precautions can reduce the risk of foodborne diseases:

- **Cook:** Make sure all meat, poultry, and eggs are cooked thoroughly. Using a thermometer to measure the internal temperature of meat is a good way to be sure that it is cooked sufficiently to kill bacteria. For example, ground beef should be cooked to an internal temperature of 160° F. Eggs should be cooked until the yolk is firm.

- **Separate:** Don't cross-contaminate one food with another. Avoid cross-contaminating foods by washing hands, utensils, and cutting boards after they have been in contact with raw meat or poultry and before they touch another food. Put cooked meat on a clean platter, rather than back on one that held the raw meat.

- **Chill:** Refrigerate leftovers promptly. Bacteria can grow quickly at room temperature, so refrigerate leftover foods if they are not going to be eaten within four hours. Large volumes of food will cool more quickly if they are divided into several shallow containers for refrigeration.

- **Clean:** Wash produce. Rinse fresh fruits and vegetables in running tap water to remove visible dirt and grime. Remove and discard the outermost leaves of a head of lettuce or cabbage. Because bacteria can grow well on the cut surface of fruits or vegetables, be careful not to contaminate these foods while slicing them up on the cutting board, and avoid leaving cut produce at room temperature for many hours. Don't be a source of foodborne illness yourself. Wash your hands with soap and water before preparing food. Avoid preparing food for others if you yourself have a diarrheal illness. Changing a baby's diaper while preparing food is a bad idea that can easily spread illness.

- **Report:** Report suspected foodborne illnesses to your local health department. The local public health department is an important part of the food safety system. Often calls from concerned citizens are how outbreaks are first detected. If a public health official contacts you to find our more about an illness you had, your cooperation is important. In public health investigations, it can be as important to talk to healthy people as to ill people. Your cooperation may be needed even if you are not ill.

Are some people more likely to contract a foodborne illness? If so, are there special precautions they should take?

Some persons at particularly high risk should take more precautions.

- Pregnant women, the elderly, and those with weakened immune systems are at higher risk for severe infections such as *Listeria* and should be particularly careful not to consume undercooked animal products. They should avoid soft French style cheeses, pates, uncooked hot dogs, and sliced deli meats, which have been sources of *Listeria* infections. Persons at high risk should also avoid alfalfa sprouts and unpasteurized juices.

- A bottle-fed infant is at higher risk for severe infections with *Salmonella* or other bacteria that can grow in a bottle of warm formula if it is left at room temperature for many hours. Particular care is needed to be sure the baby's bottle is cleaned and disinfected and that leftover milk formula or juice is not held in the bottle for many hours.

- Persons with liver disease are susceptible to infections with a rare but dangerous microbe called *Vibrio vulnificus*, found in oysters. They should avoid eating raw oysters.

What can consumers do when they eat in restaurants?

You can protect yourself first by choosing which restaurant to patronize. Restaurants are inspected by the local health department to make sure they are clean and have adequate kitchen facilities. Find out how restaurants did on their most recent inspections, and use that score to help guide your choice. In many jurisdictions, the latest inspection score is posted in the restaurant. Some restaurants have specifically trained their staff in principles of food safety. This is also good to know in deciding which restaurant to patronize.

You can also protect yourself from foodborne disease when ordering specific foods, just as you would at home. When ordering a hamburger, ask for it to be cooked to a temperature of 160°F and send it back if it is still pink in the middle. Before you order something that is made with many eggs pooled together, such as scrambled eggs, omelets, or French toast, ask the waiter whether it was made with pasteurized egg, and choose something else if it was not.

There is only so much the consumer can do. How can food be made safer in the first place?

Making food safe in the first place is a major effort, involving the farm and fishery, the production plant or factory, and many other points from the farm to the table. Many different groups in public health, industry, regulatory agencies, and academia have roles to play in making the food supply less contaminated. Consumers can promote general food safety with their dollars, by purchasing foods that have been processed for safety. For example, milk pasteurization was a major advance in food safety that was developed one hundred years ago. Buying pasteurized milk rather than raw unpasteurized milk still prevents an enormous number of foodborne diseases every day. Now juice pasteurization is a recent important step forward that prevents *E. coli O157:H7* infections and many other diseases. Consumers can look for and buy pasteurized fruit juices and ciders. In the future, meat and other foods will be available that have been treated for safety with irradiation. These new technologies are likely to be as important a step forward as the pasteurization of milk.

Foodborne diseases are largely preventable, though there is no simple one-step prevention measure like a vaccine. Instead, measures are needed to prevent or limit contamination all the way from farm to table. A variety of good agricultural and manufacturing practices can reduce the spread of microbes among animals and prevent the contamination of foods. Careful review of the whole food production process can identify the principal hazards, and the control points where contamination can be prevented, limited, or eliminated. A formal method for evaluating the control of risk in foods exists and is called the Hazard Analysis Critical Control Point, or HACCP system. This was first developed by NASA to make sure that the food eaten by astronauts was safe. HACCP safety principles are now being applied to an increasing spectrum of foods, including meat, poultry, and seafood.

For some particularly risky foods, even the most careful hygiene and sanitation are insufficient to prevent contamination, and a definitive microbe-killing step must be included in the process. For example, early in the century, large botulism outbreaks occurred when canned foods were cooked insufficiently to kill the botulism spores. After research was done to find out exactly how much heat was needed to kill the spores, the canning industry and the government regulators went to great lengths to be sure every can was sufficiently cooked. As a result, botulism related to commercial canned foods has disappeared in this country. Similarly the introduction of careful pasteurization of milk eliminated a large number of milk-borne diseases. This occurred after sanitation in dairies had already reached a high level. In the future, other foods can be made much safer by new pasteurizing technologies, such as in-shell pasteurization of eggs, and irradiation of ground beef. Just as with milk, these new technologies should be implemented in addition to good sanitation, not as a replacement for it.

In the end, it is up to the consumer to demand a safe food supply; up to industry to produce it; up to researchers to develop better ways of doing so; and up to government to see that it happens, to make sure it works, and to identify problems still in need of solutions.

Section 48.2

Campylobacter *Infections*

Reprinted from "Campylobacter Infections,"
Centers for Disease Control and Prevention, September 2003.

What is campylobacteriosis?

Campylobacteriosis is an infectious disease caused by bacteria of the genus *Campylobacter*. Most people who become ill with campylobacteriosis get diarrhea, cramping, abdominal pain, and fever within two to five days after exposure to the organism. The diarrhea may be bloody and can be accompanied by nausea and vomiting. The illness typically lasts one week. Some persons who are infected with *Campylobacter* don't have any symptoms at all. In persons with compromised immune systems, *Campylobacter* occasionally spreads to the bloodstream and causes a serious life-threatening infection.

How common is Campylobacter?

Campylobacter is one of the most common bacterial causes of diarrheal illness in the United States. Virtually all cases occur as isolated, sporadic events, not as a part of large outbreaks. Active surveillance through FoodNet indicates about fifteen cases are diagnosed each year for each one hundred thousand persons in the population. Many more cases go undiagnosed or unreported, and campylobacteriosis is estimated to affect over one million persons every year, or 0.5 percent of the general population. Campylobacteriosis occurs much more frequently in the summer months than in the winter. The organism is isolated from infants and young adults more frequently than from other age groups and from males more frequently than females. Although Campylobacter doesn't commonly cause death, it has been estimated that approximately one hundred persons with Campylobacter infections may die each year.

What sort of germ is Campylobacter?

The *Campylobacter* organism is actually a group of spiral-shaped bacteria that can cause disease in humans and animals. Most human illness is caused by one species, called *Campylobacter jejuni*, but 1 percent of human *Campylobacter* cases are caused by other species. *Campylobacter jejuni* grows best at the body temperature of a bird, and seems to be well adapted to birds, who carry it without becoming ill. The bacterium is fragile. It cannot tolerate drying and can be killed by oxygen. It grows only if there is less than the atmospheric amount of oxygen present. Freezing reduces the number of Campylobacter bacteria present on raw meat.

How is the infection diagnosed?

Many different kinds of infections can cause diarrhea and bloody diarrhea. Doctors can look for bacterial causes of diarrhea by asking a laboratory to culture a sample of stool from an ill person. Diagnosis of *Campylobacter* requires special laboratory culture procedures, which doctors may need to specifically request.

How can campylobacteriosis be treated?

Virtually all persons infected with *Campylobacter* will recover without any specific treatment. Patients should drink plenty of fluids as long as the diarrhea lasts. In more severe cases, antibiotics such as erythromycin or a fluoroquinolone can be used, and can shorten the duration of symptoms if they are given early in the illness. Your doctor will make the decision about whether antibiotics are necessary.

Are there long-term consequences?

Most people who get campylobacteriosis recover completely within two to five days, although sometimes recovery can take up to ten days. Rarely, some long-term consequences can result from a *Campylobacter* infection. Some people may have arthritis following campylobacteriosis; others may develop a rare disease that affects the nerves of the body beginning several weeks after the diarrheal illness. This disease, called Guillain-Barré syndrome, occurs when a person's immune system is "triggered" to attack the body's own nerves, and can lead to paralysis that lasts several weeks and usually requires intensive care. It is estimated that approximately one in every thousand reported campylobacteriosis cases leads to Guillain-Barré syndrome. As many as 40 percent of Guillain-Barré syndrome cases in this country may be triggered by campylobacteriosis.

How do people get infected with this germ?

Campylobacteriosis usually occurs in single, sporadic cases, but it can also occur in outbreaks, when a number of people become ill at one time. Most cases of campylobacteriosis are associated with handling raw poultry or eating raw or undercooked poultry meat. A very small number of *Campylobacter* organisms (fewer than five hundred) can cause illness in humans. Even one drop of juice from raw chicken meat can infect a person. One way to become infected is to cut poultry meat on a cutting board, and then use the unwashed cutting board or utensil to prepare vegetables or other raw or lightly cooked foods. The *Campylobacter* organisms from the raw meat can then spread to the other foods. The organism is not usually spread from person to person, but this can happen if the infected person is a small child or is producing a large volume of diarrhea. Larger outbreaks due to *Campylobacter* are not usually associated with raw poultry but are usually related to drinking unpasteurized milk or contaminated water. Animals can also be infected, and some people have acquired their infection from contact with the infected stool of an ill dog or cat.

How does food or water get contaminated with Campylobacter?

Many chicken flocks are silently infected with *Campylobacter*; that is, the chickens are infected with the organism but show no signs of illness. *Campylobacter* can be easily spread from bird to bird through a common water source or through contact with infected feces. When an infected bird is slaughtered, *Campylobacter* can be transferred from the intestines to the meat. More than half of the raw chicken in the United States market has *Campylobacter* on it. *Campylobacter* is also present in the giblets, especially the liver.

Unpasteurized milk can become contaminated if the cow has an infection with *Campylobacter* in her udder or the milk is contaminated with manure. Surface water and mountain streams can become contaminated from infected feces from cows or wild birds. This infection is common in the developing world, and travelers to foreign countries are also at risk for becoming infected with *Campylobacter*.

What can be done to prevent the infection?

There are some simple food handling practices for preventing *Campylobacter* infections. Physicians who diagnose campylobacteriosis and clinical laboratories that identify this organism should report their findings to the local health department. If many cases occur at the same time, it may mean that many people were exposed to a common contaminated food item or water source that might still be available to infect more people. When outbreaks occur, community education efforts can be directed at proper food handling techniques, especially thorough cooking of all poultry and other foods of animal origin, and common sense kitchen hygiene practices. Some data suggest that *Campylobacter* can spread through a chicken flock in their drinking water. Providing clean, chlorinated water sources for the chickens might prevent *Campylobacter* infections in poultry flocks and thereby decrease the amount of contaminated meat reaching the marketplace.

Some Tips for Preventing Campylobacteriosis

- Cook all poultry products thoroughly. Make sure that the meat is cooked throughout (no longer pink), any juices run clear, and the inside is cooked to 170°F (77°C) for breast meat, and 180°F (82°C) for thigh meat.

- If you are served undercooked poultry in a restaurant, send it back for further cooking.

- Wash hands with soap before handling raw foods of animal origin. Wash hands with soap after handling raw foods of animal origin and before touching anything else.

- Prevent cross-contamination in the kitchen:

  - Use separate cutting boards for foods of animal origin and other foods.

  - Carefully clean all cutting boards, countertops, and utensils with soap and hot water after preparing raw food of animal origin.

- Avoid consuming unpasteurized milk and untreated surface water.

- Make sure that persons with diarrhea, especially children, wash their hands carefully and frequently with soap to reduce the risk of spreading the infection.

- Wash hands with soap after having contact with pet feces.

What are public health agencies doing to prevent or control campylobacteriosis?

To learn more about how *Campylobacter* causes disease and is spread, CDC began a national surveillance program in 1982. A more detailed active surveillance system was instituted in 1996; this will provide more information on how often this disease occurs and what the risk factors are for getting it. CDC is also making an effort to inform the public about campylobacteriosis and ways to avoid getting this disease. The U.S. Department of Agriculture conducts research on how to prevent the infection in chickens. The Food and Drug Administration has produced the Model Food Code, which could decrease the risk of contaminated chicken being served in commercial food establishments.

Section 48.3

Escherichia Coli O157:H7

Reprinted from "Escherichia Coli O157:H7,"
Centers for Disease Control and Prevention, January 2004.

Escherichia coli O157:H7 is an emerging cause of foodborne illness. An estimated seventy-three thousand cases of infection and sixty-one deaths occur in the United States each year. Infection often leads to bloody diarrhea, and occasionally to kidney failure. Most illness has been associated with eating undercooked, contaminated ground beef. Person-to-person contact in families and childcare centers is also an important mode of transmission. Infection can also occur after drinking raw milk and after swimming in or drinking sewage-contaminated water.

Consumers can prevent *E. coli O157:H7* infection by thoroughly cooking ground beef, avoiding unpasteurized milk, and washing hands carefully.

Because the organism lives in the intestines of healthy cattle, preventive measures on cattle farms and during meat processing are being investigated.

What *is* Escherichia coli O157:H7?

E. coli O157:H7 is one of hundreds of strains of the bacterium *Escherichia coli*. Although most strains are harmless and live in the intestines of healthy humans and animals, this strain produces a powerful toxin and can cause severe illness.

E. coli O157:H7 was first recognized as a cause of illness in 1982 during an outbreak of severe bloody diarrhea; the outbreak was traced to contaminated hamburgers. Since then, most infections have come from eating undercooked ground beef.

The combination of letters and numbers in the name of the bacterium refers to the specific markers found on its surface and distinguishes it from other types of *E. coli*.

How *is* E. coli O157:H7 *spread?*

The organism can be found on a small number of cattle farms and can live in the intestines of healthy cattle. Meat can become contaminated during slaughter, and organisms can be thoroughly mixed into beef when it is ground. Bacteria present on the cow's udders or on equipment may get into raw milk.

Eating meat, especially ground beef that has not been cooked sufficiently to kill *E. coli O157:H7*, can cause infection. Contaminated meat looks and smells normal. Although the number of organisms required to cause disease is not known, it is suspected to be very small.

Among other known sources of infection are consumption of sprouts, lettuce, salami, and unpasteurized milk and juice, and swimming in or drinking sewage-contaminated water.

Bacteria in diarrheal stools of infected persons can be passed from one person to another if hygiene or hand washing habits are inadequate. This is particularly likely among toddlers who are not toilet trained. Family members and playmates of these children are at high risk of becoming infected.

Young children typically shed the organism in their feces for a week or two after their illness resolves. Older children rarely carry the organism without symptoms.

What *illness does* E. coli O157:H7 *cause?*

E. coli O157:H7 infection often causes severe bloody diarrhea and abdominal cramps; sometimes the infection causes nonbloody diarrhea or no symptoms. Usually little or no fever is present, and the illness resolves in five to ten days.

In some persons, particularly children under five years of age and the elderly, the infection can also cause a complication called hemolytic uremic syndrome, in which the red blood cells are destroyed and the kidneys fail. About 2 percent to 7 percent of infections lead to this complication. In the United States, hemolytic uremic syndrome is the principal cause of acute kidney failure in children, and most cases of hemolytic uremic syndrome are caused by *E. coli O157:H7*.

How is E. coli O157:H7 *infection diagnosed?*

Infection with *E. coli O157:H7* is diagnosed by detecting the bacterium in the stool. Most laboratories that culture stool do not test for *E. coli O157:H7*, so it is important to request that the stool specimen be tested on sorbitol-MacConkey (SMAC) agar for this organism. All persons who suddenly have diarrhea with blood should get their stool tested for *E. coli O157:H7*.

How is the illness treated?

Most persons recover without antibiotics or other specific treatment in five to ten days. There is no evidence that antibiotics improve the course of disease, and it is thought that treatment with some antibiotics may precipitate kidney complications. Antidiarrheal agents, such as loperamide (Imodium), should also be avoided.

Hemolytic uremic syndrome is a life-threatening condition usually treated in an intensive care unit. Blood transfusions and kidney dialysis are often required. With intensive care, the death rate for hemolytic uremic syndrome is 3 percent to 5 percent.

What are the long-term consequences of infection?

Persons who have only diarrhea usually recover completely.

About one-third of persons with hemolytic uremic syndrome have abnormal kidney function many years later, and a few require long-term dialysis. Another 8 percent of persons with hemolytic uremic syndrome have other lifelong complications, such as high blood pressure, seizures, blindness, paralysis, and the effects of having part of their bowel removed.

What can be done to prevent the infection?

E. coli O157:H7 will continue to be an important public health concern as long as it contaminates meat. Preventive measures may reduce the number of cattle that carry it and the contamination of meat during slaughter and grinding. Research into such prevention measures is just beginning.

What can you do to prevent E. coli O157:H7 *infection?*

Cook all ground beef and hamburger thoroughly. Because ground beef can turn brown before disease-causing bacteria are killed, use a digital instant-read meat thermometer to ensure thorough cooking. Ground beef should be cooked until a thermometer inserted into several parts of the patty, including the thickest part, reads at least 160° F. Persons who cook ground beef without using a thermometer can decrease their risk of illness by not eating ground beef patties that are still pink in the middle.

If you are served an undercooked hamburger or other ground beef product in a restaurant, send it back for further cooking. You may want to ask for a new bun and a clean plate, too.

Avoid spreading harmful bacteria in your kitchen. Keep raw meat separate from ready-to-eat foods. Wash hands, counters, and utensils with hot soapy water after they touch raw meat. Never place cooked hamburgers or ground beef on the unwashed plate that held raw patties. Wash meat thermometers in between tests of patties that require further cooking.

Drink only pasteurized milk, juice, or cider. Commercial juice with an extended shelf life that is sold at room temperature (e.g., juice in cardboard boxes, vacuum-sealed juice in glass containers) has been pasteurized, although this is generally not indicated on the label. Juice concentrates are also heated sufficiently to kill pathogens.

Wash fruits and vegetables thoroughly, especially those that will not be cooked. Children under five years of age, immunocompromised persons, and the elderly should avoid eating alfalfa sprouts until their safety can be assured. Methods to decontaminate alfalfa seeds and sprouts are being investigated.

Drink municipal water that has been treated with chlorine or other effective disinfectants.

Avoid swallowing lake or pool water while swimming.

Make sure that persons with diarrhea, especially children, wash their hands carefully with soap after bowel movements to reduce the risk of spreading infection, and that persons wash hands after changing soiled diapers. Anyone with a diarrheal illness should avoid swimming in public pools or lakes, sharing baths with others, and preparing food for others.

Section 48.4

Salmonellosis

Reprinted from "Salmonellosis,"
Centers for Disease Control and Prevention, September 2004.

What is salmonellosis?

Salmonellosis is an infection with a bacteria called *Salmonella*. Most persons infected with *Salmonella* develop diarrhea, fever, and abdominal cramps twelve to seventy-two hours after infection. The illness usually lasts four to seven days, and most persons recover without treatment. However, in some persons the diarrhea may be so severe that the patient needs to be hospitalized. In these patients, the *Salmonella* infection may spread from the intestines to the blood stream, and then to other body sites and can cause death unless the person is treated promptly with antibiotics. The elderly, infants, and those with impaired immune systems are more likely to have a severe illness.

What sort of germ is Salmonella?

The *Salmonella* germ is actually a group of bacteria that can cause diarrheal illness in humans. They are microscopic living creatures that pass from the feces of people or animals, to other people or other animals. There are many different kinds of *Salmonella* bacteria. *Salmonella* serotype *Typhimurium* and *Salmonella* serotype *Enteritidis* are the most common in the United States. *Salmonella* has been known to cause illness for over one hundred years. The *Salmonella* bacteria were discovered by an American scientist named Salmon, for whom they are named.

How can Salmonella *infections be diagnosed?*

Many different kinds of illnesses can cause diarrhea, fever, or abdominal cramps. Determining that *Salmonella* is the cause of the illness depends on laboratory tests that identify *Salmonella* in the stools of an infected person. These tests are sometimes not performed unless the laboratory is instructed specifically to look for the organism. Once *Salmonella* has been identified, further testing can determine its specific type, and which antibiotics could be used to treat it.

How can Salmonella *infections be treated?*

Salmonella infections usually resolve in five to seven days and often do not require treatment unless the patient becomes severely dehydrated or the infection spreads from the intestines. Persons with severe diarrhea may require rehydration, often with intravenous fluids. Antibiotics are not usually necessary unless the infection spreads from the intestines; then it can be treated with ampicillin, gentamicin, trimethoprim/sulfamethoxazole, or ciprofloxacin. Unfortunately, some *Salmonella* bacteria have become resistant to antibiotics, largely as a result of the use of antibiotics to promote the growth of feed animals.

Are there long-term consequences to a Salmonella infection?

Persons with diarrhea usually recover completely, although it may be several months before their bowel habits are entirely normal. A small number of persons who are infected with *Salmonella* will go on to develop pains in their joints, irritation of the eyes, and painful urination. This is called Reiter syndrome. It can last for months or years, and can lead to chronic arthritis, which is difficult to treat. Antibiotic treatment does not make a difference in whether or not the person later develops arthritis.

How do people catch Salmonella?

Salmonella live in the intestinal tracts of humans and other animals, including birds. *Salmonella* are usually transmitted to humans by eating foods contaminated with animal feces. Contaminated foods usually look and smell normal. Contaminated foods are often of animal origin, such as beef, poultry, milk, or eggs, but all foods, including vegetables, may become contaminated. Many raw foods of animal origin are frequently contaminated, but fortunately, thorough cooking kills *Salmonella*. Food may also become contaminated by the unwashed hands of an infected food handler, who forgot to wash his or her hands with soap after using the bathroom.

Salmonella may also be found in the feces of some pets, especially those with diarrhea, and people can become infected if they do not wash their hands after contact with these feces. Reptiles are particularly likely to harbor *Salmonella* and people should always wash their hands immediately after handling a reptile, even if the reptile is healthy. Adults should also be careful that children wash their hands after handling a reptile.

What can a person do to prevent this illness?

There is no vaccine to prevent salmonellosis. Since foods of animal origin may be contaminated with *Salmonella*, people should not eat raw or undercooked eggs, poultry, or meat. Raw eggs may be unrecognized in some foods such as homemade hollandaise sauce, caesar and other homemade salad dressings, tiramisu, homemade ice cream, homemade mayonnaise, cookie dough, and frostings. Poultry and meat, including hamburgers, should be well cooked, not pink in the middle. Persons also should not consume raw or unpasteurized milk or other dairy products. Produce should be thoroughly washed before consuming.

Cross-contamination of foods should be avoided. Uncooked meats should be keep separate from produce, cooked foods, and ready-to-eat foods. Hands, cutting boards, counters, knives, and other utensils should be washed thoroughly after handling uncooked foods. Hand should be washed before handling any food, and between handling different food items.

People who have salmonellosis should not prepare food or pour water for others until they have been shown to no longer be carrying the *Salmonella* bacterium.

People should wash their hands after contact with animal feces. Since reptiles are particularly likely to have *Salmonella*, everyone should immediately wash their hands after handling reptiles. Reptiles (including turtles) are not appropriate pets for small children and should not be in the same house as an infant.

How common is salmonellosis?

Every year, approximately forty thousand cases of salmonellosis are reported in the United States. Because many milder cases are not diagnosed or reported, the actual number of infections may be thirty or more times greater. Salmonellosis is more common in the summer than in the winter.

Children are the most likely to get salmonellosis. Young children, the elderly, and the immunocompromised are the most likely to have severe infections. It is estimated that approximately six hundred persons die each year with acute salmonellosis.

What else can be done to prevent salmonellosis?

It is important for the public health department to know about cases of salmonellosis. It is important for clinical laboratories to send isolates of *Salmonella* to the city, county, or state Public Health Laboratories so the specific type can be determined and compared with other *Salmonella* in the community. If many cases occur at the same time, it may mean that a restaurant, food, or water supply has a problem that needs correction by the public health department.

Some prevention steps occur everyday without you thinking about it. Pasteurizing milk and treating municipal water supplies are highly effective prevention measures that have been in place for many years. In the 1970s, small pet turtles were a common source of salmonellosis in the United States, and in 1975, the sale of small turtles was halted in this country. Improvements in farm animal hygiene, in slaughter plant practices, and in vegetable and fruit harvesting and packing operations may help prevent salmonellosis caused by contaminated foods. Better education of food industry workers in basic food safety and restaurant inspection procedures, may prevent cross-contamination and other food handling errors that can lead to outbreaks. Wider use of pasteurized egg in restaurants, hospitals, and nursing homes is an important prevention measure. In the future, irradiation or other treatments may greatly reduce contamination of raw meat.

What is the government doing about salmonellosis?

The Centers for Disease Control and Prevention (CDC) monitors the frequency of *Salmonella* infections in the country and assists the local and state health departments to investigate outbreaks and devise control measures. CDC also conducts research to better identify specific types of *Salmonella*. The Food and Drug Administration inspects imported foods and milk pasteurization plants, promotes better food preparation techniques in restaurants and food processing plants, and regulates the sale of turtles. The FDA also regulates the use of specific antibiotics as growth promotants in food animals. The U.S. Department of Agriculture monitors the health of food animals, inspects egg pasteurization plants, and is responsible for the quality of slaughtered and processed meat. The U.S. Environmental Protection Agency regulates and monitors the safety of our drinking water supplies.

How can I learn more about this and other public health problems?

You can discuss any medical concerns you may have with your doctor or other heath care provider. Your local city or county health department can provide more information about this and other public health problems that are occurring in your area. General information about the public health of the nation is published every week in the "Morbidity and Mortality Weekly Report," by the CDC in Atlanta, Georgia. Epidemiologists in your local and state health departments are tracking a number of important public health problems, investigating special problems that arise, and helping to prevent them from occurring in the first place, or from spreading if they do occur.

What can I do to prevent salmonellosis?

Cook poultry, ground beef, and eggs thoroughly before eating. Do not eat or drink foods containing raw eggs, or raw unpasteurized milk.

If you are served undercooked meat, poultry, or eggs in a restaurant, don't hesitate to send it back to the kitchen for further cooking.

Wash hands, kitchen work surfaces, and utensils with soap and water immediately after they have been in contact with raw meat or poultry.

Be particularly careful with foods prepared for infants, the elderly, and the immunocompromised.

Wash hands with soap after handling reptiles or birds, or after contact with pet feces.

Avoid direct or even indirect contact between reptiles (turtles, iguanas, other lizards, snakes) and infants or immunocompromised persons.

Don't work with raw poultry or meat and an infant (e.g., feed, change diaper) at the same time.

Mother's milk is the safest food for young infants. Breast-feeding prevents salmonellosis and many other health problems.

Section 48.5

Shigellosis

Reprinted from "Shigellosis,"
Centers for Disease Control and Prevention, September 2003.

What is shigellosis?

Shigellosis is an infectious disease caused by a group of bacteria called *Shigella*. Most who are infected with *Shigella* develop diarrhea, fever, and stomach cramps starting a day or two after they are exposed to the bacterium. The diarrhea is often bloody. Shigellosis usually resolves in five to seven days. In some persons, especially young children and the elderly, the diarrhea can be so severe that the patient needs to be hospitalized. A severe infection with high fever may also be associated with seizures in children less than two years old. Some persons who are infected may have no symptoms at all, but may still pass the *Shigella* bacteria to others.

What sort of germ is **Shigella?**

The *Shigella* germ is actually a family of bacteria that can cause diarrhea in humans. They are microscopic living creatures that pass from person to person. *Shigella* were discovered over one hundred years ago by a Japanese scientist named Shiga, for whom they are named. There are several different kinds of *Shigella* bacteria: *Shigella sonnei*, also known as "Group D" *Shigella*, accounts for over two-thirds of the shigellosis in the United States. A second type, *Shigella flexneri*, or "group B" *Shigella*, accounts for almost all of the rest. Other types of *Shigella* are rare in this country, though they continue to be important causes of disease in the developing world. One type found in the developing world, *Shigella dysenteriae* type 1, causes deadly epidemics there.

How can **Shigella** infections be diagnosed?

Many different kinds of diseases can cause diarrhea and bloody diarrhea, and the treatment depends on which germ is causing the diarrhea. Determining that *Shigella* is the cause of the illness depends on laboratory tests that identify *Shigella* in the stools of an infected person. These tests are sometimes not performed unless the laboratory is instructed specifically to look for the organism. The laboratory can also do special tests to tell which type of *Shigella* the person has and which antibiotics, if any, would be best to treat it.

How can Shigella *infections be treated?*

Shigellosis can usually be treated with antibiotics. The antibiotics commonly used for treatment are ampicillin, trimethoprim/sulfamethoxazole (also known as Bactrim or Septra), nalidixic acid, or ciprofloxacin. Appropriate treatment kills the *Shigella* bacteria that might be present in the patient's stools, and shortens the illness. Unfortunately, some *Shigella* bacteria have become resistant to antibiotics, and using antibiotics to treat shigellosis can actually make the germs more resistant in the future. Persons with mild infections will usually recover quickly without antibiotic treatment. Therefore, when many persons in a community are affected by shigellosis, antibiotics are sometimes used selectively to treat only the more severe cases. Antidiarrheal agents such as loperamide (Imodium) or diphenoxylate with atropine (Lomotil) are likely to make the illness worse and should be avoided.

Are there long-term consequences to a Shigella *infection?*

Persons with diarrhea usually recover completely, although it may be several months before their bowel habits are entirely normal. About 3 percent of persons who are infected with one type of *Shigella, Shigella flexneri*, will later develop pains in their joints, irritation of the eyes, and painful urination. This is called Reiter syndrome. It can last for months or years, and can lead to chronic arthritis, which is difficult to treat. Reiter syndrome is caused by a reaction to *Shigella* infection that happens only in people who are genetically predisposed to it.

Once someone has had shigellosis, they are not likely to get infected with that specific type again for at least several years. However, they can still get infected with other types of *Shigella*.

How do people catch Shigella?

The *Shigella* bacteria pass from one infected person to the next. *Shigella* are present in the diarrheal stools of infected persons while they are sick and for a week or two afterward. Most *Shigella* infections are the result of the bacterium passing from stools or soiled fingers of one person to the mouth of another person. This happens when basic hygiene and hand washing habits are inadequate. It is particularly likely to occur among toddlers who are not fully toilet-trained. Family members and playmates of such children are at high risk of becoming infected.

Shigella infections may be acquired from eating contaminated food. Contaminated food may look and smell normal. Food may become contaminated by infected food handlers who forget to wash their hands with soap after using the bathroom. Vegetables can become contaminated if they are harvested from a field with sewage in it. Flies can breed in infected feces and then contaminate food. *Shigella* infections can also be acquired by drinking or swimming in contaminated water. Water may become contaminated if sewage runs into it, or if someone with shigellosis swims in it.

What can a person do to prevent this illness?

There is no vaccine to prevent shigellosis. However, the spread of *Shigella* from an infected person to other persons can be stopped by frequent and careful hand washing with soap. Frequent and careful hand washing is important among all age groups. Frequent, supervised hand washing of all children should be followed in daycare centers and in homes with children who are not completely toilet-trained (including children in diapers). When possible, young children with a *Shigella* infection who are still in diapers should not be in contact with uninfected children.

People who have shigellosis should not prepare food or pour water for others until they have been shown to no longer be carrying the *Shigella* bacterium.

If a child in diapers has shigellosis, everyone who changes the child's diapers should be sure the diapers are disposed of properly in a closed-lid garbage can, and should wash his or her hands carefully with soap and warm water immediately after changing the diapers. After use, the diaper changing area should be wiped down with a disinfectant such as household bleach, Lysol, or bactericidal wipes.

Basic food safety precautions and regular drinking water treatment prevents shigellosis. At swimming beaches, having enough bathrooms near the swimming area helps keep the water from becoming contaminated.

Simple precautions taken while traveling to the developing world can prevent getting shigellosis. Drink only treated or boiled water, and eat only cooked hot foods or fruits you peel yourself. The same precautions prevent traveler's diarrhea in general.

How common is shigellosis?

Every year, about eighteen thousand cases of shigellosis are reported in the United States. Because many milder cases are not diagnosed or reported, the actual number of infections may be twenty times greater. Shigellosis is particularly common and causes recurrent problems in settings where hygiene is poor and can sometimes sweep through entire communities. Shigellosis is more common in summer than winter. Children, especially toddlers aged two to four, are the most likely to get shigellosis. Many cases are related to the spread of illness in childcare settings, and many more are the result of the spread of the illness in families with small children.

In the developing world, shigellosis is far more common and is present in most communities most of the time.

What else can be done to prevent shigellosis?

It is important for the public health department to know about cases of shigellosis. It is important for clinical laboratories to send isolates of *Shigella* to the city, county, or state Public Health Laboratory so the specific type can be determined and compared to other *Shigella*. If many cases occur at the same time, it may mean that a restaurant or food or water supply has a problem that needs correction by the public health department. If a number of cases occur in a daycare center, the public health department may need to coordinate efforts to improve hand washing among the staff, children, and their families. When a community-wide outbreak occurs, a community-wide approach to promote hand washing and basic hygiene among children can stop the outbreak. Improvements in hygiene for vegetables and fruit picking and packing may prevent shigellosis caused by contaminated produce.

Some prevention steps occur every day, without you thinking about it. Making municipal water supplies safe and treating sewage are highly effective prevention measures that have been in place for many years.

What is the government doing about shigellosis?

The Centers for Disease Control and Prevention (CDC) monitors the frequency of *Shigella* infections in the country, and assists local and state health departments to investigate outbreaks, determine means of transmission, and devise control measures. CDC also conducts research to better understand how to identify and treat shigellosis. The Food and Drug Administration inspects imported foods and promotes better food preparation techniques in restaurants and food processing plants. The Environmental Protection Agency regulates and monitors the safety of our drinking water supplies. The government has also maintained active research into the development of a *Shigella* vaccine.

How can I learn more about this and other public health problems?

You can discuss any medical concerns you may have with your doctor or other heath care provider. Your local city or county health department can provide more information about this and other public health problems that are occurring in your area. General information about the public health of the nation is published every week in the "Morbidity and Mortality Weekly Report" by the CDC in Atlanta, Georgia. Epidemiologists in your local and state health departments are tracking a number of important public health problems, investigating special problems that arise, and helping to prevent them form occurring in the first place, or from spreading if they do occur.

Here are some tips for preventing the spread of shigellosis:

- wash hands with soap carefully and frequently, especially after going to the bathroom, after changing diapers, and before preparing foods or beverages
- dispose of soiled diapers properly
- disinfect diaper changing areas after using them
- keep children with diarrhea out of child care settings
- supervise hand washing of toddlers and small children after they use the toilet
- persons with diarrheal illness should not prepare food for others
- if you are traveling to the developing world, "boil it, cook it, peel it, or forget it"
- avoid drinking pool water

Section 48.6

Cryptosporidium *Infection*

Reprinted from "Cryptosporidium Infection and Cryptosporidiosis,"
Centers for Disease Control and Prevention, September 2004.

What is cryptosporidiosis?

Cryptosporidiosis is a diarrheal disease caused by microscopic parasites of the genus *Cryptosporidium*. Once an animal or person is infected, the parasite lives in the intestine and passes in the stool. The parasite is protected by an outer shell that allows it to survive outside the body for long periods of time and makes it very resistant to chlorine-based disinfectants. Both the disease and the parasite are commonly known as "crypto."

During the past two decades, crypto has become recognized as one of the most common causes of waterborne disease within humans in the United States. The parasite may be found in drinking water and recreational water in every region of the United States and throughout the world.

How is cryptosporidiosis spread?

Cryptosporidium lives in the intestine of infected humans or animals. Millions of crypto germs can be released in a bowel movement from an infected human or animal. Consequently, *Cryptosporidium* is found in soil, food, water, or surfaces that have been contaminated with infected human or animal feces. If a person swallows the parasite he or she becomes infected. You cannot become infected through contact with blood. The parasite can be spread by:

- Accidentally putting something into your mouth or swallowing something that has come into contact with feces of a person or animal infected with *Cryptosporidium*.

- Swallowing recreational water contaminated with *Cryptosporidium* (Recreational water includes water in swimming pools, hot tubs, Jacuzzis, fountains, lakes, rivers, springs, ponds, or streams that can be contaminated with sewage or feces from humans or animals.) Note: *Cryptosporidium* can survive for days in swimming pools with adequate chlorine levels.

- Eating uncooked food contaminated with *Cryptosporidium*. Thoroughly wash with clean, safe water all vegetables and fruits you plan to eat raw.

- Accidentally swallowing *Cryptosporidium* picked up from surfaces (such as bathroom fixtures, changing tables, diaper pails, or toys) contaminated with feces from an infected person.

What are the symptoms of cryptosporidiosis?

The most common symptom of cryptosporidiosis is watery diarrhea. Other symptoms include the following:

- Dehydration
- Weight loss
- Stomach cramps or pain
- Fever
- Nausea
- Vomiting

Some people with crypto will have no symptoms at all. While the small intestine is the site most commonly affected, *Cryptosporidium* infections could possibly affect other areas of the digestive or the respiratory tract.

How long after infection do symptoms appear?

Symptoms of cryptosporidiosis generally begin two to ten days (average seven days) after becoming infected with the parasite.

How long will symptoms last?

In persons with healthy immune systems, symptoms usually last about one to two weeks. The symptoms may go in cycles in which you may seem to get better for a few days, then feel worse again before the illness ends.

If I have been diagnosed with Cryptosporidium, should I worry about spreading the infection to others?

Yes, *Cryptosporidium* can be very contagious. Follow these guidelines to avoid spreading the disease to others:

- Wash your hands with soap and water after using the toilet, changing diapers, and before eating or preparing food.

- Do not swim in recreational water (pools, hot tubs, lakes or rivers, the ocean, etc.) if you have cryptosporidiosis and for at least two weeks after diarrhea stops. You can pass *Cryptosporidium* in your stool and contaminate water for several weeks after your symptoms have ended. This has resulted in outbreaks of cryptosporidiosis among recreational water users. Note: *Cryptosporidium* can be spread in a chlorinated pool because it is resistant to chlorine and, therefore, can live for days in chlorine-treated swimming pools.

- Avoid fecal exposure during sexual activity.

Who is most at risk for cryptosporidiosis?

People who are most likely to become infected with *Cryptosporidium* include:

- Children who attend daycare centers, including diaper-aged children;

- Child care workers;

- Parents of infected children;

- International travelers;

- Backpackers, hikers, and campers who drink unfiltered, untreated water;

- Swimmers who swallow water while swimming in swimming pools, lakes, rivers, ponds, and streams;

- People who drink from shallow, unprotected wells;

- People who swallow water from contaminated sources.

Contaminated water includes water that has not been boiled or filtered. Several community-wide outbreaks of cryptosporidiosis have been linked to drinking municipal water or recreational water contaminated with *Cryptosporidium*.

Who is most at risk for getting seriously ill with cryptosporidiosis?

Although crypto can infect all people, some groups are more likely to develop more serious illness.

- If you have a severely weakened immune system, talk to your health care provider for additional guidance.

- Young children and pregnant women may be more susceptible to the dehydration resulting from diarrhea and should drink plenty of fluids while ill.

- If you have a severely weakened immune system, you are at risk for more serious disease. Your symptoms may be more severe and could lead to serious or life-threatening illness. Examples of persons with weakened immune systems include those with HIV/AIDS; cancer and transplant patients who are taking certain immunosuppressive drugs; and those with inherited diseases that affect the immune system.

What should I do if I think I may have cryptosporidiosis?

If you suspect that you have cryptosporidiosis, see your health care provider.

How is a cryptosporidiosis diagnosed?

Your health care provider will ask you to submit stool samples to see if you are infected. Because testing for crypto can be difficult, you may be asked to submit several stool specimens over several days. Tests for crypto are not routinely done in most laboratories; therefore, your health care provider should specifically request testing for the parasite.

What is the treatment for cryptosporidiosis?

Although there is no standard treatment for cryptosporidiosis, the symptoms can be treated. Most people who have a healthy immune system will recover without treatment. If you have diarrhea, drink plenty of fluids to prevent dehydration. Rapid loss of fluids from diarrhea may be especially life threatening to babies; therefore, parents should talk to their health care provider about fluid replacement therapy options for infants. Antidiarrheal medicine may help slow down diarrhea, but talk to your health care provider before taking it. A new drug, nitazoxanide, has been approved for treatment of diarrhea caused by *Cryptosporidium* in healthy children under the age of twelve. Consult with your health care provider for more information.

People who are in poor health or who have a weakened immune system are at higher risk for more severe and more prolonged illness.

For persons with AIDS, anti-retroviral therapy that improves immune status will also decrease or eliminate symptoms of crypto. However, even if symptoms disappear, cryptosporidiosis is usually not curable and the symptoms may return if the immune status worsens. See your health care provider to discuss anti-retroviral therapy used to improve your immune status.

How can I prevent cryptosporidiosis?

Practice good hygiene.

- Wash hands thoroughly with soap and water.
  - Wash hands after using the toilet and before handling or eating food (especially for persons with diarrhea).
  - Wash hands after every diaper change, especially if you work with diaper-aged children, even if you are wearing gloves.
- Protect others by not swimming if you are experiencing diarrhea (essential for children in diapers).

Avoid water that might be contaminated.

- Do not swallow recreational water.
- Do not drink untreated water from shallow wells, lakes, rivers, springs, ponds, and streams.
- Do not drink untreated water during community-wide outbreaks of disease caused by contaminated drinking water.
- Do not use untreated ice or drinking water when traveling in countries where the water supply might be unsafe.

In the United States, nationally distributed brands of bottled or canned carbonated soft drinks are safe to drink. Commercially packaged noncarbonated soft drinks and fruit juices that do not require refrigeration until after they are opened (those that are stored unrefrigerated on grocery shelves) also are safe.

If you are unable to avoid using or drinking water that might be contaminated, then you can make the water safe to drink by doing one of the following:

- Heat the water to a rolling boil for at least one minute; or
- Use a filter that has an absolute pore size of at least 1 micron or one that has been NSF rated for "cyst removal."

Do not rely on chemicals to disinfect water and kill *Cryptosporidium*. Because it has a thick outer shell, this particular parasite is highly resistant to disinfectants such as chlorine and iodine.

Avoid food that might be contaminated.

- Wash or peel all raw vegetables and fruits before eating.

- Use safe, uncontaminated water to wash all food that is to be eaten raw.

- Avoid eating uncooked foods when traveling in countries with minimal water treatment and sanitation systems.

Take extra care when traveling.

If you travel to developing nations, you may be at a greater risk for *Cryptosporidium* infection because of poorer water treatment and food sanitation. Warnings about food, drinks, and swimming are even more important when visiting developing countries. Avoid foods and drinks, in particular raw fruits and vegetables, tap water, or ice made from tap water, unpasteurized milk or dairy products, and items purchased from street vendors. These items may be contaminated with *Cryptosporidium*. Steaming-hot foods, fruits you peel yourself, bottled and canned processed drinks, and hot coffee or hot tea are probably safe. Talk with your health care provider about other guidelines for travel abroad.

Avoid fecal exposure during sexual activity.

Section 48.7

Giardiasis

Reprinted from "Giardiasis,"
Centers for Disease Control and Prevention, September 2004.

What is giardiasis?

Giardiasis is a diarrheal illness caused by a one-celled, microscopic parasite, *Giardia intestinalis* (also known as *Giardia lamblia*). Once an animal or person has been infected with *Giardia intestinalis*, the parasite lives in the intestine and is passed in the stool. Because the parasite is protected by an outer shell, it can survive outside the body and in the environment for long periods of time.

During the past 2 decades, *Giardia* infection has become recognized as one of the most common causes of waterborne disease (found in both drinking and recreational water) in humans in the United States. *Giardia* are found worldwide and within every region of the United States.

How do you get giardiasis and how is it spread?

The *Giardia* parasite lives in the intestine of infected humans or animals. Millions of germs can be released in a bowel movement from an infected human or animal. *Giardia* is found in soil, food, water, or surfaces that have been contaminated with the feces from infected humans or animals. You can become infected after accidentally swallowing the parasite; you cannot become infected through contact with blood. *Giardia* can be spread by:

- Accidentally putting something into your mouth or swallowing something that has come into contact with feces of a person or animal infected with *Giardia*.

- Swallowing recreational water contaminated with *Giardia*. Recreational water includes water in swimming pools, hot tubs, Jacuzzis, fountains, lakes, rivers, springs, ponds, or streams that can be contaminated with sewage or feces from humans or animals.

- Eating uncooked food contaminated with *Giardia*.

- Accidentally swallowing *Giardia* picked up from surfaces (such as bathroom fixtures, changing tables, diaper pails, or toys) contaminated with feces from an infected person.

What are the symptoms of giardiasis?

Giardia infection can cause a variety of intestinal symptoms, which include the following:

- Diarrhea
- Gas or flatulence
- Greasy stools that tend to float
- Stomach cramps
- Upset stomach or nausea

These symptoms may lead to weight loss and dehydration. Some people with giardiasis have no symptoms at all.

How long after infection do symptoms appear?

Symptoms of giardiasis normally begin one to two weeks (average seven days) after becoming infected.

How long will symptoms last?

In otherwise healthy persons, symptoms of giardiasis may last two to six weeks. Occasionally, symptoms last longer.

Who is most likely to get giardiasis?

Anyone can get giardiasis. Persons more likely to become infected include:

- Children who attend daycare centers, including diaper-aged children;
- Child care workers;
- Parents of infected children;
- International travelers;
- People who swallow water from contaminated sources;

- Backpackers, hikers, and campers who drink unfiltered, untreated water

- Swimmers who swallow water while swimming in lakes, rivers, ponds, and streams;

- People who drink from shallow wells.

Contaminated water includes water that has not been boiled, filtered, or disinfected with chemicals. Several community-wide outbreaks of giardiasis have been linked to drinking municipal water or recreational water contaminated with *Giardia*.

What should I do if I think I may have giardiasis?

See your health care provider.

How is a Giardia infection diagnosed?

Your health care provider will likely ask you to submit stool samples to check for the parasite. Because *Giardia* can be difficult to diagnose, your provider may ask you to submit several stool specimens over several days.

What is the treatment for giardiasis?

Several prescription drugs are available to treat *Giardia*. Although *Giardia* can infect all people, young children and pregnant women may be more susceptible to dehydration resulting from diarrhea and should, therefore, drink plenty of fluids while ill.

My child does not have diarrhea, but was recently diagnosed as having giardiasis. My health care provider says treatment is not necessary. Is this true?

Treatment is not necessary when the child has no symptoms. However, there are a few exceptions. If your child does not have diarrhea, but is having nausea, fatigue (very tired), weight loss, or a poor appetite, you and your health care provider may wish to consider treatment. If your child attends a daycare center where an outbreak is continuing to occur despite efforts to control it, screening and treating children who have no obvious symptoms may be a good idea. The same is true if several family members are ill, or if a family member is pregnant and therefore not able to take the most effective anti-*Giardia* medications.

If I have been diagnosed with giardiasis, should I worry about spreading the infection to others?

Yes, a *Giardia* infection can be very contagious. Follow these guidelines to avoid spreading giardiasis to others:

- Wash your hands with soap and water after using the toilet, changing diapers, and before eating or preparing food.

- Do not swim in recreational water (pools, hot tubs, lakes or rivers, the ocean, etc.) if you have *Giardia* and for at least two weeks after diarrhea stops. You can pass *Giardia* in your stool and contaminate water for several weeks after your symptoms have ended. This has resulted in outbreaks of *Giardia* among recreational water users.

- Avoid fecal exposure during sexual activity.

How can I prevent a **Giardia** *infection?*

Practice good hygiene.

- Wash hands thoroughly with soap and water.
  - Wash hands after using the toilet and before handling or eating food (especially for persons with diarrhea).
  - Wash hands after every diaper change, especially if you work with diaper-aged children, even if you are wearing gloves.
- Protect others by not swimming if you are experiencing diarrhea (essential for children in diapers).

Avoid water that might be contaminated.

- Do not swallow recreational water.
- Do not drink untreated water from shallow wells, lakes, rivers, springs, ponds, and streams.
- Do not drink untreated water during community-wide outbreaks of disease caused by contaminated drinking water.
- Do not use untreated ice or drinking water when traveling in countries where the water supply might be unsafe.

In the United States, nationally distributed brands of bottled or canned carbonated soft drinks are safe to drink. Commercially packaged noncarbonated soft drinks and fruit juices that do not require refrigeration until after they are opened (those that are stored unrefrigerated on grocery shelves) also are safe.

If you are unable to avoid using or drinking water that might be contaminated, then you can make the water safe to drink by doing one of the following:

- Heat the water to a rolling boil for at least one minute; or

- Use a filter that has an absolute pore size of at least 1 micron or one that has been NSF rated for "cyst removal."

- If you cannot heat the water to a rolling boil or use a recommended filter, then try chemically treating the water by chlorination or iodination. Using chemicals may be less effective than boiling or filtering because the amount of chemical required to make the water safe is highly dependent on the temperature, pH, and cloudiness of the water.

Avoid food that might be contaminated.

- Wash or peel all raw vegetables and fruits before eating.

- Use safe, uncontaminated water to wash all food that is to be eaten raw.

- Avoid eating uncooked foods when traveling in countries with minimal water treatment and sanitation systems.

Avoid fecal exposure during sexual activity.

If my water comes from a well, should I have my well water tested?

It depends. You should consider having your well water tested if you can answer "yes" to any of the following questions:

- Are members of your family or others who use your well water becoming ill? If yes, your well may be the source of infection.

- Is your well located at the bottom of a hill or is it considered shallow? If so, runoff from rain or floodwater may be draining directly into your well, causing contamination.

- Is your well in a rural area where animals graze? Well water can become contaminated with feces if animal waste seepage contaminates the ground water. This can occur if your well has cracked casings, is poorly constructed, or is too shallow.

Tests used to specifically identify *Giardia* are often expensive, difficult, and usually require hundreds of gallons of water to be pumped through a filter. If you answered "yes" to the above questions, consider generally testing your well for fecal contamination by testing it for the presence of coliforms or *E. coli* instead of *Giardia*. Although tests for fecal coliforms or *E. coli* do not specifically tell you whether *Giardia* is present, these tests will show whether your well water has been contaminated by fecal matter.

These tests are useful only if your well is not routinely disinfected with chlorine, since chlorine kills fecal coliforms and *E. coli*. If the tests are positive, it is possible that the water may also be contaminated with *Giardia* or other harmful bacteria and viruses. Contact your county health department, your county cooperative extension service, or a local laboratory to find out who offers water testing in your area. If the fecal coliform test comes back positive, indicating that your well is fecally contaminated, stop drinking the well water and contact your local water authority for instructions on how to disinfect your well.

Chapter 49

Viral Gastroenteritis

Viral gastroenteritis is an intestinal infection caused by several viruses. Viral gastroenteritis is highly contagious and causes millions of cases of diarrhea each year.

Anyone can get viral gastroenteritis and most people recover without any complications. However, viral gastroenteritis can be serious for people who cannot drink enough fluids to replace what is lost through vomiting and diarrhea, especially infants, young children, the elderly, and people with weak immune systems. Complications from vomiting also can occur, even in healthy people.

Symptoms

The main symptoms of viral gastroenteritis are watery diarrhea and vomiting. Other symptoms are headache, fever, chills, and abdominal pain. The symptoms may appear within hours or a few days of infection. They usually last for one to two days, but may last as long as ten days.

Causes

The viruses that cause viral gastroenteritis damage the cells in the lining of the small intestine. As a result, fluids leak from the cells into

Reprinted from "Viral Gastroenteritis," National Institute of Diabetes and Digestive and Kidney Diseases, NIH Publication No. 03-5103, April 2003.

the intestine and produce watery diarrhea. Four types of viruses cause most viral gastroenteritis.

- **Rotavirus** is the leading cause of gastroenteritis among children three to fifteen months old. Most children have been exposed to the virus by age two. Children with rotavirus have vomiting and watery diarrhea for three to eight days, along with fever and abdominal pain. Rotavirus can also infect adults who are in close contact with infected children, but the symptoms in adults are milder. Symptoms of rotavirus infection appear one to two days after exposure. In the United States, rotavirus infections are most common from November to April.

- **Adenovirus** serotypes 40 and 41 cause gastroenteritis mainly in children younger than two years old. Infections occur all year round; vomiting and diarrhea appear approximately one week after exposure.

- **Caliciviruses** cause infection in persons of all ages. This family of viruses is further divided into the noroviruses (example, Norwalk virus) and the sapoviruses (example, Sapporo virus). Caliciviruses are transmitted from person to person and also through contaminated water or food—especially oysters from contaminated waters. The noroviruses are often responsible for epidemics of viral gastroenteritis. In addition to vomiting and diarrhea, people infected with caliciviruses may have muscle aches. The symptoms appear within one to three days of exposure.

- **Astrovirus** also infects primarily infants, young children, and the elderly. This virus is most active during the winter months. Vomiting and diarrhea appear within one to three days of exposure.

Viral gastroenteritis is often mistakenly called "stomach flu," but it is not caused by the influenza virus and it does not infect the stomach. Also, viral gastroenteritis is not caused by bacteria or parasites.

Transmission

Viral gastroenteritis is highly contagious. The viruses are often transmitted on unwashed hands. People can get the viruses through close contact with infected individuals, such as sharing their food, drink, or eating utensils, or by eating food or drinking beverages that are contaminated with the virus. People who no longer have symptoms may still be contagious, since the virus can be found in the stool for up to two weeks after they recover from their illness. Also, people can become infected without having symptoms, and they can still spread the infection.

Outbreaks of viral gastroenteritis can occur in child care settings, schools, nursing homes, cruise ships, camps, dormitories, restaurants, and other places where people gather in groups. If you suspect that you were exposed to a virus in one of these settings, you may want to contact your local health department, which tracks outbreaks.

Diagnosis

If you think you have viral gastroenteritis, you may want to see your doctor, although many people don't bother. Doctors generally diagnose viral gastroenteritis based on the symptoms and a physical examination. Your doctor may ask for a stool sample to test for rotavirus or to rule out bacteria or parasites as the cause of your symptoms. No routine tests are currently available for the other types of viruses.

Treatment

Most cases of viral gastroenteritis resolve over time without specific treatment. Antibiotics are not effective against viral infections. The primary goal of treatment is to reduce the symptoms, and prompt treatment may be needed to prevent dehydration.

Your body needs fluids to function. Dehydration is the loss of fluids from the body. Important salts or minerals, known as electrolytes, can also be lost with the fluids. Dehydration can be caused by diarrhea, vomiting, excessive urination, or excessive sweating, or by not drinking enough fluids because of nausea, difficulty swallowing, or loss of appetite.

In viral gastroenteritis, the combination of diarrhea and vomiting can cause dehydration. The symptoms of dehydration include the following:

- excessive thirst

- dry mouth

- little or no urine or dark yellow urine

- decreased tears

- severe weakness or lethargy

- dizziness or lightheadedness

If you notice any of these symptoms, you should talk to your doctor. Mild dehydration can be treated by drinking liquids. Severe dehydration may require intravenous fluids and hospitalization. Untreated severe dehydration can be life threatening.

Children present special concerns. Because of their smaller body size, infants and children are at greater risk of dehydration from diarrhea and vomiting. Oral rehydration solutions such as Pedialyte can replace lost fluids, minerals, and salts.

You can take several steps to help relieve the symptoms of viral gastroenteritis.

- Allow your gastrointestinal tract to settle by not eating for a few hours.

- Sip small amounts of clear liquids or suck on ice chips if vomiting is still a problem.

- Give infants and children oral rehydration solutions to replace fluids and lost electrolytes.

- Gradually reintroduce food, starting with bland, easy-to-digest food, like toast, broth, apples, bananas, and rice.

- Avoid dairy products, caffeine, and alcohol until recovery is complete.

- Get plenty of rest.

Prevention

Prevention is the only way to avoid viral gastroenteritis. There is no vaccine available. You can avoid it by:

- washing your hands thoroughly after using the bathroom or changing diapers;

- washing your hands thoroughly before eating;

- disinfecting contaminated surfaces;

- not eating or drinking foods or liquids that might be contaminated.

Points to Remember

- Viral gastroenteritis is a highly contagious infection of the intestines caused by one of several viruses.

- Although it is sometimes called "stomach flu," viral gastroenteritis is not caused by the influenza virus and does not affect the stomach.

- The main symptoms are watery diarrhea and vomiting.

- Anyone can get viral gastroenteritis through unwashed hands, close contact with an infected person, or food and beverages that contain the virus.

- Diagnosis is based on the symptoms and a physical examination. Currently only rotavirus can be rapidly detected in a stool test.

- Viral gastroenteritis has no specific treatment; antibiotics are not effective against viruses. Treatment focuses on reducing the symptoms and preventing dehydration.

- The symptoms of dehydration are excessive thirst, dry mouth, dark yellow urine or little or no urine, decreased tears, severe weakness or lethargy, and dizziness or lightheadedness.

- Infants, young children, the elderly, and people with weak immune systems have a higher risk of developing dehydration due to vomiting and diarrhea.

- People with viral gastroenteritis should rest, drink clear liquids, and eat easy-to-digest foods.

- For infants and young children, oral rehydration solutions can replace lost fluids, minerals, and salts.

- Avoid viral gastroenteritis by washing hands thoroughly after using the bathroom or changing diapers, disinfecting contaminated surfaces, and avoiding foods or liquids that might be contaminated.

Chapter 50

Rotavirus and Norovirus

Rotavirus

Rotavirus is the most common cause of severe diarrhea among children, resulting in the hospitalization of approximately fifty-five thousand children each year in the United States and the death of over six hundred thousand children annually worldwide. The incubation period for rotavirus disease is approximately two days. The disease is characterized by vomiting and watery diarrhea for three to eight days, and fever and abdominal pain occur frequently. Immunity after infection is incomplete, but repeat infections tend to be less severe than the original infection.

The Virus

A rotavirus has a characteristic wheel-like appearance when viewed by electron microscopy (the name rotavirus is derived from the Latin *rota*, meaning "wheel"). Rotaviruses are nonenveloped, double-shelled viruses. The genome is composed of eleven segments of double-stranded RNA, which code for six structural and five nonstructural proteins. The virus is stable in the environment.

"Rotavirus" is reprinted from "Rotavirus," Centers for Disease Control and Prevention, January 2005. "Norovirus" is reprinted from "Norovirus: Q & A," Centers for Disease Control and Prevention, January 2005.

Epidemiologic Features

The primary mode of transmission is fecal-oral, although some have reported low titers of virus in respiratory tract secretions and other body fluids. Because the virus is stable in the environment, transmission can occur through ingestion of contaminated water or food and contact with contaminated surfaces. In the United States and other countries with a temperate climate, the disease has a winter seasonal pattern, with annual epidemics occurring from November to April. The highest rates of illness occur among infants and young children, and most children in the United States are infected by two years of age. Adults can also be infected, though disease tends to be mild.

Diagnosis

Diagnosis may be made by rapid antigen detection of rotavirus in stool specimens. Strains may be further characterized by enzyme immunoassay or reverse transcriptase polymerase chain reaction, but such testing is not commonly done.

Treatment

For persons with healthy immune systems, rotavirus gastroenteritis is a self-limited illness, lasting for only a few days. Treatment is nonspecific and consists of oral rehydration therapy to prevent dehydration. About one in forty children with rotavirus gastroenteritis will require hospitalization for intravenous fluids.

Prevention

In 1998, the U.S. Food and Drug Administration approved a live virus vaccine (Rotashield) for use in children. However, the Advisory Committee on Immunization Practices (ACIP) recommended that Rotashield no longer be recommended for infants in the United States because data that indicated a strong association between Rotashield and intussusception (bowel obstruction) among some infants during the first one to two weeks following vaccination.

Norovirus

Noroviruses are a group of viruses that cause the "stomach flu," or gastroenteritis, in people. The term *norovirus* was recently approved as the official name for this group of viruses. Several other names have been used for noroviruses, including the following:

- Norwalk-like viruses (NLVs)

- caliciviruses (because they belong to the virus family *Caliciviridae*)

- small round structured viruses

Viruses are very different from bacteria and parasites, some of which can cause illnesses similar to norovirus infection. Viruses are much smaller, are not affected by treatment with antibiotics, and cannot grow outside of a person's body.

Symptoms of Illness Caused by Noroviruses

The symptoms of norovirus illness usually include nausea, vomiting, diarrhea, and some stomach cramping. Sometimes people additionally have a low-grade fever, chills, headache, muscle aches, and a general sense of tiredness. The illness often begins suddenly, and the infected person may feel very sick. The illness is usually brief, with symptoms lasting only about one or two days. In general, children experience more vomiting than adults. Most people with norovirus illness have both of these symptoms.

Illness Caused by Noroviruses

Illness caused by norovirus infection has several names, including:

- stomach flu—this "stomach flu" is not related to the flu (or influenza), which is a respiratory illness caused by influenza virus.

- viral gastroenteritis—the most common name for illness caused by norovirus. Gastroenteritis refers to an inflammation of the stomach and intestines.

- acute gastroenteritis.

- nonbacterial gastroenteritis.

- food poisoning (although there are other causes of food poisoning).

- calicivirus infection.

Seriousness of Norovirus Disease

Norovirus disease is usually not serious, although people may feel very sick and vomit many times a day. Most people get better within one or two days, and they have no long-term health effects related to their illness. However, sometimes people are unable to drink enough liquids to replace the liquids they lost because of vomiting and diarrhea. These persons can become dehydrated and may need special medical attention. This problem with dehydration is usually seen only among the very young, the elderly, and persons with weakened immune systems. There is no evidence to suggest that an infected person can become a long-term carrier of norovirus.

Norovirus Transmission

Noroviruses are found in the stool or vomit of infected people. People can become infected with the virus in several ways, including:

- eating food or drinking liquids that are contaminated with norovirus;
- touching surfaces or objects contaminated with norovirus, and then placing their hand in their mouth;
- having direct contact with another person who is infected and showing symptoms (for example, when caring for someone with illness, or sharing foods or eating utensils with someone who is ill).

Persons working in daycare centers or nursing homes should pay special attention to children or residents who have norovirus illness. This virus is very contagious and can spread rapidly throughout such environments.

Appearance of Symptoms

Symptoms of norovirus illness usually begin about twenty-four to forty-eight hours after ingestion of the virus, but they can appear as early as twelve hours after exposure.

Contagiousness

Noroviruses are very contagious and can spread easily from person to person. Both stool and vomit are infectious. Particular care should be taken with young children in diapers who may have diarrhea.

People infected with norovirus are contagious from the moment they begin feeling ill to at least three days after recovery. Some people may be contagious for as long as two weeks after recovery. Therefore, it is particularly important for people to use good hand washing and other hygienic practices after they have recently recovered from norovirus illness.

People at Risk

Anyone can become infected with these viruses. There are many different strains of norovirus, which makes it difficult for a person's body to develop long-lasting immunity. Therefore, norovirus illness can recur throughout a person's lifetime. In addition, because of differences in genetic factors, some people are more likely to become infected and develop more severe illness than others.

Available Treatment

Currently, there is no antiviral medication that works against norovirus and there is no vaccine to prevent infection. Norovirus infection cannot be treated with antibiotics. This is because antibiotics work to fight bacteria and not viruses.

Norovirus illness is usually brief in healthy individuals. When people are ill with vomiting and diarrhea, they should drink plenty of fluids to prevent dehydration. Dehydration among young children, the elderly, and the sick, can be common, and it is the most serious health effect that can result from norovirus infection. By drinking oral rehydration fluids (ORF), juice, or water, people can reduce their chance of becoming dehydrated. Sports drinks do not replace the nutrients and minerals lost during this illness.

Prevention

Yes. You can decrease your chance of coming in contact with noroviruses by following these preventive steps:

- Frequently wash your hands, especially after toilet visits and changing diapers and before eating or preparing food.

- Carefully wash fruits and vegetables, and steam oysters before eating them.

- Thoroughly clean and disinfect contaminated surfaces immediately after an episode of illness by using a bleach-based household cleaner.

- Immediately remove and wash clothing or linens that may be contaminated with virus after an episode of illness (use hot water and soap).

- Flush or discard any vomitus or stool in the toilet and make sure that the surrounding area is kept clean.

Persons who are infected with norovirus should not prepare food while they have symptoms and for three days after they recover from their illness. Food that may have been contaminated by an ill person should be disposed of properly.

Chapter 51

Helicobacter Pylori
and Peptic Ulcer

What is a peptic ulcer?

A peptic ulcer is a sore on the lining of the stomach or duodenum, which is the beginning of the small intestine. Peptic ulcers are common: One in ten Americans develops an ulcer at some time in his or her life. One cause of peptic ulcer is bacterial infection, but some ulcers are caused by long-term use of nonsteroidal anti-inflammatory agents (NSAIDs), like aspirin and ibuprofen. In a few cases, cancerous tumors in the stomach or pancreas can cause ulcers. Peptic ulcers are not caused by stress or eating spicy food, but these can make ulcers worse.

What is H. pylori?

Helicobacter pylori (*H. pylori*) is a type of bacteria. Researchers believe that *H. pylori* is responsible for the majority of peptic ulcers.

H. pylori infection is common in the United States: About 20 percent of people under forty years old and half of those over sixty years have it. Most infected people, however, do not develop ulcers. Why *H. pylori* does not cause ulcers in every infected person is not known. Most likely, infection depends on characteristics of the infected person, the type of *H. pylori*, and other factors yet to be discovered.

Reprinted from "H. pylori and Peptic Ulcer," National Institute of Diabetes and Digestive and Kidney Diseases, NIH Publication No. 05-4225, October 2004.

Researchers are not certain how people contract *H. pylori*, but they think it may be through food or water.

Researchers have found *H. pylori* in the saliva of some infected people, so the bacteria may also spread through mouth-to-mouth contact such as kissing.

How does **H. pylori** *cause a peptic ulcer?*

H. pylori weakens the protective mucous coating of the stomach and duodenum, which allows acid to get through to the sensitive lining beneath. Both the acid and the bacteria irritate the lining and cause a sore, or ulcer.

H. pylori is able to survive in stomach acid because it secretes enzymes that neutralize the acid. This mechanism allows *H. pylori* to make its way to the "safe" area—the protective mucous lining. Once there, the bacterium's spiral shape helps it burrow through the lining.

What are the symptoms of an ulcer?

Abdominal discomfort is the most common symptom. This discomfort usually:

- is a dull, gnawing ache;
- comes and goes for several days or weeks;
- occurs two to three hours after a meal;
- occurs in the middle of the night (when the stomach is empty);
- is relieved by eating;
- is relieved by antacid medications.

Other symptoms include the following:

- weight loss
- poor appetite
- bloating
- burping
- nausea
- vomiting

Some people experience only very mild symptoms, or none at all.

Emergency Symptoms: If you have any of these symptoms, call your doctor right away:

- sharp, sudden, persistent stomach pain
- bloody or black stools
- bloody vomit or vomit that looks like coffee grounds

They could be signs of a serious problem, such as:

- perforation—when the ulcer burrows through the stomach or duodenal wall.
- bleeding—when acid or the ulcer breaks a blood vessel.
- obstruction—when the ulcer blocks the path of food trying to leave the stomach.

How is an H. pylori-*related ulcer diagnosed?*

Diagnosing an Ulcer: To see whether symptoms are caused by an ulcer, the doctor may do an upper gastrointestinal (GI) series or an endoscopy. An upper GI series is an x-ray of the esophagus, stomach, and duodenum. The patient drinks a chalky liquid called barium to make these organs and any ulcers show up more clearly on the x-ray.

An endoscopy is an exam that uses an endoscope, a thin, lighted tube with a tiny camera on the end. The patient is lightly sedated, and the doctor carefully eases the endoscope into the mouth and down the throat to the stomach and duodenum. This allows the doctor to see the lining of the esophagus, stomach, and duodenum. The doctor can use the endoscope to take photos of ulcers or remove a tiny piece of tissue to view under a microscope. This procedure is called a biopsy. If an ulcer is bleeding, the doctor can use the endoscope to inject drugs that promote clotting or to guide a heat probe that cauterizes the ulcer.

Diagnosing *H. pylori*: If an ulcer is found, the doctor will test the patient for *H. pylori*. This test is important because treatment for an ulcer caused by *H. pylori* is different from that for an ulcer caused by NSAIDs.

H. pylori is diagnosed through blood, breath, stool, and tissue tests. Blood tests are most common. They detect antibodies to *H. pylori* bacteria. Blood is taken at the doctor's office through a finger stick.

Urea breath tests are an effective diagnostic method for *H. pylori*. They are also used after treatment to see whether it worked. In the doctor's office, the patient drinks a urea solution that contains a special carbon atom. If *H. pylori* is present, it breaks down the urea, releasing the carbon. The blood carries the carbon to the lungs, where the patient exhales it. The breath test is 96 percent to 98 percent accurate.

Stool tests may be used to detect *H. pylori* infection in the patient's fecal matter. Studies have shown that this test, called the *Helicobacter pylori* stool antigen (HpSA) test, is accurate for diagnosing *H. pylori*.

Tissue tests are usually done using the biopsy sample that is removed with the endoscope. There are three types:

- The rapid urease test detects the enzyme urease, which is produced by *H. pylori*.

- A histology test allows the doctor to find and examine the actual bacteria.

- A culture test involves allowing *H. pylori* to grow in the tissue sample.

In diagnosing *H. pylori*, blood, breath, and stool tests are often done before tissue tests because they are less invasive. However, blood tests are not used to detect *H. pylori* following treatment because a patient's blood can show positive results even after *H. pylori* has been eliminated.

How are H. pylori *peptic ulcers treated?*

Drugs Used to Treat H. pylori *Peptic Ulcers*

- *Antibiotics:* metronidazole, tetracycline, clarithromycin, amoxicillin

- *H_2 blockers:* cimetidine, ranitidine, famotidine, nizatidine

- *Proton pump inhibitors:* omeprazole, lansoprazole, rabeprazole, esomeprazole, pantoprazole

- *Stomach-lining protector:* bismuth subsalicylate

H. pylori peptic ulcers are treated with drugs that kill the bacteria, reduce stomach acid, and protect the stomach lining. Antibiotics are used to kill the bacteria. Two types of acid-suppressing drugs might be used: H_2 blockers and proton pump inhibitors.

H_2 blockers work by blocking histamine, which stimulates acid secretion. They help reduce ulcer pain after a few weeks. Proton pump inhibitors suppress acid production by halting the mechanism that pumps the acid into the stomach. H_2 blockers and proton pump inhibitors have been prescribed alone for years as treatments for ulcers, but used alone, these drugs do not eradicate *H. pylori* and therefore do not cure *H. pylori*-related ulcers. Bismuth subsalicylate, a component of Pepto-Bismol, is used to protect the stomach lining from acid. It also kills *H. pylori.*

Treatment usually involves a combination of antibiotics, acid suppressors, and stomach protectors. Antibiotic regimens recommended for patients may differ across regions of the world because different areas have begun to show resistance to particular antibiotics.

The use of only one medication to treat *H. pylori* is not recommended. At this time, the most proven effective treatment is a two-week course of treatment called triple therapy. It involves taking two antibiotics to kill the bacteria and either an acid suppressor or stomach-lining shield. Two-week triple therapy reduces ulcer symptoms, kills the bacteria, and prevents ulcer recurrence in more than 90 percent of patients.

Unfortunately, patients may find triple therapy complicated because it involves taking as many as twenty pills a day. Also, the antibiotics used in triple therapy may cause mild side effects such as nausea, vomiting, diarrhea, dark stools, metallic taste in the mouth, dizziness, headache, and yeast infections in women. (Most side effects can be treated with medication withdrawal.) Nevertheless, recent studies show that two weeks of triple therapy is ideal.

Early results of studies in other countries suggest that one week of triple therapy may be as effective as the two-week therapy, with fewer side effects.

Another option is two weeks of dual therapy. Dual therapy involves two drugs: an antibiotic and an acid suppressor. It is not as effective as triple therapy.

Two weeks of quadruple therapy, which uses two antibiotics, an acid suppressor, and a stomach-lining shield, looks promising in research studies. It is also called bismuth triple therapy.

Can **H. pylori** *infection be prevented?*

No one knows for sure how *H. pylori* spreads, so prevention is difficult. Researchers are trying to develop a vaccine to prevent infection.

Why don't all doctors automatically check for **H. pylori?**

Changing medical belief and practice takes time. For nearly one hundred years, scientists and doctors thought that ulcers were caused by stress, spicy food, and alcohol. Treatment involved bed rest and a bland diet. Later, researchers added stomach acid to the list of causes and began treating ulcers with antacids.

Since *H. pylori* was discovered in 1982, studies conducted around the world have shown that using antibiotics to destroy *H. pylori* cures peptic ulcers. The prevalence of *H. pylori* ulcers is changing. The infection is becoming less common in people born in developed countries. The medical community, however, continues to debate *H. pylori*'s role in peptic ulcers. If you have a peptic ulcer and have not been tested for *H. pylori* infection, talk to your doctor.

Points to Remember

- A peptic ulcer is a sore in the lining of the stomach or duodenum.

- The majority of peptic ulcers are caused by the *H. pylori* bacterium. Many of the other cases are caused by NSAIDs. None are caused by spicy food or stress.

- *H. pylori* can be transmitted from person to person through close contact and exposure to vomit.

- Always wash your hands after using the bathroom and before eating.

- A combination of antibiotics and other drugs is the most effective treatment for *H. pylori* peptic ulcers.

Chapter 52

Clostridium Difficile *Infection*

What is Clostridium difficile*?*

C. difficile is a spore-forming bacteria which can be part of the normal intestinal flora in as many as 50 percent of children under age two, and less frequently in individuals over two years of age. *C. difficile* is the major cause of pseudomembranous colitis and antibiotic-associated diarrhea.

What are the risk factors for C. difficile-*associated disease?*

C. difficile-associated disease occurs when normal intestinal bacteria is altered, allowing *C. difficile* to flourish in the intestinal tract and produce a toxin that causes a watery diarrhea. Repeated enemas, prolonged nasogastric tube insertion, and gastrointestinal tract surgery increase a person's risk of developing the disease. The overuse of antibiotics, especially penicillin (ampicillin), clindamycin, and cephalosporins may also alter normal intestinal bacteria that will increase the risk of developing *C. difficile* diarrhea.

What are the symptoms of C. difficile-*associated disease?*

Mild cases of *C. difficile* disease are characterized by frequent, foul-smelling, watery stools. More severe symptoms, indicative of

Developed by the Division of Public Health, Bureau of Communicable Disease Epidemiology Section, Wisconsin Department of Health and Family Services, June 2001.

pseudomembranous colitis, include diarrhea that contains blood and mucous, and abdominal cramps. An abnormal heartbeat may also occur.

How is C. difficile-associated disease diagnosed?

C. difficile diarrhea is confirmed by the presence of a toxin in a stool specimen. A positive culture for *C. difficile* without a toxin assay is not sufficient to make the diagnosis of *C. difficile*-associated disease.

What is the treatment for C. difficile-associated disease?

As soon as *C. difficile* disease is diagnosed, current antibiotic therapy should be reassessed by the physician. Patients with severe toxicity or unresolved diarrhea may need to have their antibiotic treatment modified to use drugs not known to result in *C. difficile* diarrhea. Patients should be monitored for dehydration and electrolyte imbalance following prolonged periods of diarrhea. Antidiarrheal agents such as Lomotil or Imodium have been shown to increase the severity of symptoms and should *not* be taken.

How can C. difficile-associated disease be spread?

Individuals with *C. difficile*-associated disease shed spores in the stool that can be spread from person to person. Spores can survive up to seventy days in the environment and can be transported on the hands of health care personnel who have direct contact with infected patients or with environmental surfaces (floors, bedpans, toilets, etc.) contaminated with *C. difficile*.

How can C. difficile-associated disease be prevented?

Strict adherence to hand washing techniques and the proper handling of contaminated wastes (including diapers) are effective in preventing the spread of the disease. Environmental surfaces contaminated with *C. difficile* spores should be cleaned with an effective disinfectant (bleach). Limiting the use of antibiotics will lower the risk of developing *C. difficile* diarrhea.

Part Eight

Additional Help and Information

Chapter 53

Glossary of Gastrointestinal Terms

Absorption: The way nutrients from food move from the small intestine into the cells in the body.

Accessory Digestive Organs: Organs that help with digestion but are not part of the digestive tract. These organs are the tongue, glands in the mouth that make saliva, pancreas, liver, and gallbladder.

Achalasia: A rare disorder of the esophagus. The muscle at the end of the esophagus does not relax enough for the passage to open properly.

Aerophagia: A condition that occurs when a person swallows too much air. Causes gas and frequent belching.

Alactasia: An inherited condition causing the lack of the enzyme needed to digest milk sugar.

Alagille Syndrome: A condition of babies in their first year. The bile ducts in the liver disappear, and the bile ducts outside the liver get very narrow. May lead to a buildup of bile in the liver and damage to liver cells and other organs.

Allergy: A condition in which the body is not able to tolerate certain foods, animals, plants, or other substances.

The terms in this glossary were excerpted from "Digestive Diseases Dictionary," National Institute of Diabetes and Digestive and Kidney Diseases, February 2000.

Amebiasis: An acute or chronic infection. Symptoms vary from mild diarrhea to frequent watery diarrhea and loss of water and fluids in the body. See also Gastroenteritis.

Anal Fissure: A small tear in the anus that may cause itching, pain, or bleeding.

Anal Fistula: A channel that develops between the anus and the skin. Most fistulas are the result of an abscess (infection) that spreads to the skin.

Anastomosis: An operation to connect two body parts. An example is an operation in which a part of the colon is removed and the two remaining ends are rejoined.

Angiodysplasia: Abnormal or enlarged blood vessels in the gastrointestinal tract.

Angiography: An x-ray that uses dye to detect bleeding in the gastrointestinal tract.

Anorectal Atresia: Lack of a normal opening between the rectum and anus.

Anoscopy: A test to look for fissures, fistulae, and hemorrhoids. The doctor uses a special instrument, called an anoscope, to look into the anus.

Antacids: Medicines that balance acids and gas in the stomach. Examples are Maalox, Mylanta, and Di-Gel.

Anticholinergics: Medicines that calm muscle spasms in the intestine. Examples are dicyclomine (Bentyl) and hyoscyamine (Levsin).

Antidiarrheals: Medicines that help control diarrhea. An example is loperamide (Imodium).

Antiemetics: Medicines that prevent and control nausea and vomiting. Examples are promethazine (Phenergan) and prochlorperazine (Compazine).

Antispasmodics: Medicines that help reduce or stop muscle spasms in the intestines. Examples are dicyclomine (Bentyl) and atropine (Donnatal).

Antrectomy: An operation to remove the upper portion of the stomach, called the antrum. This operation helps reduce the amount of stomach acid. It is used when a person has complications from ulcers.

Anus: The opening at the end of the digestive tract where bowel contents leave the body.

Appendectomy: An operation to remove the appendix.

Appendicitis: Reddening, irritation (inflammation), and pain in the appendix caused by infection, scarring, or blockage.

Appendix: A four-inch pouch attached to the first part of the large intestine (cecum). No one knows what function the appendix has, if any.

Ascending Colon: The part of the colon on the right side of the abdomen.

Ascites: A buildup of fluid in the abdomen. Ascites is usually caused by severe liver disease such as cirrhosis.

Atonic Colon: Lack of normal muscle tone or strength in the colon. This is caused by the overuse of laxatives or by Hirschsprung disease. It may result in chronic constipation. Also called lazy colon. See Hirschsprung Disease.

Atresia: Lack of a normal opening from the esophagus, intestines, or anus.

Atrophic Gastritis: Chronic irritation of the stomach lining. Causes the stomach lining and glands to wither away.

Autoimmune Hepatitis: A liver disease caused when the body's immune system destroys liver cells for no known reason.

Barium: A chalky liquid used to coat the inside of organs so that they will show up on an x-ray.

Barium Enema X-Ray: See Lower GI Series.

Barium Meal: See Upper GI Series.

Barrett Esophagus: Peptic ulcer of the lower esophagus. It is caused by the presence of cells that normally stay in the stomach lining.

Bezoar: A ball of food, mucus, vegetable fiber, hair, or other material that cannot be digested in the stomach. Bezoars can cause blockage, ulcers, and bleeding.

Bile: Fluid made by the liver and stored in the gallbladder. Bile helps break down fats and gets rid of wastes in the body.

Bile Acids: Acids made by the liver that work with bile to break down fats.

Bile Ducts: Tubes that carry bile from the liver to the gallbladder for storage and to the small intestine for use in digestion.

Biliary Atresia: A condition present from birth in which the bile ducts inside or outside the liver do not have normal openings. Bile becomes trapped in the liver, causing jaundice and cirrhosis. Without surgery the condition may cause death.

Biliary Dyskinesia: See postcholecystectomy syndrome.

Biliary Stricture: A narrowing of the biliary tract from scar tissue. The scar tissue may result from injury, disease, pancreatitis, infection, or gallstones. See also Stricture.

Biliary Tract: The gallbladder and the bile ducts. Also called biliary system or biliary tree.

Bilirubin: The substance formed when hemoglobin breaks down. Bilirubin gives bile its color. Bilirubin is normally passed in stool. Too much bilirubin causes jaundice.

Bloating: Fullness or swelling in the abdomen that often occurs after meals.

Borborygmi: Rumbling sounds caused by gas moving through the intestines (stomach "growling").

Bowel: Another word for the small and large intestines.

Budd-Chiari Syndrome: A rare liver disease in which the veins that drain blood from the liver are blocked or narrowed.

Bulking Agents: Laxatives that make bowel movements soft and easy to pass.

Calculi: Stones or solid lumps such as gallstones.

Campylobacter pylori: The original name for the bacterium that causes ulcers. The new name is *Helicobacter pylori*. See also *Helicobacter pylori*.

Candidiasis: A mild infection caused by the *Candida* fungus, which lives naturally in the gastrointestinal tract. Infection occurs when a change in the body, such as surgery, causes the fungus to overgrow suddenly.

Caroli Disease: An inherited condition. Bile ducts in the liver are enlarged and may cause irritation, infection, or gallstones.

Catheter: A thin, flexible tube that carries fluids into or out of the body.

Cecostomy: A tube that goes through the skin into the beginning of the large intestine to remove gas or feces. This is a short-term way to protect part of the colon while it heals after surgery.

Cecum: The beginning of the large intestine. The cecum is connected to the lower part of the small intestine, called the ileum.

Celiac Disease: Inability to digest and absorb gliadin, the protein found in wheat. Undigested gliadin causes damage to the lining of the small intestine. This prevents absorption of nutrients from other foods. Celiac disease is also called celiac sprue, gluten intolerance, and non-tropical sprue.

Celiac Sprue: See Celiac Disease.

Cholangiography: A series of x-rays of the bile ducts.

Cholangitis: Irritated or infected bile ducts.

Cholecystectomy: An operation to remove the gallbladder.

Cholecystitis: An irritated gallbladder.

Cholecystogram, Oral: An x-ray of the gallbladder and bile ducts. The patient takes pills containing a special dye to make the organs show up in the x-ray. Also called oral cholecystography.

Cholecystokinin: A hormone released in the small intestine. Causes muscles in the gallbladder and the colon to tighten and relax.

Choledocholithiasis: Gallstones in the bile ducts.

Cholelithiasis: Gallstones in the gallbladder.

Cholestasis: Blocked bile ducts. Often caused by gallstones.

Chyme: A thick liquid made of partially digested food and stomach juices. This liquid is made in the stomach and moves into the small intestine for further digestion.

Cirrhosis: A chronic liver condition caused by scar tissue and cell damage. Cirrhosis makes it hard for the liver to remove poisons (toxins) like alcohol and drugs from the blood. These toxins build up in the blood and may affect brain function.

***Clostridium difficile* (*C. difficile*):** Bacteria naturally present in the large intestine. These bacteria make a substance that can cause a serious infection called pseudomembranous colitis in people taking antibiotics.

Colectomy: An operation to remove all or part of the colon.

Colic: Attacks of abdominal pain, caused by muscle spasms in the intestines. Colic is common in infants.

Colitis: Irritation of the colon.

Collagenous Colitis: A type of colitis. Caused by an abnormal band of collagen, a thread-like protein.

Colon: See Large Intestine.

Colon Polyps: Small, fleshy, mushroom-shaped growths in the colon.

Colonic Inertia: A condition of the colon. Colon muscles do not work properly, causing constipation.

Colonoscopy: A test to look into the rectum and colon. The doctor uses a long, flexible, narrow tube with a light and tiny lens on the end. This tube is called a colonoscope.

Colorectal Cancer: Cancer that occurs in the colon (large intestine) or the rectum (the end of the large intestine). A number of digestive diseases may increase a person's risk of colorectal cancer, including polyposis and Zollinger-Ellison Syndrome.

Colorectal Transit Study: A test to see how food moves through the colon. The patient swallows capsules that contain small markers. An x-ray tracks the movement of the capsules through the colon.

Colostomy: An operation that makes it possible for stool to leave the body after the rectum has been removed. The surgeon makes an opening in the abdomen and attaches the colon to it. A temporary colostomy may be done to let the rectum heal from injury or other surgery.

Common Bile Duct: The tube that carries bile from the liver to the small intestine.

Computed Tomography (CT) Scan: An x-ray that produces three-dimensional pictures of the body. Also known as computed axial tomography (CAT) scan.

Constipation: A condition in which the stool becomes hard and dry. A person who is constipated usually has fewer than three bowel movements in a week. Bowel movements may be painful.

Continence: The ability to hold in a bowel movement or urine.

Continent Ileostomy: An operation to create a pouch from part of the small intestine. Stool that collects in the pouch is removed by inserting a small tube through an opening made in the abdomen. See also Ileostomy.

Corticosteroids: Medicines such as cortisone and hydrocortisone. These medicines reduce irritation from Crohn disease and ulcerative colitis. They may be taken either by mouth or as suppositories.

Crohn Disease: A chronic form of inflammatory bowel disease. Crohn disease causes severe irritation in the gastrointestinal tract. It usually affects the lower small intestine (called the ileum) or the colon, but it can affect the entire gastrointestinal tract. Also called regional enteritis and ileitis. See also Inflammatory Bowel Disease (IBD) and Granuloma.

Cryptosporidia: A parasite that can cause gastrointestinal infection and diarrhea. See also Gastroenteritis.

Cyclic Vomiting Syndrome (CVS): Sudden, repeated attacks of severe vomiting (especially in children), nausea, and physical exhaustion with no apparent cause. Can last from a few hours to ten days. The episodes begin and end suddenly. Loss of fluids in the body and changes in chemicals in the body can require immediate medical attention. Also called abdominal migraine.

Cystic Duct: The tube that carries bile from the gallbladder into the common bile duct and the small intestine.

Defecography: An x-ray of the anus and rectum to see how the muscles work to move stool. The patient sits on a toilet placed inside the x-ray machine.

Dehydration: Loss of fluids from the body, often caused by diarrhea. May result in loss of important salts and minerals.

Delayed Gastric Emptying: See Gastroparesis.

Dermatitis Herpetiformis: A skin disorder associated with celiac disease. See also Celiac Disease.

Descending Colon: The part of the colon where stool is stored. Located on the left side of the abdomen.

Diarrhea: Frequent, loose, and watery bowel movements. Common causes include gastrointestinal infections, irritable bowel syndrome, medicines, and malabsorption.

Digestion: The process the body uses to break down food into simple substances for energy, growth, and cell repair.

Digestive System: The organs in the body that break down and absorb food. Organs that make up the digestive system are the mouth, esophagus, stomach, small intestine, large intestine, rectum, and anus. Organs that help with digestion but are not part of the digestive tract are the tongue, glands in the mouth that make saliva, pancreas, liver, and gallbladder.

Diverticulitis: A condition that occurs when small pouches in the colon (diverticula) become infected or irritated. Also called left-sided appendicitis.

Diverticulosis: A condition that occurs when small pouches (diverticula) push outward through weak spots in the colon.

Diverticulum: A small pouch in the colon. These pouches are not painful or harmful unless they become infected or irritated.

Dumping Syndrome: A condition that occurs when food moves too fast from the stomach into the small intestine. Symptoms are nausea, pain, weakness, and sweating. This syndrome most often affects people who have had stomach operations. Also called rapid gastric emptying.

Duodenal Ulcer: An ulcer in the lining of the first part of the small intestine (duodenum).

Duodenitis: An irritation of the first part of the small intestine (duodenum).

Duodenum: The first part of the small intestine.

Dysentery: An infectious disease of the colon. Symptoms include bloody, mucus-filled diarrhea; abdominal pain; fever; and loss of fluids from the body.

Dyspepsia: See Indigestion.

Dysphagia: Problems in swallowing food or liquid, usually caused by blockage or injury to the esophagus.

Eagle-Barrett Syndrome: See Prune Belly Syndrome.

Electrocoagulation: A procedure that uses an electrical current passed through an endoscope to stop bleeding in the digestive tract and to remove affected tissue.

Electrolytes: Chemicals such as salts and minerals needed for various functions in the body.

Encopresis: Accidental passage of a bowel movement. A common disorder in children.

Endoscope: A small, flexible tube with a light and a lens on the end. It is used to look into the esophagus, stomach, duodenum, colon, or rectum. It can also be used to take tissue from the body for testing or to take color photographs of the inside of the body. Colonoscopes and sigmoidoscopes are types of endoscopes.

Endoscopic Retrograde Cholangiopancreatography (ERCP): A test using an x-ray to look into the bile and pancreatic ducts. The doctor inserts an endoscope through the mouth into the duodenum and bile ducts. Dye is sent through the tube into the ducts. The dye makes the ducts show up on an x-ray.

Endoscopic Sphincterotomy: An operation to cut the muscle between the common bile duct and the pancreatic duct. The operation uses a catheter and a wire to remove gallstones or other blockages. Also called endoscopic papillotomy.

Endoscopy: A procedure that uses an endoscope to diagnose or treat a condition.

Enema: A liquid put into the rectum to clear out the bowel or to administer drugs or food.

Enteral Nutrition: A way to provide food through a tube placed in the nose, the stomach, or the small intestine. A tube in the nose is called a nasogastric or nasoenteral tube. A tube that goes through the skin into the stomach is called a gastrostomy or percutaneous endoscopic gastrostomy (PEG). A tube into the small intestine is called a jejunostomy or percutaneous endoscopic jejunostomy (PEJ) tube. Also called tube feeding. See also Gastrostomy and Jejunostomy.

Enteritis: An irritation of the small intestine.

Enterocele: A hernia in the intestine. See also Hernia.

Enteroscopy: An examination of the small intestine with an endoscope. The endoscope is inserted through the mouth and stomach into the small intestine.

Enterostomy: An ostomy, or opening, into the intestine through the abdominal wall.

Enzyme-Linked Immunosorbent Assay (ELISA): A blood test used to find *Helicobacter pylori* bacteria. Also used to diagnose an ulcer.

Eosinophilic Gastroenteritis: Infection and swelling of the lining of the stomach, small intestine, or large intestine. The infection is caused by white blood cells (eosinophils).

Epithelial Cells: One of many kinds of cells that form the epithelium and absorb nutrients. See also Epithelium.

Epithelium: The inner and outer tissue covering digestive tract organs.

ERCP: See Endoscopic Retrograde Cholangiopancreatography (ERCP).

Erythema Nodosum: Red swellings or sores on the lower legs during flare-ups of Crohn disease and ulcerative colitis. These sores show that the disease is active. They usually go away when the disease is treated.

Escherichia coli: Bacteria that cause infection and irritation of the large intestine. The bacteria are spread by unclean water, dirty cooking utensils, or undercooked meat. See also Gastroenteritis.

Esophageal Atresia: A birth defect. The esophagus lacks the opening to allow food to pass into the stomach.

Esophageal Manometry: A test to measure muscle tone in the esophagus.

Esophageal pH Monitoring: A test to measure the amount of acid in the esophagus.

Esophageal Stricture: A narrowing of the esophagus often caused by acid flowing back from the stomach. This condition may require surgery.

Esophageal Ulcer: A sore in the esophagus. Caused by long-term inflammation or damage from the residue of pills. The ulcer may cause chest pain.

Esophageal Varices: Stretched veins in the esophagus that occur when the liver is not working properly. If the veins burst, the bleeding can cause death.

Esophagitis: An irritation of the esophagus, usually caused by acid that flows up from the stomach.

Esophagogastroduodenoscopy (EGD): Exam of the upper digestive tract using an endoscope. See Endoscopy.

Esophagus: The organ that connects the mouth to the stomach. Also called gullet.

Extrahepatic Biliary Tree: The bile ducts located outside the liver.

Familial Polyposis: An inherited disease causing many polyps in the colon. The polyps often cause cancer.

Fatty Liver: The buildup of fat in liver cells. The most common cause is alcoholism. Other causes include obesity, diabetes, and pregnancy. Also called steatosis.

Fecal Fat Test: A test to measure the body's ability to break down and absorb fat. The patient eats a fat-free diet for two to three days before the test and collects stool samples for examination.

Fecal Incontinence: Being unable to hold stool in the colon and rectum.

Fecal Occult Blood Test (FOBT): A test to see whether there is blood in the stool that is not visible to the naked eye. A sample of stool is placed on a chemical strip that will change color if blood is present. Hidden blood in the stool is a common symptom of colorectal cancer.

Fermentation: The process of bacteria breaking down undigested food and releasing alcohols, acids, and gases.

Fiber: A substance in foods that comes from plants. Fiber helps with digestion by keeping stool soft so that it moves smoothly through the colon. Soluble fiber dissolves in water. Soluble fiber is found in beans, fruit, and oat products. Insoluble fiber does not dissolve in water. Insoluble fiber is found in whole-grain products and vegetables.

Fistula: An abnormal passage between two organs or between an organ and the outside of the body. Caused when damaged tissues come into contact with each other and join together while healing.

Flatulence: Excessive gas in the stomach or intestine. May cause bloating.

Foodborne Illness: An acute gastrointestinal infection caused by food that contains harmful bacteria. Symptoms include diarrhea, abdominal pain, fever, and chills. Also called food poisoning.

Fulminant Hepatic Failure (FHF): Liver failure that occurs suddenly in a previously healthy person. The most common causes of FHF are acute hepatitis, acetaminophen overdose, and liver damage from prescription drugs.

Functional Disorders: Disorders such as irritable bowel syndrome. These conditions result from poor nerve and muscle function. Symptoms such as gas, pain, constipation, and diarrhea come back again and again, but there are no signs of disease or damage. Emotional stress can trigger symptoms. Also called motility disorders.

Galactose: A type of sugar in milk products and sugar beets. The body also makes galactose.

Galactosemia: Buildup of galactose in the blood. Caused by lack of one of the enzymes needed to break down galactose into glucose.

Gallbladder: The organ that stores the bile made in the liver. Connected to the liver by bile ducts. The gallbladder can store about one cup of bile. Eating signals the gallbladder to empty the bile through the bile ducts to help digest fats.

Gallstones: The solid masses or stones made of cholesterol or bilirubin that form in the gallbladder or bile ducts.

Gardner Syndrome: A condition in which many polyps form throughout the digestive tract. Because these polyps are likely to cause cancer, the colon and rectum are often removed to prevent colorectal cancer.

Gastrectomy: An operation to remove all or part of the stomach.

Gastric: Related to the stomach.

Gastric Juices: Liquids produced in the stomach to help break down food and kill bacteria.

Gastric Resection: An operation to remove part or all of the stomach.

Gastric Ulcer: See Stomach Ulcer.

Gastrin: A hormone released after eating. Gastrin causes the stomach to produce more acid.

Gastritis: An inflammation of the stomach lining.

Gastrocolic Reflex: Increase of muscle movement in the gastrointestinal tract when food enters an empty stomach. May cause the urge to have a bowel movement right after eating.

Gastroenteritis: An infection or irritation of the stomach and intestines. May be caused by bacteria or parasites from spoiled food or unclean water. Other causes include eating food that irritates the stomach lining and emotional upsets such as anger, fear, or stress. Symptoms include diarrhea, nausea, vomiting, and abdominal cramping. See also Travelers' Diarrhea.

Gastroenterology: The field of medicine concerned with the function and disorders of the digestive system.

Gastroesophageal Reflux Disease (GERD): Flow of the stomach's contents back up into the esophagus. Happens when the muscle between the esophagus and the stomach (the lower esophageal sphincter) is weak or relaxes when it shouldn't. May cause esophagitis. Also called esophageal reflux or reflux esophagitis.

Gastrointestinal (GI) Tract: The large, muscular tube that extends from the mouth to the anus, where the movement of muscles and release of hormones and enzymes digest food. Also called the alimentary canal or digestive tract.

Gastroparesis: Nerve or muscle damage in the stomach. Causes slow digestion and emptying, vomiting, nausea, or bloating. Also called delayed gastric emptying.

Gastrostomy: An artificial opening from the stomach to a hole (stoma) in the abdomen where a feeding tube is inserted. See also Enteral Nutrition.

GERD: See Gastroesophageal Reflux Disease.

Giardiasis: An infection with the parasite *Giardia lamblia* from spoiled food or unclean water. May cause diarrhea. See also Gastroenteritis.

Gilbert Syndrome: A buildup of bilirubin in the blood. Caused by lack of a liver enzyme needed to break down bilirubin. See also Bilirubin.

Glucose: A simple sugar the body manufactures from carbohydrates in the diet. Glucose is the body's main source of energy.

Gluten: A protein found in wheat, rye, barley, and oats. In people who can't digest it, gluten damages the lining of the small intestine or causes sores on the skin.

Gluten Intolerance: See Celiac Disease.

Gluten Sensitive Enteropathy: A general term that refers to celiac disease and dermatitis herpetiformis.

Glycogen: A sugar stored in the liver and muscles. It releases glucose into the blood when cells need it for energy. Glycogen is the chief source of stored fuel in the body.

Glycogen Storage Diseases: A group of birth defects. These diseases change the way the liver breaks down glycogen. See also Glycogen.

Granuloma: A mass of red, irritated tissue in the GI tract found in Crohn disease.

Granulomatous Colitis: Another name for Crohn disease of the colon.

Granulomatous Enteritis: Another name for Crohn disease of the small intestine.

H$_2$-Blockers: Histamine signals the stomach to make acid. Prescription H$_2$-blockers are cimetidine (Tagamet), famotidine (Pepcid), nizatidine (Axid), and ranitidine (Zantac). They are used to treat ulcer symptoms. Nonprescription H$_2$-blockers are Zantac 75, Axid AR, Pepcid-AC, and Tagamet-HB. They are for GERD, heartburn, and acid indigestion.

Heartburn: A painful, burning feeling in the chest. Heartburn is caused by stomach acid flowing back into the esophagus. Changing the diet and other habits can help to prevent heartburn. Heartburn may be a symptom of GERD. See also Gastroesophageal Reflux Disease (GERD).

***Helicobacter pylori* (*H. pylori*):** A spiral-shaped bacterium found in the stomach. *H. pylori* damages stomach and duodenal tissue, causing ulcers. Previously called *Campylobacter pylori.*

Hemochromatosis: A disease that occurs when the body absorbs too much iron. The body stores the excess iron in the liver, pancreas, and other organs. May cause cirrhosis of the liver. Also called iron overload disease.

Hemorrhoidectomy: An operation to remove hemorrhoids.

Hemorrhoids: Swollen blood vessels in and around the anus and lower rectum. Continual straining to have a bowel movement causes them to stretch and swell. They cause itching, pain, and sometimes bleeding.

Hepatic: Related to the liver.

Hepatitis: Irritation of the liver that sometimes causes permanent damage. Hepatitis may be caused by viruses or by medicines or alcohol.

Hepatitis A: A virus most often spread by unclean food and water.

Hepatitis B: A virus commonly spread by sexual intercourse or blood transfusion, or from mother to newborn at birth. Another way it spreads is by using a needle that was used by an infected person. Hepatitis B is more common and much more easily spread than the AIDS virus and may lead to cirrhosis and liver cancer.

Hepatitis B Immunoglobulin (HBIg): A shot that gives short-term protection from the hepatitis B virus.

Hepatitis B Vaccine: A shot to prevent hepatitis B. The vaccine tells the body to make its own protection (antibodies) against the virus.

Hepatitis C: A virus spread by blood transfusion and possibly by sexual intercourse or sharing needles with infected people. Hepatitis C may lead to cirrhosis and liver cancer. Hepatitis C used to be called non-A, non-B hepatitis.

Hepatitis D (Delta): A virus that occurs mostly in people who take illegal drugs by using needles. Only people who have hepatitis B can get hepatitis D.

Hepatitis E: A virus spread mostly through unclean water. This type of hepatitis is common in developing countries. It has not occurred in the United States.

Hernia: The part of an internal organ that pushes through an opening in the organ's wall. Most hernias occur in the abdominal area.

Hiatal Hernia (Hiatus Hernia): A small opening in the diaphragm that allows the upper part of the stomach to move up into the chest. Causes heartburn from stomach acid flowing back up through the opening.

Hirschsprung Disease: A birth defect in which some nerve cells are lacking in the large intestine. The intestine cannot move stool through, so the intestine gets blocked. Causes the abdomen to swell. See also Megacolon.

Hormone: A substance in the body that regulates certain organs. Hormones such as gastrin help in breaking down food. Some hormones come from cells in the stomach and small intestine.

Hydrogen Breath Test: A test for lactose intolerance. It measures breath samples for too much hydrogen. The body makes too much hydrogen when lactose is not broken down properly in the small intestine.

Hyperbilirubinemia: Too much bilirubin in the blood. Symptoms include jaundice. This condition occurs when the liver does not work normally. See also Jaundice.

IBD: See Inflammatory Bowel Disease (IBD).

IBS: See Irritable Bowel Syndrome (IBS).

Ileal: Related to the ileum, the lowest end of the small intestine.

Ileal Pouch: See Ileoanal Reservoir.

Ileitis: See Crohn Disease.

Ileoanal Anastomosis: See Ileoanal Pull-Through.

Ileoanal Pull-Through: An operation to remove the colon and inner lining of the rectum. The outer muscle of the rectum is not touched. The bottom end of the small intestine (ileum) is pulled through the remaining rectum and joined to the anus. Stool can be passed normally. Also called ileoanal anastomosis.

Ileoanal Reservoir: An operation to remove the colon, upper rectum, and part of the lower rectum. An internal pouch is created from the remaining intestine to hold stool. The operation may be done in two stages. The pouch may also be called a J-pouch or W-pouch.

Ileocecal Valve: A valve that connects the lower part of the small intestine and the upper part of the large intestine (ileum and cecum). Controls the flow of fluid in the intestines and prevents backflow.

Ileocolitis: Irritation of the lower part of the small intestine (ileum) and colon.

Ileostomy: An operation that makes it possible for stool to leave the body after the colon and rectum are removed. The surgeon makes an opening in the abdomen and attaches the bottom of the small intestine (ileum) to it.

Ileum: The lower end of the small intestine.

Imperforate Anus: A birth defect in which the anal canal fails to develop. The condition is treated with an operation.

Indigestion: Poor digestion. Symptoms include heartburn, nausea, bloating, and gas. Also called dyspepsia.

Inflammatory Bowel Disease (IBD): Long-lasting problems that cause irritation and ulcers in the GI tract. The most common disorders are ulcerative colitis and Crohn disease.

Inguinal Hernia: A small part of the large or small intestine or bladder that pushes into the groin. May cause pain and feelings of pressure or burning in the groin. Often requires surgery.

Intestinal Flora: The bacteria, yeasts, and fungi that grow normally in the intestines.

Intestinal Mucosa: The surface lining of the intestines where the cells absorb nutrients.

Intestinal Pseudo-Obstruction: A disorder that causes symptoms of blockage, but no actual blockage. Causes constipation, vomiting, and pain. See also Obstruction.

Intestines: See Large Intestine and Small Intestine. Also called gut.

Intolerance: Allergy to a food, drug, or other substance.

Intussusception: A rare disorder. A part of the intestines folds into another part of the intestines, causing blockage. Most common in infants. Can be treated with an operation.

Irritable Bowel Syndrome (IBS): A disorder that comes and goes. Nerves that control the muscles in the GI tract are too active. The GI tract becomes sensitive to food, stool, gas, and stress. Causes abdominal pain, bloating, and constipation or diarrhea. Also called spastic colon or mucous colitis.

Ischemic Colitis: Decreased blood flow to the colon. Causes fever, pain, and bloody diarrhea.

Jaundice: A symptom of many disorders. Jaundice causes the skin and eyes to turn yellow from too much bilirubin in the blood. See also Hyperbilirubinemia.

Jejunostomy: An operation to create an opening of the jejunum to a hole (stoma) in the abdomen. See also Enteral Nutrition.

Jejunum: The middle section of the small intestine between the duodenum and ileum.

Kupffer Cells: Cells that line the liver. These cells remove waste such as bacteria from the blood.

Lactase: An enzyme in the small intestine needed to digest milk sugar (lactose).

Lactose: The sugar found in milk. The body breaks lactose down into galactose and glucose.

Lactose Intolerance: Being unable to digest lactose, the sugar in milk. This condition occurs because the body does not produce the lactase enzyme.

Laparoscope: A thin tube with a tiny video camera attached. Used to look inside the body and see the surface of organs. See also Endoscope.

Laparoscopic Cholecystectomy: An operation to remove the gallbladder. The doctor inserts a laparoscope and other surgical instruments through small holes in the abdomen. The camera allows the doctor to see the gallbladder on a television screen. The doctor removes the gallbladder through the holes.

Laparoscopy: A test that uses a laparoscope to look at and take tissue from the inside of the body.

Large Intestine: The part of the intestine that goes from the cecum to the rectum. The large intestine absorbs water from stool and changes it from a liquid to a solid form. The large intestine is five feet long and includes the appendix, cecum, colon, and rectum. Also called colon.

Laxatives: Medicines to relieve long-term constipation. Used only if other methods fail. Also called cathartics.

Lazy Colon: See Atonic Colon.

Levator Syndrome: Feeling of fullness in the anus and rectum with occasional pain. Caused by muscle spasms.

Liver: The largest organ in the body. The liver carries out many important functions, such as making bile, changing food into energy, and cleaning alcohol and poisons from the blood.

Liver Enzyme Tests: Blood tests that look at how well the liver and biliary system are working. Also called liver function tests.

Liver Function Tests: See Liver Enzyme Tests.

Lower Esophageal Ring: An abnormal ring of tissue that may partially block the lower esophagus. Also called Schatzki ring.

Lower Esophageal Sphincter: The muscle between the esophagus and stomach. When a person swallows, this muscle relaxes to let food pass from the esophagus to the stomach. It stays closed at other times to keep stomach contents from flowing back into the esophagus.

Lower GI Series: X-rays of the rectum, colon, and lower part of the small intestine. A barium enema is given first. Barium coats the organs so they will show up on the x-ray. Also called barium enema x-ray.

Magnetic Resonance Imaging (MRI): A test that takes pictures of the soft tissues in the body. The pictures are clearer than x-rays.

Malabsorption Syndromes: Conditions that happen when the small intestine cannot absorb nutrients from foods.

Mallory-Weiss Tear: A tear in the lower end of the esophagus. Caused by severe vomiting. Common in alcoholics.

Manometry: Tests that measure muscle pressure and movements in the GI tract. See also Esophageal Manometry and Rectal Manometry.

Meckel Diverticulum: A birth defect in which a small sac forms in the ileum.

Megacolon: A huge, swollen colon. Results from severe constipation. In children, megacolon is more common in boys than girls. See also Hirschsprung Disease.

Ménétrier Disease: A long-term disorder that causes large, coiled folds in the stomach. Also called giant hypertrophic gastritis.

Motility: The movement of food through the digestive tract.

Motility Disorders: See Functional Disorders.

Mucosal Lining: The lining of GI tract organs that makes mucus.

Mucosal Protective Drugs: Medicines that protect the stomach lining from acid. Examples are sucralfate (Carafate), misoprostol (Cytotec), antacids (Mylanta and Maalox), and bismuth subsalicylate (Pepto-Bismol).

Mucous Colitis: See Irritable Bowel Syndrome.

Mucus: A clear liquid made by the intestines. Mucus coats and protects tissues in the GI tract.

Necrotizing Enterocolitis: A condition in which part of the tissue in the intestines is destroyed. Occurs mainly in underweight newborn babies. A temporary ileostomy may be necessary.

Neonatal Hepatitis: Irritation of the liver with no known cause. Occurs in newborn babies. Symptoms include jaundice and liver cell changes.

Nissen Fundoplication: An operation to sew the top of the stomach (fundus) around the esophagus. Used to stop stomach contents from flowing back into the esophagus (reflux) and to repair a hiatal hernia.

Norwalk Virus: A virus that may cause GI infection and diarrhea. See also Gastroenteritis.

Obstruction: A blockage in the GI tract that prevents the flow of liquids or solids.

Occult Bleeding: Blood in stool that is not visible to the naked eye. May be a sign of disease such as diverticulosis or colorectal cancer.

Oral Dissolution Therapy: A method of dissolving cholesterol gallstones. The patient takes the oral medications chenodiol (Chenix) and ursodiol (Actigall). These medicines are most often used for people who cannot have an operation.

Ostomy: An operation that makes it possible for stool to leave the body through an opening made in the abdomen. An ostomy is necessary when part or all of the intestines are removed. Colostomy and ileostomy are types of ostomy.

Pancreas: A gland that makes enzymes for digestion and the hormone insulin.

Pancreatitis: Irritation of the pancreas that can make it stop working. Most often caused by gallstones or alcohol abuse.

Papillary Stenosis: A condition in which the openings of the bile ducts and pancreatic ducts narrow.

Parenteral Nutrition: A way to provide a liquid food mixture through a special tube in the chest. Also called hyperalimentation or total parenteral nutrition.

Parietal Cells: Cells in the stomach wall that make hydrochloric acid.

Pepsin: An enzyme made in the stomach that breaks down proteins.

Peptic: Related to the stomach and the duodenum, where pepsin is present.

Peptic Ulcer: A sore in the lining of the esophagus, stomach, or duodenum. Usually caused by the bacterium *Helicobacter pylori*. An ulcer in the stomach is a gastric ulcer; an ulcer in the duodenum is a duodenal ulcer.

Percutaneous Transhepatic Cholangiography: X-rays of the gallbladder and bile ducts. A dye is injected through the abdomen to make the organs show up on the x-ray.

Perforated Ulcer: An ulcer that breaks through the wall of the stomach or the duodenum. Causes stomach contents to leak into the abdominal cavity.

Perianal: The area around the anus.

Perineal: Related to the perineum.

Perineum: The area between the anus and the sex organs.

Peristalsis: A wavelike movement of muscles in the GI tract. Peristalsis moves food and liquid through the GI tract.

Peritoneum: The lining of the abdominal cavity.

Peritonitis: Infection of the peritoneum.

Polyp: Tissue bulging from the surface of an organ. Although these growths are not normal, they often are not cause for concern. However, people who have polyps in the colon may have an increased risk of colorectal cancer.

Polyposis: The presence of many polyps.

Porphyria: A group of rare, inherited blood disorders. When a person has porphyria, cells fail to change chemicals (porphyrins) to the substance (heme) that gives blood its color. Porphyrins then build up in the body. They show up in large amounts in stool and urine, causing the urine to be colored reddish-purple.

Portal Vein: The large vein that carries blood from the intestines and spleen to the liver.

Postcholecystectomy Syndrome: A condition that occurs after gallbladder removal. The muscle between the gallbladder and the small intestine does not work properly, causing pain, nausea, and indigestion. Also called biliary dyskinesia.

Postgastrectomy Syndrome: A condition that occurs after an operation to remove the stomach (gastrectomy). See also Dumping Syndrome.

Primary Biliary Cirrhosis: A chronic liver disease. Slowly destroys the bile ducts in the liver. This prevents release of bile. Long-term irritation of the liver may cause scarring and cirrhosis in later stages of the disease.

Primary Sclerosing Cholangitis: Irritation, scarring, and narrowing of the bile ducts inside and outside the liver. Bile builds up in the liver and may damage its cells. Many people with this condition also have ulcerative colitis.

Proctalgia Fugax: Intense pain in the rectum that occasionally happens at night. Caused by muscle spasms around the anus.

Proctectomy: An operation to remove the rectum.

Proctitis: Irritation of the rectum.

Proctocolectomy: An operation to remove the colon and rectum. Also called coloproctectomy.

Proctocolitis: Irritation of the colon and rectum.

Proctoscope: A short, rigid metal tube used to look into the rectum and anus.

Proctoscopy: Looking into the rectum and anus with a proctoscope.

Proctosigmoiditis: Irritation of the rectum and the sigmoid colon.

Proctosigmoidoscopy: An endoscopic examination of the rectum and sigmoid colon. See also Endoscopy.

Prokinetic Drugs: Medicines that cause muscles in the GI tract to move food. An example is cisapride (Propulsid).

Prolapse: A condition that occurs when a body part slips from its normal position.

Proton Pump Inhibitors: Medicines that stop the stomach's acid pump. Examples are omeprazole (Prilosec) and lansoprazole (Prevacid).

Prune Belly Syndrome: A condition of newborn babies. The baby has no abdominal muscles, so the stomach looks like a shriveled prune. Also called Eagle-Barrett syndrome.

Pruritus Ani: Itching around the anus.

Pseudomembranous Colitis: Severe irritation of the colon. Caused by *Clostridium difficile* bacteria. Occurs after taking oral antibiotics, which kill bacteria that normally live in the colon.

Pyloric Sphincter: The muscle between the stomach and the small intestine.

Pyloric Stenosis: A narrowing of the opening between the stomach and the small intestine.

Pylorus: The opening from the stomach into the top of the small intestine (duodenum).

Radionuclide Scans: Tests to find GI bleeding. Radioactive material is injected to highlight organs on a special camera. Also called scintigraphy.

Rapid Gastric Emptying: See Dumping Syndrome.

Rectal Manometry: A test that uses a thin tube and balloon to measure pressure and movements of the rectal and anal sphincter muscles. Usually used to diagnose chronic constipation and fecal incontinence.

Rectal Prolapse: A condition in which the rectum slips so that it protrudes from the anus.

Rectum: The lower end of the large intestine, leading to the anus.

Reflux: A condition that occurs when gastric juices or small amounts of food from the stomach flow back into the esophagus and mouth. Also called regurgitation.

Reflux Esophagitis: Irritation of the esophagus because stomach contents flow back into the esophagus.

Retching: Dry vomiting.

Rotavirus: The most common cause of infectious diarrhea in the United States, especially in children under age two.

Saliva: A mixture of water, protein, and salts that makes food easy to swallow and begins digestion.

Salmonella: A bacterium that may cause intestinal infection and diarrhea. See also Gastroenteritis.

Sarcoidosis: A condition that causes small, fleshy swellings in the liver, lungs, and spleen.

Schatzki Ring: See Lower Esophageal Ring.

Sclerotherapy: A method of stopping upper GI bleeding. A needle is inserted through an endoscope to bring hardening agents to the place that is bleeding.

Secretin: A hormone made in the duodenum. Causes the stomach to make pepsin, the liver to make bile, and the pancreas to make a digestive juice.

Segmentation: The process by which muscles in the intestines move food and wastes through the body.

Shigellosis: Infection with the bacterium *Shigella*. Usually causes a high fever, acute diarrhea, and dehydration. See also Gastroenteritis.

Short Bowel Syndrome: Problems related to absorbing nutrients after removal of part of the small intestine. Symptoms include diarrhea, weakness, and weight loss. Also called short gut syndrome.

Short Gut Syndrome: See Short Bowel Syndrome.

Shwachman Syndrome: A digestive and respiratory disorder of children. Certain digestive enzymes are missing and white blood cells are few. Symptoms may include diarrhea and short stature.

Sigmoid Colon: The lower part of the colon that empties into the rectum.

Sigmoidoscopy: Looking into the sigmoid colon and rectum with a flexible or rigid tube, called a sigmoidoscope.

Small Bowel Enema: X-rays of the small intestine taken as barium liquid passes through the organ. Also called small bowel follow-through. See also Lower GI Series.

Small Intestine: Organ where most digestion occurs. It measures about twenty feet and includes the duodenum, jejunum, and ileum.

Somatostatin: A hormone in the pancreas. Somatostatin helps tell the body when to make the hormones insulin, glucagon, gastrin, secretin, and renin.

Spasms: Muscle movements such as those in the colon that cause pain, cramps, and diarrhea.

Spastic Colon: See Irritable Bowel Syndrome (IBS).

Sphincter: A ring-like band of muscle that opens and closes an opening in the body. An example is the muscle between the esophagus and the stomach known as the lower esophageal sphincter.

Sphincter of Oddi: The muscle between the common bile duct and pancreatic ducts.

Spleen: The organ that cleans blood and makes white blood cells. White blood cells attack bacteria and other foreign cells.

Splenic Flexure Syndrome: A condition that occurs when air or gas collects in the upper parts of the colon. Causes pain in the upper left abdomen. The pain often moves to the left chest and may be confused with heart problems.

Steatorrhea: A condition in which the body cannot absorb fat. Causes a buildup of fat in the stool and loose, greasy, and foul bowel movements.

Steatosis: See Fatty Liver.

Stoma: An opening in the abdomen that is created by an operation (ostomy). Must be covered at all times by a bag that collects stool.

Stomach: The organ between the esophagus and the small intestine. The stomach is where digestion of protein begins.

Stomach Ulcer: An open sore in the lining of the stomach. Also called gastric ulcer.

Stool: The solid wastes that pass through the rectum as bowel movements. Stools are undigested foods, bacteria, mucus, and dead cells. Also called feces.

Stress Ulcer: An upper GI ulcer from physical injury such as surgery, major burns, or critical head injury.

Stricture: The abnormal narrowing of a body opening. Also called stenosis. See also Esophageal Stricture and Pyloric Stenosis.

Tenesmus: Straining to have a bowel movement. May be painful and continue for a long time without result.

Tracheoesophageal Fistula (TEF): A condition that occurs when there is a gap between the upper and lower segments of the esophagus. Food and saliva cannot pass through.

Transverse Colon: The part of the colon that goes across the abdomen from right to left.

Travelers' Diarrhea: An infection caused by unclean food or drink. Often occurs during travel outside one's own country. See also Gastroenteritis.

Triple Therapy: Drugs that stop the body from making acid are often added to relieve symptoms.

Tropical Sprue: A condition of unknown cause. Abnormalities in the lining of the small intestine prevent the body from absorbing food normally.

Ulcer: A sore on the skin surface or on the stomach lining.

Ulcerative Colitis: A serious disease that causes ulcers and irritation in the inner lining of the colon and rectum. See also Inflammatory Bowel Disease (IBD).

Upper GI Endoscopy: Looking into the esophagus, stomach, and duodenum with an endoscope. See also Endoscopy.

Upper GI Series: X-rays of the esophagus, stomach, and duodenum. The patient swallows barium first. Barium makes the organs show up on x-rays. Also called barium meal.

Urea Breath Test: A test used to detect *Helicobacter pylori* infection. The test measures breath samples for urease, an enzyme *H. pylori* makes.

Vagotomy: An operation to cut the vagus nerve. This causes the stomach to make less acid.

Vagus Nerve: The nerve in the stomach that controls the making of stomach acid.

Varices: Stretched veins such as those that form in the esophagus from cirrhosis.

Villi: The tiny, finger-like projections on the surface of the small intestine. Villi help absorb nutrients.

Viral Hepatitis: Hepatitis caused by a virus. Five different viruses (A, B, C, D, and E) most commonly cause this form of hepatitis. Other rare viruses may also cause hepatitis. See Hepatitis.

Volvulus: A twisting of the stomach or large intestine. May be caused by the stomach being in the wrong position, a foreign substance, or abnormal joining of one part of the stomach or intestine to another. Volvulus can lead to blockage, perforation, peritonitis, and poor blood flow.

Watermelon Stomach: Parallel red sores in the stomach that look like the stripes on a watermelon. Frequently seen with cirrhosis.

Wilson Disease: An inherited disorder. Too much copper builds up in the liver and is slowly released into other parts of the body. The overload can cause severe liver and brain damage if not treated with medication.

Zenker Diverticulum: Pouches in the esophagus from increased pressure in and around the esophagus.

Zollinger-Ellison Syndrome: A group of symptoms that occur when a tumor called a gastrinoma forms in the pancreas. The tumor, which may cause cancer, releases large amounts of the hormone gastrin. The gastrin causes too much acid in the duodenum, resulting in ulcers, bleeding, and perforation.

Chapter 54

Resources for Information about Gastrointestinal Conditions

General Information

American Academy of Family Physicians
11400 Tomahawk Creek Parkway
Leawood, KS 66211-2672
Toll-Free: 800-274-2237
Phone: 913-906-6000
Website: http://www.aafp.org
E-mail: fp@aafp.org

American College of Gastroenterology (ACG)
P.O. Box 342260
Bethesda, MD 20827-2260
Phone: 301-263-9000
Website: http://www.acg.gi.org
E-mail: info@acg.gi.org

American College of Surgeons
633 North Saint Clair Street
Chicago, IL 60611-3211
Phone: 312-202-5000
Fax: 312-202-5001
Website: http://www.facs.org
E-mail: postmaster@facs.org

American Gastroenterological Association
National Office
4930 Del Ray Avenue
Bethesda, MD 20814
Phone: 301-654-2055
Fax: 301-654-5920
Website: http://www.gastro.org
E-mail: info@gastro.org or webmaster@gastro.org

Resources listed in this chapter were compiled from several sources deemed accurate; inclusion does not constitute endorsement and this list is not considered complete. All contact information was verified and updated in August 2005.

American Society of Colon and Rectal Surgeons (ASCRS)
85 West Algonquin Road, Suite 550
Arlington Heights, IL 60005
Phone: 847-290-9184
Fax: 847-290-9203
Website: http://www.fascrs.org
E-mail: ascrs@fascrs.org

Cleveland Clinic
Department of Patient Education and Health Information
9500 Euclid Ave. NA31
Cleveland, OH 44195
Toll-Free: 800-223-2273 ext. 43771
Phone: 216-444-3771
TTY: 216-444-0261
Website: http://www.clevelandclinic.org
E-mail: healthl@ccf.org

Digestive Disorders Foundation (CORE)
3 St. Andrews Place
London, England NW1 4LB
Phone: 011-020-7486-0341
Fax: 011-020-7224-2012
Website: http://www.digestivedisorders.org.uk
E-mail: info@corecharity.org.uk

International Foundation for Functional Gastrointestinal Disorders (IFFGD)
P.O. Box 170864
Milwaukee, WI 53217-8076
Toll-Free: 888-964-2001
Phone: 414-964-1799
Fax: 414-964-7176
Website: http://www.iffgd.org
E-mail: iffgd@iffgd.org

Intestinal Disease Foundation, Inc.
The Landmarks Bldg., Suite 525
One Station Square
Pittsburgh, PA 15219
Toll Free: 877-587-9606
Phone: 412-261-5888
Fax: 412-471-2722
Website: http://www.intestinalfoundation.org
E-mail: intdis@stargate.net

Mayo Clinic
Health Information Division
200 First St., SW, Centerplace 5
Rochester, MN 55905
Fax: 507-266-0230
Website: http://www.mayoclinic.com

National Organization for Rare Disorders Inc. (NORD)
55 Kenosia Avenue
P.O. Box 1968
Danbury, CT 06813-1968
Toll-Free: 800-999-6673
Phone: 203-744-0100
Fax: 203-798-2291
TDD: 203-797-9590
Website: http://www.rarediseases.org
E-mail: orphan@rarediseases.org

Government Associations

Centers for Disease Control and Prevention (CDC)
1600 Clifton Road, NE.
Mail Stop G37
Atlanta, GA 30333
Toll-Free: 800-311-3435
Phone: 404-639-3311
Website: http://www.cdc.gov

National Cancer Institute (NCI)

National Institutes of Health
31 Center Drive
Building 31, Room 10A-19
Bethesda, MD 20892
Toll-Free: 800-422-6237
Phone: 301-496-6641
Fax: 301-496-0846
Website: http://www.nci.nih.gov

National Digestive Diseases Information Clearinghouse

Building 31
Room 9A04 Center Drive
MSC 260
Bethesda, MD 20892-2560
Phone: 301-496-3583
Website: http://
www.niddk.nih.gov
E-mail:
nddic@info.niddk.nih.gov

National Institutes of Health Osteoporosis and Related Bone Diseases National Resource Center

2 AMS Circle
Bethesda, MD 20892-3676
Toll-Free: 800-624-BONE
Phone: 202-223-0344
Fax: 202-293-2356
TTY: 202-466-4315
Website: http://www.osteo.org
E-mail:
niamsboneinfo@mail.nih.gov

National Library of Medicine—MEDLINEplus

Website: http://
www.nlm.nih.gov/medlineplus

Anorectal Disorders

Pull-thru Network

2312 Savoy Street
Hoover, AL 35226
Phone: 205-978-2930
Website: http://
www.pullthrough.org
E-mail: info@pullthrough.org

Barrett Esophagus

Barrett's Oesophagus Foundation

University Dept. of Surgery
Royal Free Campus
Royal Free & University College
Medical School
Rowland Hill Street
London, England NW3 2PF
Phone: 011-020-7472-6223
Fax: 011-020-7472-6224
Website: http://
www.barrettsfoundation.org.uk
E-mail:
enquiries@barrettsfoundation.org.uk

Barrettsinfo.com

http://www.barrettsinfo.com

Cancer

American Cancer Society

Toll-Free: 800-ACS-2345
Website: http://www.cancer.org

Colon Cancer Alliance

175 Ninth Avenue
New York, NY 10011
Toll-Free: 877-422-2030
Fax: 425-940-6147
Website: http://www.ccalliance.org

Colorectal Cancer Network
P.O. Box 182
Kensington, MD 20895-0182
Phone: 301-879-1500
Fax: 301-821-7080
Website: http://www
.colorectal-cancer.net

**National Cancer Institute
(NCI)**
National Institutes of Health
31 Center Drive
Building 31, Room 10A-19
Bethesda, MD 20892
Toll-Free: 800-422-6237
Phone: 301-496-6641
Fax: 301-496-0846
Website: http://www.nci.nih.gov

Celiac Disease/Allergies

**American Celiac Society—
Dietary Support Coalition**
58 Musano Court
West Orange, NJ 07052
Phone: 973-352-8837
E-mail:
amerceliacsoc@netscape.net

**American Dietetic
Association**
120 South Riverside Plaza,
Suite 2000
Chicago, IL 60606-6995
Toll-Free: 800-877-1600
Website: http://www.eatright.org
E-mail: hotline@eatright.org

**Canadian Celiac
Association**
5170 Dixie Road, Suite 204
Mississauga, Ontario L4W 1E3
Toll-Free: 800-363-7296
Phone: 905-507-6208
Fax: 905-507-4673
Website: http://www.celiac.ca/
englishcca.html
E-mail: celiac@look.ca

Celiac Disease Foundation
13251 Ventura Blvd. #1
Studio City, Ca. 91604
Phone: 818-990-2354
Fax: 818-990-2379
Website: http://www.celiac.org
E-mail: cdf@celiac.org

Celiac Sprue Association
P.O. Box 31700
Omaha, NE 68131-0700
Toll Free: 877-CSA-4CSA
Phone: 402-558-0600
Fax: 402-558-1347
Website: http://
www.csaceliacs.org
E-mail: celiacs@csaceliacs.org

**Food Allergy and
Anaphylaxis Network**
11781 Lee Jackson Highway,
Suite 160
Fairfax, VA 22033-3309
Toll-Free: 800-929-4040
Fax: 703-691-2713
Website: http://
www.foodallergy.org
E-mail: faan@foodallergy.org

Gluten-Free Living
(a bimonthly newsletter)
19 A Broadway
Hawthorne, NY 10532
Phone: 914-741-5420
Website: http://
www.glutenfreeliving.com
E-mail:
info@glutenfreeliving.com

Gluten Intolerance Group of
North America
15110 10th Ave SW, Suite A
Seattle, WA 98166
Phone: 206-246-6652
Fax : 206-246-6531
Website: http://www.gluten.net
E-mail: info@gluten.net

University of Maryland
School of Medicine
Center for Celiac Research
20 Penn Street, Room S303B
Baltimore, MD 21201
Phone: 410-706-8021
Fax: 410-706-5508
Website: http://www.celiaccenter.org

Children's Issues

Children's Digestive Health
and Nutrition Foundation
Toll-Free: 800-344-8888
Website: http://www.cdhnf.org

Children's Liver Association
for Support Services
27023 McBean Parkway #126
Valencia, CA 91355
Toll-Free: 877-679-8256
Phone: 661-263-9099
Website: http://www.classkids.org

North American Society for
Pediatric Gastroenterology,
Hepatology, and Nutrition
P.O. Box 6
Flourtown, PA 19031
Phone: 215-233-0808
Fax: 215-233-3918
Website: http://
www.NASPGHAN.org
E-mail:
naspghan@naspghan.org

Pediatric/Adolescent
Gastroesophageal Reflux
Association Inc. (PAGER)
P.O. Box 486
Buckeystown, MD 21717-1486
Phone: 301-601-9541
Website: http://www.reflux.org
E-mail: gergroup@aol.com

Pediatric Crohn's & Colitis
Association Inc.
P.O. Box 188
Newton, MA 02468
Phone: 617-489-5854
Website: http://
pcca.hypermart.net

Reach Out for Youth With
Ileitis and Colitis Inc.
84 Northgate Circle
Melville, NY 11747
Phone: 631-293-3102
Fax: 631-293-3103
Website: http://
www.reachoutforyouth.org
E-mail:
reachoutforyouth@reachoutfor
youth.org

Crohn Disease and Ulcerative Colitis

Crohn's & Colitis Foundation of America Inc.
386 Park Avenue South,
17th Floor
New York, NY 10016-8804
Toll-Free: 800-932-2423
Phone: 212-685-3440
Fax: 212-779-4098
Website: http://www.ccfa.org
E-mail: info@ccfa.org

Pediatric Crohn's & Colitis Association Inc.
P.O. Box 188
Newton, MA 02468
Phone: 617-489-5854
Website: http://
pcca.hypermart.net

Reach Out for Youth With Ileitis and Colitis Inc.
84 Northgate Circle
Melville, NY 11747
Phone: 631-293-3102
Fax: 631-293-3103
Website: http://
www.reachoutforyouth.org
E-mail:
reachoutforyouth@reachoutfor
youth.org

United Ostomy Association Inc.
19772 MacArthur Boulevard,
Suite 200
Irvine, CA 92612-2405
Toll-Free: 800-826-0826
Phone: 949-660-8624
Fax: 949-660-9262
Website: http://www.uoa.org
E-mail: info@uoa.org

Cyclic Vomiting Syndrome

Cyclic Vomiting Syndrome Association
3585 Cedar Hill Road, NW
Canal Winchester, OH 43110
Phone: 614-837-2586
Fax: 614-837-2586
Website: http://
www.cvsaonline.org
E-mail: waitesd@cvsaonline.org

Cystic Fibrosis

Cystic Fibrosis Foundation
6931 Arlington Road
Bethesda, Maryland 20814
Toll-Free: 800-FIGHT CF (344-4823)
Phone: 301-951-4422
Fax: 301-951-6378
Website: http://www.cff.org
E-mail: info@cff.org

Diagnostic Testing

American Society for Gastrointestinal Endoscopy
1520 Kensington Rd., Suite 202
Oak Brook, IL 60523
Phone: 630-570-5601
Fax: 630-573-0691
Website: http://www.asge.org
E-mail: info@asge.org

Society of American Gastrointestinal and Endoscopic Surgeons (SAGES)
11300 W. Olympic Blvd., Suite 600
Los Angeles, CA 90064
Phone: 310-437-0544
Fax: 310-437-0585
Website: http://www.sages.org
E-mail: sagesweb@sages.org

Irritable Bowel Syndrome (IBS)

IBS Association
1440 Whalley Ave. #145
New Haven, CT 06515
Website: http://
www.ibsassociation.org
E-mail: ibsa@ibsassociation.org

Liver Disease

American Association for the Study of Liver Disease (AASLD)
1729 King Street, Suite 200
Alexandria, Virginia 22314
Phone: 703-299-9766
Fax: 703-299-9622
Website: http://www.aasld.org
E-mail:aasld@aasld.org

American Liver Foundation (ALF)
75 Maiden Lane, Suite 603
New York, NY 10038
Toll-Free: 800-465-4837 or 888-443-7872
Phone: 212-668-1000
Fax: 212-483-8179
Website: http://
www.liverfoundation.org
E-mail: info@liverfoundation.org

Children's Liver Association for Support Services
27023 McBean Parkway #126
Valencia, CA 91355
Toll-Free: 877-679-8256
Phone: 661-263-9099
Website: http://
www.classkids.org

Hepatitis B Foundation
700 East Butler Avenue
Doylestown, PA 18901-2697
Phone: 215-489-4900
Fax: 215-489-4920
Website: http://www.hepb.org
E-mail: info@hepb.org

Hepatitis Foundation International (HFI)
504 Blick Drive
Silver Spring, MD 20904-2901
Toll-Free: 800-891-0707
Phone: 301-622-4200
Fax: 301-622-4702
Website: http://www.hepfi.org
E-mail: hfi@comcast.net

United Network for Organ Sharing
P.O. Box 2484
Richmond, VA 23218
Toll-Free: 888-894-6361
Phone: 804-782-4800
Fax: 804-782-4817
Website: http://www.unos.org

Wilson's Disease Association
1802 Brookside Drive
Wooster, OH 44691
Toll-Free: 800-399-0266
Phone: 330-264-1450
Fax: 509-757-6418
Website: http://www.wilsonsdisease.org
E-mail: info@wilsondisease.org

Index

Index

Health Reference Series

COMPLETE CATALOG

List price $87 per volume. **School and library price $78 per volume.**

Adolescent Health Sourcebook

Basic Consumer Health Information about Common Medical, Mental, and Emotional Concerns in Adolescents, Including Facts about Acne, Body Piercing, Mononucleosis, Nutrition, Eating Disorders, Stress, Depression, Behavior Problems, Peer Pressure, Violence, Gangs, Drug Use, Puberty, Sexuality, Pregnancy, Learning Disabilities, and More

Along with a Glossary of Terms and Other Resources for Further Help and Information

Edited by Chad T. Kimball. 658 pages. 2002. 0-7808-0248-9.

"It is written in clear, nontechnical language aimed at general readers. . . . Recommended for public libraries, community colleges, and other agencies serving health care consumers."
— *American Reference Books Annual, 2003*

"Recommended for school and public libraries. Parents and professionals dealing with teens will appreciate the easy-to-follow format and the clearly written text. This could become a 'must have' for every high school teacher." — *E-Streams, Jan '03*

"A good starting point for information related to common medical, mental, and emotional concerns of adolescents." — *School Library Journal, Nov '02*

"This book provides accurate information in an easy to access format. It addresses topics that parents and caregivers might not be aware of and provides practical, useable information." — *Doody's Health Sciences Book Review Journal, Sep-Oct '02*

"Recommended reference source."
— *Booklist, American Library Association, Sep '02*

AIDS Sourcebook, 3rd Edition

Basic Consumer Health Information about Acquired Immune Deficiency Syndrome (AIDS) and Human Immunodeficiency Virus (HIV) Infection, Including Facts about Transmission, Prevention, Diagnosis, Treatment, Opportunistic Infections, and Other Complications, with a Section for Women and Children, Including Details about Associated Gynecological Concerns, Pregnancy, and Pediatric Care

Along with Updated Statistical Information, Reports on Current Research Initiatives, a Glossary, and Directories of Internet, Hotline, and Other Resources

Edited by Dawn D. Matthews. 664 pages. 2003. 0-7808-0631-X.

ALSO AVAILABLE: *AIDS Sourcebook, 1st Edition.* Edited by Karen Bellenir and Peter D. Dresser. 831 pages. 1995. 0-7808-0031-1.

AIDS Sourcebook, 2nd Edition. Edited by Karen Bellenir. 751 pages. 1999. 0-7808-0225-X.

"The 3rd edition of the *AIDS Sourcebook,* part of Omnigraphics' *Health Reference Series,* is a welcome update. . . . This resource is highly recommended for academic and public libraries."
— *American Reference Books Annual, 2004*

"Excellent sourcebook. This continues to be a highly recommended book. There is no other book that provides as much information as this book provides."
— *AIDS Book Review Journal, Dec-Jan 2000*

"Recommended reference source."
— *Booklist, American Library Association, Dec '99*

"A solid text for college-level health libraries."
— *The Bookwatch, Aug '99*

Cited in *Reference Sources for Small and Medium-Sized Libraries, American Library Association, 1999*

Alcoholism Sourcebook

Basic Consumer Health Information about the Physical and Mental Consequences of Alcohol Abuse, Including Liver Disease, Pancreatitis, Wernicke-Korsakoff Syndrome (Alcoholic Dementia), Fetal Alcohol Syndrome, Heart Disease, Kidney Disorders, Gastrointestinal Problems, and Immune System Compromise and Featuring Facts about Addiction, Detoxification, Alcohol Withdrawal, Recovery, and the Maintenance of Sobriety

Along with a Glossary and Directories of Resources for Further Help and Information

Edited by Karen Bellenir. 613 pages. 2000. 0-7808-0325-6.

"This title is one of the few reference works on alcoholism for general readers. For some readers this will be a welcome complement to the many self-help books on the market. Recommended for collections serving general readers and consumer health collections."
— *E-Streams, Mar '01*

"This book is an excellent choice for public and academic libraries."
— *American Reference Books Annual, 2001*

"Recommended reference source."
— *Booklist, American Library Association, Dec '00*

"Presents a wealth of information on alcohol use and abuse and its effects on the body and mind, treatment, and prevention." — *SciTech Book News, Dec '00*

"Important new health guide which packs in the latest consumer information about the problems of alcoholism." — *Reviewer's Bookwatch, Nov '00*

SEE ALSO *Drug Abuse Sourcebook, Substance Abuse Sourcebook*

Allergies Sourcebook, 2nd Edition

Basic Consumer Health Information about Allergic Disorders, Triggers, Reactions, and Related Symptoms, Including Anaphylaxis, Rhinitis, Sinusitis, Asthma, Dermatitis, Conjunctivitis, and Multiple Chemical Sensitivity

Along with Tips on Diagnosis, Prevention, and Treatment, Statistical Data, a Glossary, and a Directory of Sources for Further Help and Information

Edited by Annemarie S. Muth. 598 pages. 2002. 0-7808-0376-0.

ALSO AVAILABLE: *Allergies Sourcebook, 1st Edition.* Edited by Allan R. Cook. 611 pages. 1997. 0-7808-0036-2.

"This book brings a great deal of useful material together. . . . This is an excellent addition to public and consumer health library collections."
— *American Reference Books Annual, 2003*

"This second edition would be useful to laypersons with little or advanced knowledge of the subject matter. This book would also serve as a resource for nursing and other health care professions students. It would be useful in public, academic, and hospital libraries with consumer health collections." — *E-Streams, Jul '02*

■

Alternative Medicine Sourcebook, 2nd Edition

Basic Consumer Health Information about Alternative and Complementary Medical Practices, Including Acupuncture, Chiropractic, Herbal Medicine, Homeopathy, Naturopathic Medicine, Mind-Body Interventions, Ayurveda, and Other Non-Western Medical Traditions

Along with Facts about such Specific Therapies as Massage Therapy, Aromatherapy, Qigong, Hypnosis, Prayer, Dance, and Art Therapies, a Glossary, and Resources for Further Information

Edited by Dawn D. Matthews. 618 pages. 2002. 0-7808-0605-0.

ALSO AVAILABLE: *Alternative Medicine Sourcebook, 1st Edition.* Edited by Allan R. Cook. 737 pages. 1999. 0-7808-0200-4.

"Recommended for public, high school, and academic libraries that have consumer health collections. Hospital libraries that also serve the public will find this to be a useful resource." — *E-Streams, Feb '03*

"Recommended reference source."
— *Booklist, American Library Association, Jan '03*

"An important alternate health reference."
— *MBR Bookwatch, Oct '02*

"A great addition to the reference collection of every type of library." — *American Reference Books Annual, 2000*

Alzheimer's Disease Sourcebook, 3rd Edition

Basic Consumer Health Information about Alzheimer's Disease, Other Dementias, and Related Disorders, Including Multi-Infarct Dementia, AIDS Dementia Complex, Dementia with Lewy Bodies, Huntington's Disease, Wernicke-Korsakoff Syndrome (Alcohol-Reated Dementia), Delirium, and Confusional States

Along with Information for People Newly Diagnosed with Alzheimer's Disease and Caregivers, Reports Detailing Current Research Efforts in Prevention, Diagnosis, and Treatment, Facts about Long-Term Care Issues, and Listings of Sources for Additional Information

Edited by Karen Bellenir. 645 pages. 2003. 0-7808-0666-2.

ALSO AVAILABLE: *Alzheimer's, Stroke & 29 Other Neurological Disorders Sourcebook, 1st Edition.* Edited by Frank E. Bair. 579 pages. 1993. 1-55888-748-2.

ALSO AVAILABLE: *Alzheimer's Disease Sourcebook, 2nd Edition.* Edited by Karen Bellenir. 524 pages. 1999. 0-7808-0223-3.

"This very informative and valuable tool will be a great addition to any library serving consumers, students and health care workers."
— *American Reference Books Annual, 2004*

"This is a valuable resource for people affected by dementias such as Alzheimer's. It is easy to navigate and includes important information and resources."
— *Doody's Review Service, Feb. 2004*

"Recommended reference source."
— *Booklist, American Library Association, Oct '99*

SEE ALSO *Brain Disorders Sourcebook*

■

Arthritis Sourcebook, 2nd Edition

Basic Consumer Health Information about Osteoarthritis, Rheumatoid Arthritis, Other Rheumatic Disorders, Infectious Forms of Arthritis, and Diseases with Symptoms Linked to Arthritis, Featuring Facts about Diagnosis, Pain Management, and Surgical Therapies

Along with Coping Strategies, Research Updates, a Glossary, and Resources for Additional Help and Information

Edited by Amy L. Sutton. 593 pages. 2004. 0-7808-0667-0.

ALSO AVAILABLE: *Arthritis Sourcebook, 1st Edition.* Edited by Allan R. Cook. 550 pages. 1998. 0-7808-0201-2.

". . . accessible to the layperson."
— *Reference and Research Book News, Feb '99*

■

Asthma Sourcebook

Basic Consumer Health Information about Asthma, Including Symptoms, Traditional and Nontraditional Remedies, Treatment Advances, Quality-of-Life Aids,

Medical Research Updates, and the Role of Allergies, Exercise, Age, the Environment, and Genetics in the Development of Asthma

Along with Statistical Data, a Glossary, and Directories of Support Groups, and Other Resources for Further Information

Edited by Annemarie S. Muth. 628 pages. 2000. 0-7808-0381-7.

"A worthwhile reference acquisition for public libraries and academic medical libraries whose readers desire a quick introduction to the wide range of asthma information." — *Choice, Association of College & Research Libraries, Jun '01*

"Recommended reference source." — *Booklist, American Library Association, Feb '01*

"Highly recommended." — *The Bookwatch, Jan '01*

"There is much good information for patients and their families who deal with asthma daily." — *American Medical Writers Association Journal, Winter '01*

"This informative text is recommended for consumer health collections in public, secondary school, and community college libraries and the libraries of universities with a large undergraduate population." — *American Reference Books Annual, 2001*

∎

Attention Deficit Disorder Sourcebook

Basic Consumer Health Information about Attention Deficit/Hyperactivity Disorder in Children and Adults, Including Facts about Causes, Symptoms, Diagnostic Criteria, and Treatment Options Such as Medications, Behavior Therapy, Coaching, and Homeopathy

Along with Reports on Current Research Initiatives, Legal Issues, and Government Regulations, and Featuring a Glossary of Related Terms, Internet Resources, and a List of Additional Reading Material

Edited by Dawn D. Matthews. 470 pages. 2002. 0-7808-0624-7.

"Recommended reference source." — *Booklist, American Library Association, Jan '03*

"This book is recommended for all school libraries and the reference or consumer health sections of public libraries." — *American Reference Books Annual, 2003*

∎

Back & Neck Sourcebook, 2nd Edition

Basic Consumer Health Information about Spinal Pain, Spinal Cord Injuries, and Related Disorders, Such as Degenerative Disk Disease, Osteoarthritis, Scoliosis, Sciatica, Spina Bifida, and Spinal Stenosis, and Featuring Facts about Maintaining Spinal Health, Self-Care, Pain Management, Rehabilitative Care, Chiropractic Care, Spinal Surgeries, and Complementary Therapies

Along with Suggestions for Preventing Back and Neck Pain, a Glossary of Related Terms, and a Directory of Resources

Edited by Amy L. Sutton. 633 pages. 2004. 0-7808-0738-3

ALSO AVAILABLE: *Back & Neck Disorders Sourcebook, 1st Edition.* Edited by Karen Bellenir. 548 pages. 1997. 0-7808-0202-0.

"The strength of this work is its basic, easy-to-read format. Recommended." — *Reference and User Services Quarterly, American Library Association, Winter '97*

∎

Blood & Circulatory Disorders Sourcebook, 2nd Edition

Basic Consumer Health Information about the Blood and Circulatory System and Related Disorders, Such as Anemia and Other Hemoglobin Diseases, Cancer of the Blood and Associated Bone Marrow Disorders, Clotting and Bleeding Problems, and Conditions That Affect the Veins, Blood Vessels, and Arteries, Including Facts about the Donation and Transplantation of Bone Marrow, Stem Cells, and Blood and Tips for Keeping the Blood and Circulatory System Healthy

Along with a Glossary of Related Terms and Resources for Additional Help and Information

Edited by Amy L. Sutton. 659 pages. 2005. 0-7808-0746-4.

ALSO AVAILABLE: *Blood and Circulatory Disorders Sourcebook, 1st Edition.* Edited by Karen Bellenir and Linda M. Shin. 554 pages. 1998. 0-7808-0203-9.

"Recommended reference source." — *Booklist, American Library Association, Feb '99*

"An important reference sourcebook written in simple language for everyday, non-technical users. " — *Reviewer's Bookwatch, Jan '99*

∎

Brain Disorders Sourcebook, 2nd Edition

Basic Consumer Health Information about Acquired and Traumatic Brain Injuries, Infections of the Brain, Epilepsy and Seizure Disorders, Cerebral Palsy, and Degenerative Neurological Disorders, Including Amyotrophic Lateral Sclerosis (ALS), Dementias, Multiple Sclerosis, and More

Along with Information on the Brain's Structure and Function, Treatment and Rehabilitation Options, Reports on Current Research Initiatives, a Glossary of Terms Related to Brain Disorders and Injuries, and a Directory of Sources for Further Help and Information

Edited by Sandra J. Judd. 625 pages. 2005. 0-7808-0744-8.

ALSO AVAILABLE: *Brain Disorders Sourcebook, 1st Edition.* Edited by Karen Bellenir. 481 pages. 1999. 0-7808-0229-2.

"Belongs on the shelves of any library with a consumer health collection." — *E-Streams, Mar '00*

SEE ALSO *Alzheimer's Disease Sourcebook*

![separator]

Breast Cancer Sourcebook, 2nd Edition

Basic Consumer Health Information about Breast Cancer, Including Facts about Risk Factors, Prevention, Screening and Diagnostic Methods, Treatment Options, Complementary and Alternative Therapies, Post-Treatment Concerns, Clinical Trials, Special Risk Populations, and New Developments in Breast Cancer Research

Along with Breast Cancer Statistics, a Glossary of Related Terms, and a Directory of Resources for Additional Help and Information

Edited by Sandra J. Judd. 595 pages. 2004. 0-7808-0668-9.

ALSO AVAILABLE: *Breast Cancer Sourcebook, 1st Edition.* Edited by Edward J. Prucha and Karen Bellenir. 580 pages. 2001. 0-7808-0244-6.

"It would be a useful reference book in a library or on loan to women in a support group."
— *Cancer Forum*, Mar '03

"Recommended reference source."
— *Booklist, American Library Association*, Jan '02

"This reference source is highly recommended. It is quite informative, comprehensive and detailed in nature, and yet it offers practical advice in easy-to-read language. It could be thought of as the 'bible' of breast cancer for the consumer." — *E-Streams*, Jan '02

"The broad range of topics covered in lay language make the *Breast Cancer Sourcebook* an excellent addition to public and consumer health library collections."
— *American Reference Books Annual 2002*

"From the pros and cons of different screening methods and results to treatment options, *Breast Cancer Sourcebook* provides the latest information on the subject."
— *Library Bookwatch*, Dec '01

"This thoroughgoing, very readable reference covers all aspects of breast health and cancer. . . . Readers will find much to consider here. Recommended for all public and patient health collections."
— *Library Journal*, Sep '01

SEE ALSO *Cancer Sourcebook for Women, Women's Health Concerns Sourcebook*

![separator]

Breastfeeding Sourcebook

Basic Consumer Health Information about the Benefits of Breastmilk, Preparing to Breastfeed, Breastfeeding as a Baby Grows, Nutrition, and More, Including Information on Special Situations and Concerns Such as Mastitis, Illness, Medications, Allergies, Multiple Births, Prematurity, Special Needs, and Adoption

Along with a Glossary and Resources for Additional Help and Information

Edited by Jenni Lynn Colson. 388 pages. 2002. 0-7808-0332-9.

SEE ALSO *Pregnancy & Birth Sourcebook*

"Particularly useful is the information about professional lactation services and chapters on breastfeeding when returning to work. . . . *Breastfeeding Sourcebook* will be useful for public libraries, consumer health libraries, and technical schools offering nurse assistant training, especially in areas where Internet access is problematic."
— *American Reference Books Annual*, 2003

![separator]

Burns Sourcebook

Basic Consumer Health Information about Various Types of Burns and Scalds, Including Flame, Heat, Cold, Electrical, Chemical, and Sun Burns

Along with Information on Short-Term and Long-Term Treatments, Tissue Reconstruction, Plastic Surgery, Prevention Suggestions, and First Aid

Edited by Allan R. Cook. 604 pages. 1999. 0-7808-0204-7.

"This is an exceptional addition to the series and is highly recommended for all consumer health collections, hospital libraries, and academic medical centers."
— *E-Streams*, Mar '00

"This key reference guide is an invaluable addition to all health care and public libraries in confronting this ongoing health issue."
— *American Reference Books Annual*, 2000

"Recommended reference source."
— *Booklist, American Library Association*, Dec '99

SEE ALSO *Skin Disorders Sourcebook*

![separator]

Cancer Sourcebook, 4th Edition

Basic Consumer Health Information about Major Forms and Stages of Cancer, Featuring Facts about Head and Neck Cancers, Lung Cancers, Gastrointestinal Cancers, Genitourinary Cancers, Lymphomas, Blood Cell Cancers, Endocrine Cancers, Skin Cancers, Bone Cancers, Sarcomas, and Others, and Including Information about Cancer Treatments and Therapies, Identifying and Reducing Cancer Risks, and Strategies for Coping with Cancer and the Side Effects of Treatment

Along with a Cancer Glossary, Statistical and Demographic Data, and a Directory of Sources for Additional Help and Information

Edited by Karen Bellenir. 1,119 pages. 2003. 0-7808-0633-6.

ALSO AVAILABLE: *Cancer Sourcebook, 1st Edition.* Edited by Frank E. Bair. 932 pages. 1990. 1-55888-888-8.

New Cancer Sourcebook, 2nd Edition. Edited by Allan R. Cook. 1,313 pages. 1996. 0-7808-0041-9.

Cancer Sourcebook, 3rd Edition. Edited by Edward J. Prucha. 1,069 pages. 2000. 0-7808-0227-6.

"With cancer being the second leading cause of death for Americans, a prodigious work such as this one, which locates centrally so much cancer-related information, is clearly an asset to this nation's citizens and others."
— *Journal of the National Medical Association, 2004*

"This title is recommended for health sciences and public libraries with consumer health collections."
— *E-Streams, Feb '01*

". . . can be effectively used by cancer patients and their families who are looking for answers in a language they can understand. Public and hospital libraries should have it on their shelves."
— *American Reference Books Annual, 2001*

"Recommended reference source."
— *Booklist, American Library Association, Dec '00*

Cited in *Reference Sources for Small and Medium-Sized Libraries*, American Library Association, 1999

"The amount of factual and useful information is extensive. The writing is very clear, geared to general readers. Recommended for all levels." — *Choice, Association of College & Research Libraries, Jan '97*

SEE ALSO Breast Cancer Sourcebook, Cancer Sourcebook for Women, Pediatric Cancer Sourcebook, Prostate Cancer Sourcebook

■

Cancer Sourcebook for Women, 2nd Edition

Basic Consumer Health Information about Gynecologic Cancers and Related Concerns, Including Cervical Cancer, Endometrial Cancer, Gestational Trophoblastic Tumor, Ovarian Cancer, Uterine Cancer, Vaginal Cancer, Vulvar Cancer, Breast Cancer, and Common Non-Cancerous Uterine Conditions, with Facts about Cancer Risk Factors, Screening and Prevention, Treatment Options, and Reports on Current Research Initiatives

Along with a Glossary of Cancer Terms and a Directory of Resources for Additional Help and Information

Edited by Karen Bellenir. 604 pages. 2002. 0-7808-0226-8.

ALSO AVAILABLE: *Cancer Sourcebook for Women, 1st Edition.* Edited by Allan R. Cook and Peter D. Dresser. 524 pages. 1996. 0-7808-0076-1.

"An excellent addition to collections in public, consumer health, and women's health libraries."
— *American Reference Books Annual, 2003*

"Overall, the information is excellent, and complex topics are clearly explained. As a reference book for the consumer it is a valuable resource to assist them to make informed decisions about cancer and its treatments." — *Cancer Forum, Nov '02*

"Highly recommended for academic and medical reference collections." — *Library Bookwatch, Sep '02*

"This is a highly recommended book for any public or consumer library, being reader friendly and containing accurate and helpful information."
— *E-Streams, Aug '02*

"Recommended reference source."
— *Booklist, American Library Association, Jul '02*

SEE ALSO Breast Cancer Sourcebook, Women's Health Concerns Sourcebook

■

Cardiovascular Diseases & Disorders Sourcebook, 3rd Edition

Basic Consumer Health Information about Heart and Vascular Diseases and Disorders, Such as Angina, Heart Attacks, Arrhythmias, Cardiomyopathy, Valve Disease, Atherosclerosis, and Aneurysms, with Information about Managing Cardiovascular Risk Factors and Maintaining Heart Health, Medications and Procedures Used to Treat Cardiovascular Disorders, and Concerns of Special Significance to Women

long with Reports on Current Research Initiatives, a Glossary of Related Medical Terms, and a Directory of Sources for Further Help and Information

Edited by Sandra J. Judd. 713 pages. 2005. 0-7808-0739-1.

ALSO AVAILABLE: *Heart Diseases & Disorders Sourcebook, 2nd Edition.* Edited by Karen Bellenir. 612 pages. 2000. 0-7808-0238-1.

Cardiovascular Diseases & Disorders Sourcebook, 1st Edition. Edited by Karen Bellenir and Peter D. Dresser. 683 pages. 1995. 0-7808-0032-X.

"This work stands out as an imminently accessible resource for the general public. It is recommended for the reference and circulating shelves of school, public, and academic libraries."
— *American Reference Books Annual, 2001*

"Recommended reference source."
— *Booklist, American Library Association, Dec '00*

"Provides comprehensive coverage of matters related to the heart. This title is recommended for health sciences and public libraries with consumer health collections."
— *E-Streams, Oct '00*

SEE ALSO Healthy Heart Sourcebook for Women

■

Caregiving Sourcebook

Basic Consumer Health Information for Caregivers, Including a Profile of Caregivers, Caregiving Responsibilities and Concerns, Tips for Specific Conditions, Care Environments, and the Effects of Caregiving

Along with Facts about Legal Issues, Financial Information, and Future Planning, a Glossary, and a Listing of Additional Resources

Edited by Joyce Brennfleck Shannon. 600 pages. 2001. 0-7808-0331-0.

"Essential for most collections."
— *Library Journal, Apr 1, 2002*

"An ideal addition to the reference collection of any public library. Health sciences information professionals may also want to acquire the *Caregiving Source-*

659

book for their hospital or academic library for use as a ready reference tool by health care workers interested in aging and caregiving." —*E-Streams, Jan '02*

"Recommended reference source."
—*Booklist, American Library Association, Oct '01*

■

Child Abuse Sourcebook

Basic Consumer Health Information about the Physical, Sexual, and Emotional Abuse of Children, with Additional Facts about Neglect, Munchausen Syndrome by Proxy (MSBP), Shaken Baby Syndrome, and Controversial Issues Related to Child Abuse, Such as Withholding Medical Care, Corporal Punishment, and Child Maltreatment in Youth Sports, and Featuring Facts about Child Protective Services, Foster Care, Adoption, Parenting Challenges, and Other Abuse Prevention Efforts

Along with a Glossary of Related Terms and Resources for Additional Help and Information

Edited by Dawn D. Matthews. 620 pages. 2004. 0-7808-0705-7.

■

Childhood Diseases & Disorders Sourcebook

Basic Consumer Health Information about Medical Problems Often Encountered in Pre-Adolescent Children, Including Respiratory Tract Ailments, Ear Infections, Sore Throats, Disorders of the Skin and Scalp, Digestive and Genitourinary Diseases, Infectious Diseases, Inflammatory Disorders, Chronic Physical and Developmental Disorders, Allergies, and More

Along with Information about Diagnostic Tests, Common Childhood Surgeries, and Frequently Used Medications, with a Glossary of Important Terms and Resource Directory

Edited by Chad T. Kimball. 662 pages. 2003. 0-7808-0458-9.

"This is an excellent book for new parents and should be included in all health care and public libraries."
—*American Reference Books Annual, 2004*

■

Colds, Flu & Other Common Ailments Sourcebook

Basic Consumer Health Information about Common Ailments and Injuries, Including Colds, Coughs, the Flu, Sinus Problems, Headaches, Fever, Nausea and Vomiting, Menstrual Cramps, Diarrhea, Constipation, Hemorrhoids, Back Pain, Dandruff, Dry and Itchy Skin, Cuts, Scrapes, Sprains, Bruises, and More

Along with Information about Prevention, Self-Care, Choosing a Doctor, Over-the-Counter Medications, Folk Remedies, and Alternative Therapies, and Including a Glossary of Important Terms and a Directory of Resources for Further Help and Information

Edited by Chad T. Kimball. 638 pages. 2001. 0-7808-0435-X.

"A good starting point for research on common illnesses. It will be a useful addition to public and consumer health library collections."
—*American Reference Books Annual 2002*

"Will prove valuable to any library seeking to maintain a current, comprehensive reference collection of health resources. . . . Excellent reference."
—*The Bookwatch, Aug '01*

"Recommended reference source."
—*Booklist, American Library Association, July '01*

■

Communication Disorders Sourcebook

Basic Information about Deafness and Hearing Loss, Speech and Language Disorders, Voice Disorders, Balance and Vestibular Disorders, and Disorders of Smell, Taste, and Touch

Edited by Linda M. Ross. 533 pages. 1996. 0-7808-0077-X.

"This is skillfully edited and is a welcome resource for the layperson. It should be found in every public and medical library." —*Booklist Health Sciences Supplement, American Library Association, Oct '97*

■

Congenital Disorders Sourcebook

Basic Information about Disorders Acquired during Gestation, Including Spina Bifida, Hydrocephalus, Cerebral Palsy, Heart Defects, Craniofacial Abnormalities, Fetal Alcohol Syndrome, and More

Along with Current Treatment Options and Statistical Data

Edited by Karen Bellenir. 607 pages. 1997. 0-7808-0205-5.

"Recommended reference source."
—*Booklist, American Library Association, Oct '97*

SEE ALSO Pregnancy & Birth Sourcebook

■

Consumer Issues in Health Care Sourcebook

Basic Information about Health Care Fundamentals and Related Consumer Issues, Including Exams and Screening Tests, Physician Specialties, Choosing a Doctor, Using Prescription and Over-the-Counter Medications Safely, Avoiding Health Scams, Managing Common Health Risks in the Home, Care Options for Chronically or Terminally Ill Patients, and a List of Resources for Obtaining Help and Further Information

Edited by Karen Bellenir. 618 pages. 1998. 0-7808-0221-7.

"Both public and academic libraries will want to have a copy in their collection for readers who are interested in self-education on health issues."
—*American Reference Books Annual, 2000*

"The editor has researched the literature from government agencies and others, saving readers the time and effort of having to do the research themselves. Recommended for public libraries."
— *Reference and User Services Quarterly, American Library Association, Spring '99*

"Recommended reference source."
— *Booklist, American Library Association, Dec '98*

■

Contagious Diseases Sourcebook

Basic Consumer Health Information about Infectious Diseases Spread by Person-to-Person Contact through Direct Touch, Airborne Transmission, Sexual Contact, or Contact with Blood or Other Body Fluids, Including Hepatitis, Herpes, Influenza, Lice, Measles, Mumps, Pinworm, Ringworm, Severe Acute Respiratory Syndrome (SARS), Streptococcal Infections, Tuberculosis, and Others

Along with Facts about Disease Transmission, Antimicrobial Resistance, and Vaccines, with a Glossary and Directories of Resources for More Information

Edited by Karen Bellenir. 643 pages. 2004. 0-7808-0736-7.

■

Contagious & Non-Contagious Infectious Diseases Sourcebook

Basic Information about Contagious Diseases like Measles, Polio, Hepatitis B, and Infectious Mononucleosis, and Non-Contagious Infectious Diseases like Tetanus and Toxic Shock Syndrome, and Diseases Occurring as Secondary Infections Such as Shingles and Reye Syndrome

Along with Vaccination, Prevention, and Treatment Information, and a Section Describing Emerging Infectious Disease Threats

Edited by Karen Bellenir and Peter D. Dresser. 566 pages. 1996. 0-7808-0075-3.

■

Death & Dying Sourcebook

Basic Consumer Health Information for the Layperson about End-of-Life Care and Related Ethical and Legal Issues, Including Chief Causes of Death, Autopsies, Pain Management for the Terminally Ill, Life Support Systems, Insurance, Euthanasia, Assisted Suicide, Hospice Programs, Living Wills, Funeral Planning, Counseling, Mourning, Organ Donation, and Physician Training

Along with Statistical Data, a Glossary, and Listings of Sources for Further Help and Information

Edited by Annemarie S. Muth. 641 pages. 1999. 0-7808-0230-6.

"Public libraries, medical libraries, and academic libraries will all find this sourcebook a useful addition to their collections."
— *American Reference Books Annual, 2001*

"An extremely useful resource for those concerned with death and dying in the United States."
— *Respiratory Care, Nov '00*

"Recommended reference source."
— *Booklist, American Library Association, Aug '00*

"This book is a definite must for all those involved in end-of-life care." — *Doody's Review Service, 2000*

■

Dental Care & Oral Health Sourcebook, 2nd Edition

Basic Consumer Health Information about Dental Care, Including Oral Hygiene, Dental Visits, Pain Management, Cavities, Crowns, Bridges, Dental Implants, and Fillings, and Other Oral Health Concerns, Such as Gum Disease, Bad Breath, Dry Mouth, Genetic and Developmental Abnormalities, Oral Cancers, Orthodontics, and Temporomandibular Disorders

Along with Updates on Current Research in Oral Health, a Glossary, a Directory of Dental and Oral Health Organizations, and Resources for People with Dental and Oral Health Disorders

Edited by Amy L. Sutton. 609 pages. 2003. 0-7808-0634-4.

ALSO AVAILABLE: *Oral Health Sourcebook, 1st Edition.* Edited by Allan R. Cook. 558 pages. 1997. 0-7808-0082-6.

"This book could serve as a turning point in the battle to educate consumers in issues concerning oral health."
— *American Reference Books Annual, 2004*

"Unique source which will fill a gap in dental sources for patients and the lay public. A valuable reference tool even in a library with thousands of books on dentistry. Comprehensive, clear, inexpensive, and easy to read and use. It fills an enormous gap in the health care literature." — *Reference and User Services Quarterly, American Library Association, Summer '98*

"Recommended reference source."
— *Booklist, American Library Association, Dec '97*

■

Depression Sourcebook

Basic Consumer Health Information about Unipolar Depression, Bipolar Disorder, Postpartum Depression, Seasonal Affective Disorder, and Other Types of Depression in Children, Adolescents, Women, Men, the Elderly, and Other Selected Populations

Along with Facts about Causes, Risk Factors, Diagnostic Criteria, Treatment Options, Coping Strategies, Suicide Prevention, a Glossary, and a Directory of Sources for Additional Help and Information

Edited by Karen Belleni. 602 pages. 2002. 0-7808-0611-5.

"*Depression Sourcebook* is of a very high standard. Its purpose, which is to serve as a reference source to the lay reader, is very well served."
— *Journal of the National Medical Association, 2004*

"Invaluable reference for public and school library collections alike." — *Library Bookwatch, Apr '03*

"Recommended for purchase."
— *American Reference Books Annual, 2003*

Dermatological Disorders Sourcebook, 2nd Edition

Basic Consumer Health Information about Conditions and Disorders Affecting the Skin, Hair, and Nails, Such as Acne, Rosacea, Rashes, Dermatitis, Pigmentation Disorders, Birthmarks, Skin Cancer, Skin Injuries, Psoriasis, Scleroderma, and Hair Loss, Including Facts about Medications and Treatments for Dermatological Disorders and Tips for Maintaining Healthy Skin, Hair, and Nails

Along with Information about How Aging Affects the Skin, a Glossary of Related Terms, and a Directory of Resources for Additional Help and Information

Edited by Amy L. Sutton. 645 pages. 2005. 0-7808-0795-2.

ALSO AVAILABLE: *Skin Disorders Sourcebook, 1st Edition.* Edited by Allan R. Cook. 647 pages. 1997. 0-7808-0080-X.

". . . comprehensive, easily read reference book."
— *Doody's Health Sciences Book Reviews, Oct '97*

∎

Diabetes Sourcebook, 3rd Edition

Basic Consumer Health Information about Type 1 Diabetes (Insulin-Dependent or Juvenile-Onset Diabetes), Type 2 Diabetes (Noninsulin-Dependent or Adult-Onset Diabetes), Gestational Diabetes, Impaired Glucose Tolerance (IGT), and Related Complications, Such as Amputation, Eye Disease, Gum Disease, Nerve Damage, and End-Stage Renal Disease, Including Facts about Insulin, Oral Diabetes Medications, Blood Sugar Testing, and the Role of Exercise and Nutrition in the Control of Diabetes

Along with a Glossary and Resources for Further Help and Information

Edited by Dawn D. Matthews. 622 pages. 2003. 0-7808-0629-8.

ALSO AVAILABLE: *Diabetes Sourcebook, 1st Edition.* Edited by Karen Bellenir and Peter D. Dresser. 827 pages. 1994. 1-55888-751-2.

Diabetes Sourcebook, 2nd Edition. Edited by Karen Bellenir. 688 pages. 1998. 0-7808-0224-1.

"This edition is even more helpful than earlier versions. . . . It is a truly valuable tool for anyone seeking readable and authoritative information on diabetes."
— *American Reference Books Annual, 2004*

"An invaluable reference." — *Library Journal, May '00*

Selected as one of the 250 "Best Health Sciences Books of 1999." — *Doody's Rating Service, Mar-Apr 2000*

"Provides useful information for the general public."
— *Healthlines, University of Michigan Health Management Research Center, Sep/Oct '99*

". . . provides reliable mainstream medical information . . . belongs on the shelves of any library with a consumer health collection." — *E-Streams, Sep '99*

"Recommended reference source."
— *Booklist, American Library Association, Feb '99*

Diet & Nutrition Sourcebook, 2nd Edition

Basic Consumer Health Information about Dietary Guidelines, Recommended Daily Intake Values, Vitamins, Minerals, Fiber, Fat, Weight Control, Dietary Supplements, and Food Additives

Along with Special Sections on Nutrition Needs throughout Life and Nutrition for People with Such Specific Medical Concerns as Allergies, High Blood Cholesterol, Hypertension, Diabetes, Celiac Disease, Seizure Disorders, Phenylketonuria (PKU), Cancer, and Eating Disorders, and Including Reports on Current Nutrition Research and Source Listings for Additional Help and Information

Edited by Karen Bellenir. 650 pages. 1999. 0-7808-0228-4.

ALSO AVAILABLE: *Diet & Nutrition Sourcebook, 1st Edition.* Edited by Dan R. Harris. 662 pages. 1996. 0-7808-0084-2.

"This book is an excellent source of basic diet and nutrition information." — *Booklist Health Sciences Supplement, American Library Association, Dec '00*

"This reference document should be in any public library, but it would be a very good guide for beginning students in the health sciences. If the other books in this publisher's series are as good as this, they should all be in the health sciences collections."
— *American Reference Books Annual, 2000*

"This book is an excellent general nutrition reference for consumers who desire to take an active role in their health care for prevention. Consumers of all ages who select this book can feel confident they are receiving current and accurate information." — *Journal of Nutrition for the Elderly, Vol. 19, No. 4, '00*

"Recommended reference source."
— *Booklist, American Library Association, Dec '99*

SEE ALSO *Digestive Diseases & Disorders Sourcebook, Eating Disorders Sourcebook, Gastrointestinal Diseases & Disorders Sourcebook, Vegetarian Sourcebook*

∎

Digestive Diseases & Disorders Sourcebook

Basic Consumer Health Information about Diseases and Disorders that Impact the Upper and Lower Digestive System, Including Celiac Disease, Constipation, Crohn's Disease, Cyclic Vomiting Syndrome, Diarrhea, Diverticulosis and Diverticulitis, Gallstones, Heartburn, Hemorrhoids, Hernias, Indigestion (Dyspepsia), Irritable Bowel Syndrome, Lactose Intolerance, Ulcers, and More

Along with Information about Medications and Other Treatments, Tips for Maintaining a Healthy Digestive Tract, a Glossary, and Directory of Digestive Diseases Organizations

Edited by Karen Bellenir. 335 pages. 2000. 0-7808-0327-2.

"This title would be an excellent addition to all public or patient-research libraries."
— *American Reference Books Annual, 2001*

"This title is recommended for public, hospital, and health sciences libraries with consumer health collections."   — E-Streams, Jul-Aug '00

"Recommended reference source."
— Booklist, American Library Association, May '00

SEE ALSO Diet & Nutrition Sourcebook, Eating Disorders Sourcebook, Gastrointestinal Diseases & Disorders Sourcebook

■

Disabilities Sourcebook

Basic Consumer Health Information about Physical and Psychiatric Disabilities, Including Descriptions of Major Causes of Disability, Assistive and Adaptive Aids, Workplace Issues, and Accessibility Concerns

Along with Information about the Americans with Disabilities Act, a Glossary, and Resources for Additional Help and Information

Edited by Dawn D. Matthews. 616 pages. 2000. 0-7808-0389-2.

"It is a must for libraries with a consumer health section."   — American Reference Books Annual 2002

"A much needed addition to the Omnigraphics Health Reference Series. A current reference work to provide people with disabilities, their families, caregivers or those who work with them, a broad range of information in one volume, has not been available until now. . . . It is recommended for all public and academic library reference collections."   — E-Streams, May '01

"An excellent source book in easy-to-read format covering many current topics; highly recommended for all libraries."   — Choice, Association of College and Research Libraries, Jan '01

"Recommended reference source."
— Booklist, American Library Association, Jul '00

■

Domestic Violence Sourcebook, 2nd Edition

Basic Consumer Health Information about the Causes and Consequences of Abusive Relationships, Including Physical Violence, Sexual Assault, Battery, Stalking, and Emotional Abuse, and Facts about the Effects of Violence on Women, Men, Young Adults, and the Elderly, with Reports about Domestic Violence in Selected Populations, and Featuring Facts about Medical Care, Victim Assistance and Protection, Prevention Strategies, Mental Health Services, and Legal Issues

Along with a Glossary of Related Terms and Resources for Additional Help and Information

Edited by Dawn D. Matthews. 628 pages. 2004. 0-7808-0669-7.

ALSO AVAILABLE: Domestic Violence & Child Abuse Sourcebook, 1st Edition. Edited by Helene Henderson. 1,064 pages. 2001. 0-7808-0235-7.

"Interested lay persons should find the book extremely beneficial. . . . A copy of Domestic Violence and Child

Abuse Sourcebook should be in every public library in the United States."
— Social Science & Medicine, No. 56, 2003

"This is important information. The Web has many resources but this sourcebook fills an important societal need. I am not aware of any other resources of this type."   — Doody's Review Service, Sep '01

"Recommended for all libraries, scholars, and practitioners."   — Choice, Association of College & Research Libraries, Jul '01

"Recommended reference source."
— Booklist, American Library Association, Apr '01

"Important pick for college-level health reference libraries."   — The Bookwatch, Mar '01

"Because this problem is so widespread and because this book includes a lot of issues within one volume, this work is recommended for all public libraries."
— American Reference Books Annual, 2001

■

Drug Abuse Sourcebook, 2nd Edition

Basic Consumer Health Information about Illicit Substances of Abuse and the Misuse of Prescription and Over-the-Counter Medications, Including Depressants, Hallucinogens, Inhalants, Marijuana, Stimulants, and Anabolic Steroids

Along with Facts about Related Health Risks, Treatment Programs, Prevention Programs, a Glossary of Abuse and Addiction Terms, a Glossary of Drug-Related Street Terms, and a Directory of Resources for More Information

Edited by Catherine Ginther. 607 pages. 2004. 0-7808-0740-5.

ALSO AVAILABLE: Drug Abuse Sourcebook, 1st Edition. Edited by Karen Bellenir. 629 pages. 2000. 0-7808-0242-X.

"Containing a wealth of information . . . . This resource belongs in libraries that serve a lower-division undergraduate or community college clientele as well as the general public."   — Choice, Association of College and Research Libraries, Jun '01

"Recommended reference source."
— Booklist, American Library Association, Feb '01

"Highly recommended."   — The Bookwatch, Jan '01

"Even though there is a plethora of books on drug abuse, this volume is recommended for school, public, and college libraries."
— American Reference Books Annual, 2001

SEE ALSO Alcoholism Sourcebook, Substance Abuse Sourcebook

Ear, Nose & Throat Disorders Sourcebook

Basic Information about Disorders of the Ears, Nose, Sinus Cavities, Pharynx, and Larynx, Including Ear Infections, Tinnitus, Vestibular Disorders, Allergic and Non-Allergic Rhinitis, Sore Throats, Tonsillitis, and Cancers That Affect the Ears, Nose, Sinuses, and Throat

Along with Reports on Current Research Initiatives, a Glossary of Related Medical Terms, and a Directory of Sources for Further Help and Information

Edited by Karen Bellenir and Linda M. Shin. 576 pages. 1998. 0-7808-0206-3.

"Overall, this sourcebook is helpful for the consumer seeking information on ENT issues. It is recommended for public libraries."
—American Reference Books Annual, 1999

"Recommended reference source."
—Booklist, American Library Association, Dec '98

■

Eating Disorders Sourcebook

Basic Consumer Health Information about Eating Disorders, Including Information about Anorexia Nervosa, Bulimia Nervosa, Binge Eating, Body Dysmorphic Disorder, Pica, Laxative Abuse, and Night Eating Syndrome

Along with Information about Causes, Adverse Effects, and Treatment and Prevention Issues, and Featuring a Section on Concerns Specific to Children and Adolescents, a Glossary, and Resources for Further Help and Information

Edited by Dawn D. Matthews. 322 pages. 2001. 0-7808-0335-3.

"Recommended for health science libraries that are open to the public, as well as hospital libraries. This book is a good resource for the consumer who is concerned about eating disorders." *— E-Streams, Mar '02*

"This volume is another convenient collection of excerpted articles. Recommended for school and public library patrons; lower-division undergraduates; and two-year technical program students." *— Choice, Association of College & Research Libraries, Jan '02*

"Recommended reference source." *— Booklist, American Library Association, Oct '01*

SEE ALSO *Diet & Nutrition Sourcebook, Digestive Diseases & Disorders Sourcebook, Gastrointestinal Diseases & Disorders Sourcebook*

■

Emergency Medical Services Sourcebook

Basic Consumer Health Information about Preventing, Preparing for, and Managing Emergency Situations, When and Who to Call for Help, What to Expect in the Emergency Room, the Emergency Medical Team, Patient Issues, and Current Topics in Emergency Medicine

Along with Statistical Data, a Glossary, and Sources of Additional Help and Information

Edited by Jenni Lynn Colson. 494 pages. 2002. 0-7808-0420-1.

"Handy and convenient for home, public, school, and college libraries. Recommended."
— Choice, Association of College and Research Libraries, Apr '03

"This reference can provide the consumer with answers to most questions about emergency care in the United States, or it will direct them to a resource where the answer can be found."
—American Reference Books Annual, 2003

"Recommended reference source."
— Booklist, American Library Association, Feb '03

■

Endocrine & Metabolic Disorders Sourcebook

Basic Information for the Layperson about Pancreatic and Insulin-Related Disorders Such as Pancreatitis, Diabetes, and Hypoglycemia; Adrenal Gland Disorders Such as Cushing's Syndrome, Addison's Disease, and Congenital Adrenal Hyperplasia; Pituitary Gland Disorders Such as Growth Hormone Deficiency, Acromegaly, and Pituitary Tumors; Thyroid Disorders Such as Hypothyroidism, Graves' Disease, Hashimoto's Disease, and Goiter; Hyperparathyroidism; and Other Diseases and Syndromes of Hormone Imbalance or Metabolic Dysfunction

Along with Reports on Current Research Initiatives

Edited by Linda M. Shin. 574 pages. 1998. 0-7808-0207-1.

"Omnigraphics has produced another needed resource for health information consumers."
—American Reference Books Annual, 2000

"Recommended reference source."
— Booklist, American Library Association, Dec '98

■

Environmental Health Sourcebook, 2nd Edition

Basic Consumer Health Information about the Environment and Its Effect on Human Health, Including the Effects of Air Pollution, Water Pollution, Hazardous Chemicals, Food Hazards, Radiation Hazards, Biological Agents, Household Hazards, Such as Radon, Asbestos, Carbon Monoxide, and Mold, and Information about Associated Diseases and Disorders, Including Cancer, Allergies, Respiratory Problems, and Skin Disorders

Along with Information about Environmental Concerns for Specific Populations, a Glossary of Related Terms, and Resources for Further Help and Information

Edited by Dawn D. Matthews. 673 pages. 2003. 0-7808-0632-8.

ALSO AVAILABLE: *Environmentally Induced Disorders Sourcebook, 1st Edition.* Edited by Allan R. Cook. 620 pages. 1997. 0-7808-0083-4.

"This recently updated edition continues the level of quality and the reputation of the numerous other volumes in Omnigraphics' *Health Reference Series.*"
— *American Reference Books Annual, 2004*

"Recommended reference source."
— *Booklist, American Library Association, Sep '98*

"This book will be a useful addition to anyone's library." — *Choice Health Sciences Supplement, Association of College and Research Libraries, May '98*

". . . a good survey of numerous environmentally induced physical disorders . . . a useful addition to anyone's library."
— *Doody's Health Sciences Book Reviews, Jan '98*

". . . provide[s] introductory information from the best authorities around. Since this volume covers topics that potentially affect everyone, it will surely be one of the most frequently consulted volumes in the *Health Reference Series.*" — *Rettig on Reference, Nov '97*

■

Environmentally Induced Disorders Sourcebook, 1st Edition

SEE *Environmental Health Sourcebook, 2nd Edition*

■

Ethnic Diseases Sourcebook

Basic Consumer Health Information for Ethnic and Racial Minority Groups in the United States, Including General Health Indicators and Behaviors, Ethnic Diseases, Genetic Testing, the Impact of Chronic Diseases, Women's Health, Mental Health Issues, and Preventive Health Care Services

Along with a Glossary and a Listing of Additional Resources

Edited by Joyce Brennfleck Shannon. 664 pages. 2001. 0-7808-0336-1.

"Recommended for health sciences libraries where public health programs are a priority."
— *E-Streams, Jan '02*

"Not many books have been written on this topic to date, and the *Ethnic Diseases Sourcebook* is a strong addition to the list. It will be an important introductory resource for health consumers, students, health care personnel, and social scientists. It is recommended for public, academic, and large hospital libraries."
— *American Reference Books Annual 2002*

"Recommended reference source."
— *Booklist, American Library Association, Oct '01*

"Will prove valuable to any library seeking to maintain a current, comprehensive reference collection of health resources. . . . An excellent source of health information about genetic disorders which affect particular ethnic and racial minorities in the U.S."
— *The Bookwatch, Aug '01*

Eye Care Sourcebook, 2nd Edition

Basic Consumer Health Information about Eye Care and Eye Disorders, Including Facts about the Diagnosis, Prevention, and Treatment of Common Refractive Problems Such as Myopia, Hyperopia, Astigmatism, and Presbyopia, and Eye Diseases, Including Glaucoma, Cataract, Age-Related Macular Degeneration, and Diabetic Retinopathy

Along with a Section on Vision Correction and Refractive Surgeries, Including LASIK and LASEK, a Glossary, and Directories of Resources for Additional Help and Information

Edited by Amy L. Sutton. 543 pages. 2003. 0-7808-0635-2.

ALSO AVAILABLE: Ophthalmic Disorders Sourcebook, 1st Edition. Edited by Linda M. Ross. 631 pages. 1996. 0-7808-0081-8.

". . . a solid reference tool for eye care and a valuable addition to a collection."
— *American Reference Books Annual, 2004*

■

Family Planning Sourcebook

Basic Consumer Health Information about Planning for Pregnancy and Contraception, Including Traditional Methods, Barrier Methods, Hormonal Methods, Permanent Methods, Future Methods, Emergency Contraception, and Birth Control Choices for Women at Each Stage of Life

Along with Statistics, a Glossary, and Sources of Additional Information

Edited by Amy Marcaccio Keyzer. 520 pages. 2001. 0-7808-0379-5.

"Recommended for public, health, and undergraduate libraries as part of the circulating collection."
— *E-Streams, Mar '02*

"Information is presented in an unbiased, readable manner, and the sourcebook will certainly be a necessary addition to those public and high school libraries where Internet access is restricted or otherwise problematic." — *American Reference Books Annual 2002*

"Recommended reference source."
— *Booklist, American Library Association, Oct '01*

"Will prove valuable to any library seeking to maintain a current, comprehensive reference collection of health resources. . . . Excellent reference."
— *The Bookwatch, Aug '01*

SEE ALSO *Pregnancy & Birth Sourcebook*

■

Fitness & Exercise Sourcebook, 2nd Edition

Basic Consumer Health Information about the Fundamentals of Fitness and Exercise, Including How to Begin and Maintain a Fitness Program, Fitness as a Lifestyle, the Link between Fitness and Diet, Advice for Specific Groups of People, Exercise as It Relates to Specific Medical Conditions, and Recent Research in Fitness and Exercise

Along with a Glossary of Important Terms and Resources for Additional Help and Information

Edited by Kristen M. Gledhill. 646 pages. 2001. 0-7808-0334-5.

ALSO AVAILABLE: Fitness & Exercise Sourcebook, 1st Edition. Edited by Dan R. Harris. 663 pages. 1996. 0-7808-0186-5.

"This work is recommended for all general reference collections."
— American Reference Books Annual 2002

"Highly recommended for public, consumer, and school grades fourth through college."
—E-Streams, Nov '01

"Recommended reference source."   — Booklist, American Library Association, Oct '01

"The information appears quite comprehensive and is considered reliable. . . . This second edition is a welcomed addition to the series."
—Doody's Review Service, Sep '01

"This reference is a valuable choice for those who desire a broad source of information on exercise, fitness, and chronic-disease prevention through a healthy lifestyle."   —American Medical Writers Association Journal, Fall '01

"Will prove valuable to any library seeking to maintain a current, comprehensive reference collection of health resources. . . . Excellent reference."
— The Bookwatch, Aug '01

■

Food & Animal Borne Diseases Sourcebook

Basic Information about Diseases That Can Be Spread to Humans through the Ingestion of Contaminated Food or Water or by Contact with Infected Animals and Insects, Such as Botulism, E. Coli, Hepatitis A, Trichinosis, Lyme Disease, and Rabies

Along with Information Regarding Prevention and Treatment Methods, and Including a Special Section for International Travelers Describing Diseases Such as Cholera, Malaria, Travelers' Diarrhea, and Yellow Fever, and Offering Recommendations for Avoiding Illness

Edited by Karen Bellenir and Peter D. Dresser. 535 pages. 1995. 0-7808-0033-8.

"Targeting general readers and providing them with a single, comprehensive source of information on selected topics, this book continues, with the excellent caliber of its predecessors, to catalog topical information on health matters of general interest. Readable and thorough, this valuable resource is highly recommended for all libraries."
— Academic Library Book Review, Summer '96

"A comprehensive collection of authoritative information."   — Emergency Medical Services, Oct '95

Food Safety Sourcebook

Basic Consumer Health Information about the Safe Handling of Meat, Poultry, Seafood, Eggs, Fruit Juices, and Other Food Items, and Facts about Pesticides, Drinking Water, Food Safety Overseas, and the Onset, Duration, and Symptoms of Foodborne Illnesses, Including Types of Pathogenic Bacteria, Parasitic Protozoa, Worms, Viruses, and Natural Toxins

Along with the Role of the Consumer, the Food Handler, and the Government in Food Safety; a Glossary, and Resources for Additional Help and Information

Edited by Dawn D. Matthews. 339 pages. 1999. 0-7808-0326-4.

"This book is recommended for public libraries and universities with home economic and food science programs."   —E-Streams, Nov '00

"Recommended reference source."
—Booklist, American Library Association, May '00

"This book takes the complex issues of food safety and foodborne pathogens and presents them in an easily understood manner. [It does] an excellent job of covering a large and often confusing topic."
—American Reference Books Annual, 2000

■

Forensic Medicine Sourcebook

Basic Consumer Information for the Layperson about Forensic Medicine, Including Crime Scene Investigation, Evidence Collection and Analysis, Expert Testimony, Computer-Aided Criminal Identification, Digital Imaging in the Courtroom, DNA Profiling, Accident Reconstruction, Autopsies, Ballistics, Drugs and Explosives Detection, Latent Fingerprints, Product Tampering, and Questioned Document Examination

Along with Statistical Data, a Glossary of Forensics Terminology, and Listings of Sources for Further Help and Information

Edited by Annemarie S. Muth. 574 pages. 1999. 0-7808-0232-2.

"Given the expected widespread interest in its content and its easy to read style, this book is recommended for most public and all college and university libraries."
— E-Streams, Feb '01

"Recommended for public libraries."
—Reference & User Services Quarterly, American Library Association, Spring 2000

"Recommended reference source."
—Booklist, American Library Association, Feb '00

"A wealth of information, useful statistics, references are up-to-date and extremely complete. This wonderful collection of data will help students who are interested in a career in any type of forensic field. It is a great resource for attorneys who need information about types of expert witnesses needed in a particular case. It also offers useful information for fiction and nonfiction writers whose work involves a crime. A fascinating compilation. All levels."   — Choice, Association of College and Research Libraries, Jan 2000

■

Gastrointestinal Diseases & Disorders Sourcebook, 2nd Edition

Basic Consumer Health Information about the Upper and Lower Gastrointestinal (GI) Tract, Including the Esophagus, Stomach, Intestines, Rectum, Liver, and Pancreas, with Facts about Gastroesophageal Reflux Disease, Gastritis, Hernias, Ulcers, Celiac Disease, Diverticulitis, Irritable Bowel Syndrome, Hemorrhoids, Gastrointestinal Cancers, and Other Diseases and Disorders Related to the Digestive Process

Along with Information about Commonly Used Diagnostic and Surgical Procedures, Statistics, Reports on Current Research Initiatives and Clinical Trials, a Glossary, and Resources for Additional Help and Information

Edited by Sandra J. Judd. 682 pages. 2006. 0-7808-0798-7.

ALSO AVAILABLE: Gastrointestinal Diseases & Disorders Sourcebook, 1st Edition. Edited by Linda M. Ross. 413 pages. 1996. 0-7808-0078-8.

SEE ALSO *Diet & Nutrition Sourcebook, Digestive Diseases & Disorders, Eating Disorders Sourcebook*

■

Genetic Disorders Sourcebook, 3rd Edition

Basic Consumer Health Information about Hereditary Diseases and Disorders, Including Facts about the Human Genome, Genetic Inheritance Patterns, Disorders Associated with Specific Genes, Such as Sickle Cell Disease, Hemophilia, and Cystic Fibrosis, Chromosome Disorders, Such as Down Syndrome, Fragile X Syndrome, and Turner Syndrome, and Complex Diseases and Disorders Resulting from the Interaction of Environmental and Genetic Factors, Such as Allergies, Cancer, and Obesity

Along with Facts about Genetic Testing, Suggestions for Parents of Children with Special Needs, Reports on Current Research Initiatives, a Glossary of Genetic Terminology, and Resources for Additional Help and Information

Edited by Karen Bellenir. 777 pages. 2004. 0-7808-0742-1.

ALSO AVAILABLE: Genetic Disorders Sourcebook, 1st Edition. Edited by Karen Bellenir. 642 pages. 1996. 0-7808-0034-6.

Genetic Disorders Sourcebook, 2nd Edition. Edited by Kathy Massimini. 768 pages. 2001. 0-7808-0241-1.

■

Head Trauma Sourcebook

Basic Information for the Layperson about Open-Head and Closed-Head Injuries, Treatment Advances, Recovery, and Rehabilitation

Along with Reports on Current Research Initiatives

Edited by Karen Bellenir. 414 pages. 1997. 0-7808-0208-X.

■

Headache Sourcebook

Basic Consumer Health Information about Migraine, Tension, Cluster, Rebound and Other Types of Headaches, with Facts about the Cause and Prevention of Headaches, the Effects of Stress and the Environment, Headaches during Pregnancy and Menopause, and Childhood Headaches

Along with a Glossary and Other Resources for Additional Help and Information

Edited by Dawn D. Matthews. 362 pages. 2002. 0-7808-0337-X.

■

Health Insurance Sourcebook

Basic Information about Managed Care Organizations, Traditional Fee-for-Service Insurance, Insurance Portability and Pre-Existing Conditions Clauses, Medicare, Medicaid, Social Security, and Military Health Care

Along with Information about Insurance Fraud

Edited by Wendy Wilcox. 530 pages. 1997. 0-7808-0222-5.

Health Reference Series Cumulative Index 1999

A Comprehensive Index to the Individual Volumes of the Health Reference Series, Including a Subject Index, Name Index, Organization Index, and Publication Index

Along with a Master List of Acronyms and Abbreviations

Edited by Edward J. Prucha, Anne Holmes, and Robert Rudnick. 990 pages. 2000. 0-7808-0382-5.

"This volume will be most helpful in libraries that have a relatively complete collection of the Health Reference Series." —*American Reference Books Annual, 2001*

"Essential for collections that hold any of the numerous *Health Reference Series* titles."
— *Choice, Association of College and Research Libraries, Nov '00*

■

Healthy Aging Sourcebook

Basic Consumer Health Information about Maintaining Health through the Aging Process, Including Advice on Nutrition, Exercise, and Sleep, Help in Making Decisions about Midlife Issues and Retirement, and Guidance Concerning Practical and Informed Choices in Health Consumerism

Along with Data Concerning the Theories of Aging, Different Experiences in Aging by Minority Groups, and Facts about Aging Now and Aging in the Future; and Featuring a Glossary, a Guide to Consumer Help, Additional Suggested Reading, and Practical Resource Directory

Edited by Jenifer Swanson. 536 pages. 1999. 0-7808-0390-6.

"Recommended reference source."
—*Booklist, American Library Association, Feb '00*

SEE ALSO *Physical & Mental Issues in Aging Sourcebook*

■

Healthy Children Sourcebook

Basic Consumer Health Information about the Physical and Mental Development of Children between the Ages of 3 and 12, Including Routine Health Care, Preventative Health Services, Safety and First Aid, Healthy Sleep, Dental Care, Nutrition, and Fitness, and Featuring Parenting Tips on Such Topics as Bedwetting, Choosing Day Care, Monitoring TV and Other Media, and Establishing a Foundation for Substance Abuse Prevention

Along with a Glossary of Commonly Used Pediatric Terms and Resources for Additional Help and Information.

Edited by Chad T. Kimball. 647 pages. 2003. 0-7808-0247-0.

"It is hard to imagine that any other single resource exists that would provide such a comprehensive guide of timely information on health promotion and disease prevention for children aged 3 to 12."
— *American Reference Books Annual, 2004*

"The strengths of this book are many. It is clearly written, presented and structured."
— *Journal of the National Medical Association, 2004*

■

Healthy Heart Sourcebook for Women

Basic Consumer Health Information about Cardiac Issues Specific to Women, Including Facts about Major Risk Factors and Prevention, Treatment and Control Strategies, and Important Dietary Issues

Along with a Special Section Regarding the Pros and Cons of Hormone Replacement Therapy and Its Impact on Heart Health, and Additional Help, Including Recipes, a Glossary, and a Directory of Resources

Edited by Dawn D. Matthews. 336 pages. 2000. 0-7808-0329-9.

"A good reference source and recommended for all public, academic, medical, and hospital libraries."
— *Medical Reference Services Quarterly, Summer '01*

"Because of the lack of information specific to women on this topic, this book is recommended for public libraries and consumer libraries."
—*American Reference Books Annual, 2001*

"Contains very important information about coronary artery disease that all women should know. The information is current and presented in an easy-to-read format. The book will make a good addition to any library." — *American Medical Writers Association Journal, Summer '00*

"Important, basic reference."
— *Reviewer's Bookwatch, Jul '00*

SEE ALSO *Heart Diseases & Disorders Sourcebook, Women's Health Concerns Sourcebook*

■

Heart Diseases & Disorders Sourcebook, 2nd Edition

SEE *Cardiovascular Diseases & Disorders Sourcebook, 3rd Edition*

■

Hepatitis Sourcebook

Basic Consumer Health Information about Hepatitis A, Hepatitis B, Hepatitis C, and Other Forms of Hepatitis, Including Autoimmune Hepatitis, Alcoholic Hepatitis, Nonalcoholic Steatohepatitis, and Toxic Hepatitis, with Facts about Risk Factors, Screening Methods, Diagnostic Tests, and Treatment Options

Along with Information on Liver Health, Tips for People Living with Chronic Hepatitis, Reports on Current Research Initiatives, a Glossary of Terms Related to Hepatitis, and a Directory of Sources for Further Help and Information

Edited by Sandra J. Judd. 597 pages. 2005. 0-7808-0749-9.

Household Safety Sourcebook

Basic Consumer Health Information about Household Safety, Including Information about Poisons, Chemicals, Fire, and Water Hazards in the Home

Along with Advice about the Safe Use of Home Maintenance Equipment, Choosing Toys and Nursery Furniture, Holiday and Recreation Safety, a Glossary, and Resources for Further Help and Information

Edited by Dawn D. Matthews. 606 pages. 2002. 0-7808-0338-8.

"This work will be useful in public libraries with large consumer health and wellness departments."
— *American Reference Books Annual, 2003*

"As a sourcebook on household safety this book meets its mark. It is encyclopedic in scope and covers a wide range of safety issues that are commonly seen in the home." — *E-Streams, Jul '02*

Hypertension Sourcebook

Basic Consumer Health Information about the Causes, Diagnosis, and Treatment of High Blood Pressure, with Facts about Consequences, Complications, and Co-Occurring Disorders, Such as Coronary Heart Disease, Diabetes, Stroke, Kidney Disease, and Hypertensive Retinopathy, and Issues in Blood Pressure Control, Including Dietary Choices, Stress Management, and Medications

Along with Reports on Current Research Initiatives and Clinical Trials, a Glossary, and Resources for Additional Help and Information

Edited by Dawn D. Matthews and Karen Bellenir. 613 pages. 2004. 0-7808-0674-3.

Immune System Disorders Sourcebook, 2nd Edition

Basic Consumer Health Information about Disorders of the Immune System, Including Immune System Function and Response, Diagnosis of Immune Disorders, Information about Inherited Immune Disease, Acquired Immune Disease, and Autoimmune Diseases, Including Primary Immune Deficiency, Acquired Immunodeficiency Syndrome (AIDS), Lupus, Multiple Sclerosis, Type 1 Diabetes, Rheumatoid Arthritis, and Graves Disease

Along with Treatments, Tips for Coping with Immune Disorders, a Glossary, and a Directory of Additional Resources

Edited by Joyce Brennfleck Shannon. 671 pages. 2005. 0-7808-0748-0.

ALSO AVAILABLE: *Immune System Disorders Sourcebook. Edited by Allan R. Cook. 608 pages. 1997. 0-7808-0209-8.*

Infant & Toddler Health Sourcebook

Basic Consumer Health Information about the Physical and Mental Development of Newborns, Infants, and Toddlers, Including Neonatal Concerns, Nutrition Recommendations, Immunization Schedules, Common Pediatric Disorders, Assessments and Milestones, Safety Tips, and Advice for Parents and Other Caregivers

Along with a Glossary of Terms and Resource Listings for Additional Help

Edited by Jenifer Swanson. 585 pages. 2000. 0-7808-0246-2.

"As a reference for the general public, this would be useful in any library." — *E-Streams, May '01*

"Recommended reference source."
— *Booklist, American Library Association, Feb '01*

"This is a good source for general use."
— *American Reference Books Annual, 2001*

Infectious Diseases Sourcebook

Basic Consumer Health Information about Non-Contagious Bacterial, Viral, Prion, Fungal, and Parasitic Diseases Spread by Food and Water, Insects and Animals, or Environmental Contact, Including Botulism, E. Coli, Encephalitis, Legionnaires' Disease, Lyme Disease, Malaria, Plague, Rabies, Salmonella, Tetanus, and Others, and Facts about Newly Emerging Diseases, Such as Hantavirus, Mad Cow Disease, Monkeypox, and West Nile Virus

Along with Information about Preventing Disease Transmission, the Threat of Bioterrorism, and Current Research Initiatives, with a Glossary and Directory of Resources for More Information

Edited by Karen Bellenir. 634 pages. 2004. 0-7808-0675-1.

Injury & Trauma Sourcebook

Basic Consumer Health Information about the Impact of Injury, the Diagnosis and Treatment of Common and Traumatic Injuries, Emergency Care, and Specific Injuries Related to Home, Community, Workplace, Transportation, and Recreation

Along with Guidelines for Injury Prevention, a Glossary, and a Directory of Additional Resources

Edited by Joyce Brennfleck Shannon. 696 pages. 2002. 0-7808-0421-X.

"This publication is the most comprehensive work of its kind about injury and trauma."
— *American Reference Books Annual, 2003*

"This sourcebook provides concise, easily readable, basic health information about injuries. . . . This book is well organized and an easy to use reference resource suitable for hospital, health sciences and public libraries with consumer health collections."
— *E-Streams, Nov '02*

Kidney & Urinary Tract Diseases & Disorders Sourcebook, 1st Edition

SEE *Urinary Tract & Kidney Diseases & Disorders Sourcebook, 2nd Edition*

Learning Disabilities Sourcebook, 2nd Edition

Basic Consumer Health Information about Learning Disabilities, Including Dyslexia, Developmental Speech and Language Disabilities, Non-Verbal Learning Disorders, Developmental Arithmetic Disorder, Developmental Writing Disorder, and Other Conditions That Impede Learning Such as Attention Deficit/ Hyperactivity Disorder, Brain Injury, Hearing Impairment, Klinefelter Syndrome, Dyspraxia, and Tourette Syndrome

Along with Facts about Educational Issues and Assistive Technology, Coping Strategies, a Glossary of Related Terms, and Resources for Further Help and Information

Edited by Dawn D. Matthews. 621 pages. 2003. 0-7808-0626-3.

ALSO AVAILABLE: *Learning Disabilities Sourcebook, 1st Edition.* Edited by Linda M. Shin. 579 pages. 1998. 0-7808-0210-1.

Leukemia Sourcebook

Basic Consumer Health Information about Adult and Childhood Leukemias, Including Acute Lymphocytic Leukemia (ALL), Chronic Lymphocytic Leukemia (CLL), Acute Myelogenous Leukemia (AML), Chronic Myelogenous Leukemia (CML), and Hairy Cell Leukemia, and Treatments Such as Chemotherapy, Radiation Therapy, Peripheral Blood Stem Cell and Marrow Transplantation, and Immunotherapy

Along with Tips for Life During and After Treatment, a Glossary, and Directories of Additional Resources

Edited by Joyce Brennfleck Shannon. 587 pages. 2003. 0-7808-0627-1.

Liver Disorders Sourcebook

Basic Consumer Health Information about the Liver and How It Works; Liver Diseases, Including Cancer, Cirrhosis, Hepatitis, and Toxic and Drug Related Diseases; Tips for Maintaining a Healthy Liver; Laboratory Tests, Radiology Tests, and Facts about Liver Transplantation

Along with a Section on Support Groups, a Glossary, and Resource Listings

Edited by Joyce Brennfleck Shannon. 591 pages. 2000. 0-7808-0383-3.

Lung Disorders Sourcebook

Basic Consumer Health Information about Emphysema, Pneumonia, Tuberculosis, Asthma, Cystic Fibrosis, and Other Lung Disorders, Including Facts about Diagnostic Procedures, Treatment Strategies, Disease Prevention Efforts, and Such Risk Factors as Smoking, Air Pollution, and Exposure to Asbestos, Radon, and Other Agents

Along with a Glossary and Resources for Additional Help and Information

Edited by Dawn D. Matthews. 678 pages. 2002. 0-7808-0339-6.

"This title is a great addition for public and school libraries because it provides concise health information on the lungs."
— *American Reference Books Annual, 2003*

"Highly recommended for academic and medical reference collections."   — *Library Bookwatch, Sep '02*

Medical Tests Sourcebook, 2nd Edition

Basic Consumer Health Information about Medical Tests, Including Age-Specific Health Tests, Important Health Screenings and Exams, Home-Use Tests, Blood and Specimen Tests, Electrical Tests, Scope Tests, Genetic Testing, and Imaging Tests, Such as X-Rays, Ultrasound, Computed Tomography, Magnetic Resonance Imaging, Angiography, and Nuclear Medicine

Along with a Glossary and Directory of Additional Resources

Edited by Joyce Brennfleck Shannon. 654 pages. 2004. 0-7808-0670-0.

ALSO AVAILABLE: *Medical Tests, 1st Edition.* Edited by Joyce Brennfleck Shannon. 691 pages. 1999. 0-7808-0243-8.

"Recommended for hospital and health sciences libraries with consumer health collections."
— *E-Streams, Mar '00*

"This is an overall excellent reference with a wealth of general knowledge that may aid those who are reluctant to get vital tests performed."
— *Today's Librarian, Jan 2000*

"A valuable reference guide."
— *American Reference Books Annual, 2000*

Men's Health Concerns Sourcebook, 2nd Edition

Basic Consumer Health Information about the Medical and Mental Concerns of Men, Including Theories about the Shorter Male Lifespan, the Leading Causes of Death and Disability, Physical Concerns of Special Significance to Men, Reproductive and Sexual Concerns, Sexually Transmitted Diseases, Men's Mental and Emotional Health, and Lifestyle Choices That Affect Wellness, Such as Nutrition, Fitness, and Substance Use

Along with a Glossary of Related Terms and a Directory of Organizational Resources in Men's Health

Edited by Robert Aquinas McNally. 644 pages. 2004. 0-7808-0671-9.

ALSO AVAILABLE: *Men's Health Concerns Sourcebook, 1st Edition.* Edited by Allan R. Cook. 738 pages. 1998. 0-7808-0212-8.

"This comprehensive resource and the series are highly recommended."
— *American Reference Books Annual, 2000*

"Recommended reference source."
— *Booklist, American Library Association, Dec '98*

Mental Health Disorders Sourcebook, 3rd Edition

Basic Consumer Health Information about Mental and Emotional Health and Mental Illness, Including Facts about Depression, Bipolar Disorder, and Other Mood Disorders, Phobias, Post-Traumatic Stress Disorder (PTSD), Obsessive-Compulsive Disorder, and Other Anxiety Disorders, Impulse Control Disorders, Eating Disorders, Personality Disorders, and Psychotic Disorders, Including Schizophrenia and Dissociative Disorders

Along with Statistical Information, a Special Section Concerning Mental Health Issues in Children and Adolescents, a Glossary, and Directories of Resources for Additional Help and Information

Edited by Karen Bellenir. 661 pages. 2005. 0-7808-0747-2.

ALSO AVAILABLE: *Mental Health Disorders Sourcebook, 1st Edition.* Edited by Karen Bellenir. 548 pages. 1995. 0-7808-0040-0.

ALSO AVAILABLE: *Mental Health Disorders Sourcebook, 2nd Edition.* Edited by Karen Bellenir. 605 pages. 2000. 0-7808-0240-3.

"Well organized and well written."
— *American Reference Books Annual, 2001*

"Recommended reference source."
— *Booklist, American Library Association, Jun '00*

Mental Retardation Sourcebook

Basic Consumer Health Information about Mental Retardation and Its Causes, Including Down Syndrome, Fetal Alcohol Syndrome, Fragile X Syndrome, Genetic Conditions, Injury, and Environmental Sources

Along with Preventive Strategies, Parenting Issues, Educational Implications, Health Care Needs, Employment and Economic Matters, Legal Issues, a Glossary, and a Resource Listing for Additional Help and Information

Edited by Joyce Brennfleck Shannon. 642 pages. 2000. 0-7808-0377-9.

"Public libraries will find the book useful for reference and as a beginning research point for students, parents, and caregivers."
— *American Reference Books Annual, 2001*

"The strength of this work is that it compiles many basic fact sheets and addresses for further information in one volume. It is intended and suitable for the general public. This sourcebook is relevant to any collection providing health information to the general public."
— *E-Streams, Nov '00*

"From preventing retardation to parenting and family challenges, this covers health, social and legal issues and will prove an invaluable overview."
— *Reviewer's Bookwatch, Jul '00*

Movement Disorders Sourcebook

Basic Consumer Health Information about Neurological Movement Disorders, Including Essential Tremor, Parkinson's Disease, Dystonia, Cerebral Palsy, Huntington's Disease, Myasthenia Gravis, Multiple Sclerosis, and Other Early-Onset and Adult-Onset Movement Disorders, Their Symptoms and Causes, Diagnostic Tests, and Treatments

Along with Mobility and Assistive Technology Information, a Glossary, and a Directory of Additional Resources

Edited by Joyce Brennfleck Shannon. 655 pages. 2003. 0-7808-0628-X.

". . . a good resource for consumers and recommended for public, community college and undergraduate libraries."
— *American Reference Books Annual, 2004*

Muscular Dystrophy Sourcebook

Basic Consumer Health Information about Congenital, Childhood-Onset, and Adult-Onset Forms of Muscular Dystrophy, Such as Duchenne, Becker, Emery-Dreifuss, Distal, Limb-Girdle, Facioscapulohumeral (FSHD), Myotonic, and Ophthalmoplegic Muscular Dystrophies, Including Facts about Diagnostic Tests, Medical and Physical Therapies, Management of Co-Occurring Conditions, and Parenting Guidelines

Along with Practical Tips for Home Care, a Glossary, and Directories of Additional Resources

Edited by Joyce Brennfleck Shannon. 577 pages. 2004. 0-7808-0676-X.

Obesity Sourcebook

Basic Consumer Health Information about Diseases and Other Problems Associated with Obesity, and Including Facts about Risk Factors, Prevention Issues, and Management Approaches

Along with Statistical and Demographic Data, Information about Special Populations, Research Updates, a Glossary, and Source Listings for Further Help and Information

Edited by Wilma Caldwell and Chad T. Kimball. 376 pages. 2001. 0-7808-0333-7.

"The book synthesizes the reliable medical literature on obesity into one easy-to-read and useful resource for the general public."
— *American Reference Books Annual 2002*

"This is a very useful resource book for the lay public."
—*Doody's Review Service, Nov '01*

"Well suited for the health reference collection of a public library or an academic health science library that serves the general population." —*E-Streams, Sep '01*

"Recommended reference source."
—*Booklist, American Library Association, Apr '01*

" Recommended pick both for specialty health library collections and any general consumer health reference collection." — *The Bookwatch, Apr '01*

Ophthalmic Disorders Sourcebook, 1st Edition
SEE Eye Care Sourcebook, 2nd Edition

Oral Health Sourcebook
SEE Dental Care & Oral Health Sourcebook, 2nd Ed.

Osteoporosis Sourcebook

Basic Consumer Health Information about Primary and Secondary Osteoporosis and Juvenile Osteoporosis and Related Conditions, Including Fibrous Dysplasia, Gaucher Disease, Hyperthyroidism, Hypophosphatasia, Myeloma, Osteopetrosis, Osteogenesis Imperfecta, and Paget's Disease

Along with Information about Risk Factors, Treatments, Traditional and Non-Traditional Pain Management, a Glossary of Related Terms, and a Directory of Resources

Edited by Allan R. Cook. 584 pages. 2001. 0-7808-0239-X.

"This would be a book to be kept in a staff or patient library. The targeted audience is the layperson, but the therapist who needs a quick bit of information on a particular topic will also find the book useful."
— *Physical Therapy, Jan '02*

"This resource is recommended as a great reference source for public, health, and academic libraries, and is another triumph for the editors of Omnigraphics."
— *American Reference Books Annual 2002*

"Recommended for all public libraries and general health collections, especially those supporting patient education or consumer health programs."
— *E-Streams, Nov '01*

"Will prove valuable to any library seeking to maintain a current, comprehensive reference collection of health resources. . . . From prevention to treatment and associated conditions, this provides an excellent survey."
— *The Bookwatch, Aug '01*

"Recommended reference source."
— *Booklist, American Library Association, July '01*

SEE ALSO Women's Health Concerns Sourcebook

Pain Sourcebook, 2nd Edition

Basic Consumer Health Information about Specific Forms of Acute and Chronic Pain, Including Muscle and Skeletal Pain, Nerve Pain, Cancer Pain, and Disorders Characterized by Pain, Such as Fibromyalgia, Shingles, Angina, Arthritis, and Headaches

Along with Information about Pain Medications and Management Techniques, Complementary and Alternative Pain Relief Options, Tips for People Living with Chronic Pain, a Glossary, and a Directory of Sources for Further Information

Edited by Karen Bellenir. 670 pages. 2002. 0-7808-0612-3.

"A source of valuable information. . . . This book offers help to nonmedical people who need information about pain and pain management. It is also an excellent reference for those who participate in patient education."
— Doody's Review Service, Sep '02

"The text is readable, easily understood, and well indexed. This excellent volume belongs in all patient education libraries, consumer health sections of public libraries, and many personal collections."
— American Reference Books Annual, 1999

"A beneficial reference." — Booklist Health Sciences Supplement, American Library Association, Oct '98

"The information is basic in terms of scholarship and is appropriate for general readers. Written in journalistic style . . . intended for non-professionals. Quite thorough in its coverage of different pain conditions and summarizes the latest clinical information regarding pain treatment." — Choice, Association of College and Research Libraries, Jun '98

"Recommended reference source."
— Booklist, American Library Association, Mar '98

Pediatric Cancer Sourcebook

Basic Consumer Health Information about Leukemias, Brain Tumors, Sarcomas, Lymphomas, and Other Cancers in Infants, Children, and Adolescents, Including Descriptions of Cancers, Treatments, and Coping Strategies

Along with Suggestions for Parents, Caregivers, and Concerned Relatives, a Glossary of Cancer Terms, and Resource Listings

Edited by Edward J. Prucha. 587 pages. 1999. 0-7808-0245-4.

"An excellent source of information. Recommended for public, hospital, and health science libraries with consumer health collections." — E-Streams, Jun '00

"Recommended reference source."
— Booklist, American Library Association, Feb '00

"A valuable addition to all libraries specializing in health services and many public libraries."
— American Reference Books Annual, 2000

Physical & Mental Issues in Aging Sourcebook

Basic Consumer Health Information on Physical and Mental Disorders Associated with the Aging Process, Including Concerns about Cardiovascular Disease, Pulmonary Disease, Oral Health, Digestive Disorders, Musculoskeletal and Skin Disorders, Metabolic Changes, Sexual and Reproductive Issues, and Changes in Vision, Hearing, and Other Senses

Along with Data about Longevity and Causes of Death, Information on Acute and Chronic Pain, Descriptions of Mental Concerns, a Glossary of Terms, and Resource Listings for Additional Help

Edited by Jenifer Swanson. 660 pages. 1999. 0-7808-0233-0.

"This is a treasure of health information for the layperson." — Choice Health Sciences Supplement, Association of College & Research Libraries, May 2000

"Recommended for public libraries."
— American Reference Books Annual, 2000

"Recommended reference source."
— Booklist, American Library Association, Oct '99

SEE ALSO Healthy Aging Sourcebook

Podiatry Sourcebook

Basic Consumer Health Information about Foot Conditions, Diseases, and Injuries, Including Bunions, Corns, Calluses, Athlete's Foot, Plantar Warts, Hammertoes and Clawtoes, Clubfoot, Heel Pain, Gout, and More

Along with Facts about Foot Care, Disease Prevention, Foot Safety, Choosing a Foot Care Specialist, a Glossary of Terms, and Resource Listings for Additional Information

Edited by M. Lisa Weatherford. 380 pages. 2001. 0-7808-0215-2.

"Recommended reference source."
— Booklist, American Library Association, Feb '02

"There is a lot of information presented here on a topic that is usually only covered sparingly in most larger comprehensive medical encyclopedias."
— American Reference Books Annual 2002

Pregnancy & Birth Sourcebook, 2nd Edition

Basic Consumer Health Information about Conception and Pregnancy, Including Facts about Fertility, Infertility, Pregnancy Symptoms and Complications, Fetal Growth and Development, Labor, Delivery, and the Postpartum Period, as Well as Information about Maintaining Health and Wellness during Pregnancy and Caring for a Newborn

Along with Information about Public Health Assistance for Low-Income Pregnant Women, a Glossary, and Directories of Agencies and Organizations Providing Help and Support

Edited by Amy L. Sutton. 626 pages. 2004. 0-7808-0672-7.

ALSO AVAILABLE: Pregnancy & Birth Sourcebook, 1st Edition. Edited by Heather E. Aldred. 737 pages. 1997. 0-7808-0216-0.

"A well-organized handbook. Recommended."
— Choice, Association of College and Research Libraries, Apr '98

"Recommended reference source."
— Booklist, American Library Association, Mar '98

"Recommended for public libraries."
— American Reference Books Annual, 1998

SEE ALSO Congenital Disorders Sourcebook, Family Planning Sourcebook

Prostate Cancer Sourcebook

Basic Consumer Health Information about Prostate Cancer, Including Information about the Associated Risk Factors, Detection, Diagnosis, and Treatment of Prostate Cancer

Along with Information on Non-Malignant Prostate Conditions, and Featuring a Section Listing Support and Treatment Centers and a Glossary of Related Terms

Edited by Dawn D. Matthews. 358 pages. 2001. 0-7808-0324-8.

"Recommended reference source."
— *Booklist, American Library Association, Jan '02*

"A valuable resource for health care consumers seeking information on the subject. . . . All text is written in a clear, easy-to-understand language that avoids technical jargon. Any library that collects consumer health resources would strengthen their collection with the addition of the *Prostate Cancer Sourcebook*."
— *American Reference Books Annual 2002*

∎

Prostate & Urological Disorders Sourcebook

Basic Consumer Health Information about Urogenital and Sexual Disorders in Men, Including Prostate and Other Andrological Cancers, Prostatitis, Benign Prostatic Hyperplasia, Testicular and Penile Trauma, Cryptorchidism, Peyronie Disease, Erectile Dysfunction, and Male Factor Infertility, and Facts about Commonly Used Tests and Procedures, Such as Prostatectomy, Vasectomy, Vasectomy Reversal, Penile Implants, and Semen Analysis

Along with a Glossary of Andrological Terms and a Directory of Resources for Additional Information

Edited by Karen Bellenir. 631 pages. 2005. 0-7808-0797-9.

∎

Public Health Sourcebook

Basic Information about Government Health Agencies, Including National Health Statistics and Trends, Healthy People 2000 Program Goals and Objectives, the Centers for Disease Control and Prevention, the Food and Drug Administration, and the National Institutes of Health

Along with Full Contact Information for Each Agency

Edited by Wendy Wilcox. 698 pages. 1998. 0-7808-0220-9.

"Recommended reference source."
— *Booklist, American Library Association, Sep '98*

"This consumer guide provides welcome assistance in navigating the maze of federal health agencies and their data on public health concerns."
— *SciTech Book News, Sep '98*

Reconstructive & Cosmetic Surgery Sourcebook

Basic Consumer Health Information on Cosmetic and Reconstructive Plastic Surgery, Including Statistical Information about Different Surgical Procedures, Things to Consider Prior to Surgery, Plastic Surgery Techniques and Tools, Emotional and Psychological Considerations, and Procedure-Specific Information

Along with a Glossary of Terms and a Listing of Resources for Additional Help and Information

Edited by M. Lisa Weatherford. 374 pages. 2001. 0-7808-0214-4.

"An excellent reference that addresses cosmetic and medically necessary reconstructive surgeries. . . . The style of the prose is calm and reassuring, discussing the many positive outcomes now available due to advances in surgical techniques."
— *American Reference Books Annual 2002*

"Recommended for health science libraries that are open to the public, as well as hospital libraries that are open to the patients. This book is a good resource for the consumer interested in plastic surgery."
— *E-Streams, Dec '01*

"Recommended reference source."
— *Booklist, American Library Association, July '01*

∎

Rehabilitation Sourcebook

Basic Consumer Health Information about Rehabilitation for People Recovering from Heart Surgery, Spinal Cord Injury, Stroke, Orthopedic Impairments, Amputation, Pulmonary Impairments, Traumatic Injury, and More, Including Physical Therapy, Occupational Therapy, Speech/ Language Therapy, Massage Therapy, Dance Therapy, Art Therapy, and Recreational Therapy

Along with Information on Assistive and Adaptive Devices, a Glossary, and Resources for Additional Help and Information

Edited by Dawn D. Matthews. 531 pages. 1999. 0-7808-0236-5.

"This is an excellent resource for public library reference and health collections."
— *American Reference Books Annual, 2001*

"Recommended reference source."
— *Booklist, American Library Association, May '00*

∎

Respiratory Diseases & Disorders Sourcebook

Basic Information about Respiratory Diseases and Disorders, Including Asthma, Cystic Fibrosis, Pneumonia, the Common Cold, Influenza, and Others, Featuring Facts about the Respiratory System, Statistical and Demographic Data, Treatments, Self-Help Management Suggestions, and Current Research Initiatives

Edited by Allan R. Cook and Peter D. Dresser. 771 pages. 1995. 0-7808-0037-0.

"Designed for the layperson and for patients and their families coping with respiratory illness. . . . an extensive array of information on diagnosis, treatment, management, and prevention of respiratory illnesses for the general reader." — *Choice, Association of College and Research Libraries, Jun '96*

"A highly recommended text for all collections. It is a comforting reminder of the power of knowledge that good books carry between their covers." — *Academic Library Book Review, Spring '96*

"A comprehensive collection of authoritative information presented in a nontechnical, humanitarian style for patients, families, and caregivers." — *Association of Operating Room Nurses, Sep/Oct '95*

SEE ALSO Lung Disorders Sourcebook

■

Sexually Transmitted Diseases Sourcebook, 2nd Edition

Basic Consumer Health Information about Sexually Transmitted Diseases, Including Information on the Diagnosis and Treatment of Chlamydia, Gonorrhea, Hepatitis, Herpes, HIV, Mononucleosis, Syphilis, and Others

Along with Information on Prevention, Such as Condom Use, Vaccines, and STD Education; And Featuring a Section on Issues Related to Youth and Adolescents, a Glossary, and Resources for Additional Help and Information

Edited by Dawn D. Matthews. 538 pages. 2001. 0-7808-0249-7.

ALSO AVAILABLE: Sexually Transmitted Diseases Sourcebook, 1st Edition. Edited by Linda M. Ross. 550 pages. 1997. 0-7808-0217-9.

"Recommended for consumer health collections in public libraries, and secondary school and community college libraries."
 — *American Reference Books Annual 2002*

"Every school and public library should have a copy of this comprehensive and user-friendly reference book."
 — *Choice, Association of College & Research Libraries, Sep '01*

"This is a highly recommended book. This is an especially important book for all school and public libraries." — *AIDS Book Review Journal, Jul-Aug '01*

"Recommended reference source."
 — *Booklist, American Library Association, Apr '01*

"Recommended pick both for specialty health library collections and any general consumer health reference collection." — *The Bookwatch, Apr '01*

■

Skin Disorders Sourcebook, 1st Edition

SEE Dermatological Disorders Sourcebook, 2nd Edition

Sleep Disorders Sourcebook, 2nd Edition

Basic Consumer Health Information about Sleep and Sleep Disorders, Including Insomnia, Sleep Apnea, Restless Legs Syndrome, Narcolepsy, Parasomnias, and Other Health Problems That Affect Sleep, Plus Facts about Diagnostic Procedures, Treatment Strategies, Sleep Medications, and Tips for Improving Sleep Quality

Along with a Glossary of Related Terms and Resources for Additional Help and Information

Edited by Amy L. Sutton. 567 pages. 2005. 0-7808-0745-6.

ALSO AVAILABLE: Sleep Disorders Sourcebook, 1st Edition. Edited by Jenifer Swanson. 439 pages. 1998. 0-7808-0234-9.

"This text will complement any home or medical library. It is user-friendly and ideal for the adult reader."
 — *American Reference Books Annual, 2000*

"A useful resource that provides accurate, relevant, and accessible information on sleep to the general public. Health care providers who deal with sleep disorders patients may also find it helpful in being prepared to answer some of the questions patients ask."
 — *Respiratory Care, Jul '99*

"Recommended reference source."
 — *Booklist, American Library Association, Feb '99*

■

Smoking Concerns Sourcebook

Basic Consumer Health Information about Nicotine Addiction and Smoking Cessation, Featuring Facts about the Health Effects of Tobacco Use, Including Lung and Other Cancers, Heart Disease, Stroke, and Respiratory Disorders, Such as Emphysema and Chronic Bronchitis

Along with Information about Smoking Prevention Programs, Suggestions for Achieving and Maintaining a Smoke-Free Lifestyle, Statistics about Tobacco Use, Reports on Current Research Initiatives, a Glossary of Related Terms, and Directories of Resources for Additional Help and Information

Edited by Karen Bellenir. 621 pages. 2004. 0-7808-0323-X.

■

Sports Injuries Sourcebook, 2nd Edition

Basic Consumer Health Information about the Diagnosis, Treatment, and Rehabilitation of Common Sports-Related Injuries in Children and Adults

Along with Suggestions for Conditioning and Training, Information and Prevention Tips for Injuries Frequently Associated with Specific Sports and Special Populations, a Glossary, and a Directory of Additional Resources

Edited by Joyce Brennfleck Shannon. 614 pages. 2002. 0-7808-0604-2.

ALSO AVAILABLE: Sports Injuries Sourcebook, 1st Edition. Edited by Heather E. Aldred. 624 pages. 1999. 0-7808-0218-7.

"This is an excellent reference for consumers and it is recommended for public, community college, and undergraduate libraries."
— *American Reference Books Annual, 2003*

"Recommended reference source."
— *Booklist, American Library Association, Feb '03*

▪

Stress-Related Disorders Sourcebook

Basic Consumer Health Information about Stress and Stress-Related Disorders, Including Stress Origins and Signals, Environmental Stress at Work and Home, Mental and Emotional Stress Associated with Depression, Post-Traumatic Stress Disorder, Panic Disorder, Suicide, and the Physical Effects of Stress on the Cardiovascular, Immune, and Nervous Systems

Along with Stress Management Techniques, a Glossary, and a Listing of Additional Resources

Edited by Joyce Brennfleck Shannon. 610 pages. 2002. 0-7808-0560-7.

"**Well written for a general readership, the *Stress-Related Disorders Sourcebook* is a useful addition to the health reference literature.**"
— *American Reference Books Annual, 2003*

"**I am impressed by the amount of information. It offers a thorough overview of the causes and consequences of stress for the layperson. . . . A well-done and thorough reference guide for professionals and nonprofessionals alike.**" — *Doody's Review Service, Dec '02*

▪

Stroke Sourcebook

Basic Consumer Health Information about Stroke, Including Ischemic, Hemorrhagic, Transient Ischemic Attack (TIA), and Pediatric Stroke, Stroke Triggers and Risks, Diagnostic Tests, Treatments, and Rehabilitation Information

Along with Stroke Prevention Guidelines, Legal and Financial Information, a Glossary, and a Directory of Additional Resources

Edited by Joyce Brennfleck Shannon. 606 pages. 2003. 0-7808-0630-1.

"**This volume is highly recommended and should be in every medical, hospital, and public library.**"
— *American Reference Books Annual, 2004*

▪

Substance Abuse Sourcebook

Basic Health-Related Information about the Abuse of Legal and Illegal Substances Such as Alcohol, Tobacco, Prescription Drugs, Marijuana, Cocaine, and Heroin; and Including Facts about Substance Abuse Prevention Strategies, Intervention Methods, Treatment and Recovery Programs, and a Section Addressing the Special Problems Related to Substance Abuse during Pregnancy

Edited by Karen Bellenir. 573 pages. 1996. 0-7808-0038-9.

"A valuable addition to any health reference section. Highly recommended."
— *The Book Report, Mar/Apr '97*

". . . a comprehensive collection of substance abuse information that's both highly readable and compact. Families and caregivers of substance abusers will find the information enlightening and helpful, while teachers, social workers and journalists should benefit from the concise format. Recommended."
— *Drug Abuse Update, Winter '96/'97*

SEE ALSO *Alcoholism Sourcebook, Drug Abuse Sourcebook*

▪

Surgery Sourcebook

Basic Consumer Health Information about Inpatient and Outpatient Surgeries, Including Cardiac, Vascular, Orthopedic, Ocular, Reconstructive, Cosmetic, Gynecologic, and Ear, Nose, and Throat Procedures and More

Along with Information about Operating Room Policies and Instruments, Laser Surgery Techniques, Hospital Errors, Statistical Data, a Glossary, and Listings of Sources for Further Help and Information

Edited by Annemarie S. Muth and Karen Bellenir. 596 pages. 2002. 0-7808-0380-9.

"**Large public libraries and medical libraries would benefit from this material in their reference collections.**"
— *American Reference Books Annual, 2004*

"**Invaluable reference for public and school library collections alike.**" — *Library Bookwatch, Apr '03*

▪

Thyroid Disorders Sourcebook

Basic Consumer Health Information about Disorders of the Thyroid and Parathyroid Glands, Including Hypothyroidism, Hyperthyroidism, Graves Disease, Hashimoto Thyroiditis, Thyroid Cancer, and Parathyroid Disorders, Featuring Facts about Symptoms, Risk Factors, Tests, and Treatments

Along with Information about the Effects of Thyroid Imbalance on Other Body Systems, Environmental Factors That Affect the Thyroid Gland, a Glossary, and a Directory of Additional Resources

Edited by Joyce Brennfleck Shannon. 599 pages. 2005. 0-7808-0745-6.

▪

Transplantation Sourcebook

Basic Consumer Health Information about Organ and Tissue Transplantation, Including Physical and Financial Preparations, Procedures and Issues Relating to Specific Solid Organ and Tissue Transplants, Rehabilitation, Pediatric Transplant Information, the Future of Transplantation, and Organ and Tissue Donation

Along with a Glossary and Listings of Additional Resources

Edited by Joyce Brennfleck Shannon. 628 pages. 2002. 0-7808-0322-1.

"Along with these advances [in transplantation technology] have come a number of daunting questions for potential transplant patients, their families, and their health care providers. This reference text is the best single tool to address many of these questions. . . . It will be a much-needed addition to the reference collections in health care, academic, and large public libraries."
— *American Reference Books Annual, 2003*

"Recommended for libraries with an interest in offering consumer health information." — *E-Streams, Jul '02*

"This is a unique and valuable resource for patients facing transplantation and their families."
— *Doody's Review Service, Jun '02*

■

Traveler's Health Sourcebook

Basic Consumer Health Information for Travelers, Including Physical and Medical Preparations, Transportation Health and Safety, Essential Information about Food and Water, Sun Exposure, Insect and Snake Bites, Camping and Wilderness Medicine, and Travel with Physical or Medical Disabilities

Along with International Travel Tips, Vaccination Recommendations, Geographical Health Issues, Disease Risks, a Glossary, and a Listing of Additional Resources

Edited by Joyce Brennfleck Shannon. 613 pages. 2000. 0-7808-0384-1.

"Recommended reference source."
— *Booklist, American Library Association, Feb '01*

"This book is recommended for any public library, any travel collection, and especially any collection for the physically disabled."
— *American Reference Books Annual, 2001*

■

Urinary Tract & Kidney Diseases & Disorders Sourcebook, 2nd Edition

Basic Consumer Health Information about the Urinary System, Including the Bladder, Urethra, Ureters, and Kidneys, with Facts about Urinary Tract Infections, Incontinence, Congenital Disorders, Kidney Stones, Cancers of the Urinary Tract and Kidneys, Kidney Failure, Dialysis, and Kidney Transplantation

Along with Statistical and Demographic Information, Reports on Current Research in Kidney and Urologic Health, a Summary of Commonly Used Diagnostic Tests, a Glossary of Related Terms, and a Directory of Resources for Additional Help and Information

Edited by Ivy L. Alexander. 649 pages. 2005. 0-7808-0750-2.

ALSO AVAILABLE: Kidney & Urinary Tract Diseases & Disorders Sourcebook, 1st Ed. Edited by Linda M. Ross. 602 pages. 1997. 0-7808-0079-6.

Vegetarian Sourcebook

Basic Consumer Health Information about Vegetarian Diets, Lifestyle, and Philosophy, Including Definitions of Vegetarianism and Veganism, Tips about Adopting Vegetarianism, Creating a Vegetarian Pantry, and Meeting Nutritional Needs of Vegetarians, with Facts Regarding Vegetarianism's Effect on Pregnant and Lactating Women, Children, Athletes, and Senior Citizens

Along with a Glossary of Commonly Used Vegetarian Terms and Resources for Additional Help and Information

Edited by Chad T. Kimball. 360 pages. 2002. 0-7808-0439-2.

"Organizes into one concise volume the answers to the most common questions concerning vegetarian diets and lifestyles. This title is recommended for public and secondary school libraries." — *E-Streams, Apr '03*

"Invaluable reference for public and school library collections alike." — *Library Bookwatch, Apr '03*

"The articles in this volume are easy to read and come from authoritative sources. The book does not necessarily support the vegetarian diet but instead provides the pros and cons of this important decision. The *Vegetarian Sourcebook* is recommended for public libraries and consumer health libraries."
— *American Reference Books Annual, 2003*

■

Women's Health Concerns Sourcebook, 2nd Edition

Basic Consumer Health Information about the Medical and Mental Concerns of Women, Including Maintaining Health and Wellness, Gynecological Concerns, Breast Health, Sexuality and Reproductive Issues, Menopause, Cancer in Women, the Leading Causes of Death and Disability among Women, Physical Concerns of Special Significance to Women, and Women's Mental and Emotional Health

Along with a Glossary of Related Terms and Directories of Resources for Additional Help and Information

Edited by Amy L. Sutton. 748 pages. 2004. 0-7808-0673-5.

ALSO AVAILABLE: Women's Health Concerns Sourcebook, 1st Edition. Edited by Heather E. Aldred. 567 pages. 1997. 0-7808-0219-5.

"Handy compilation. There is an impressive range of diseases, devices, disorders, procedures, and other physical and emotional issues covered . . . well organized, illustrated, and indexed." — *Choice, Association of College and Research Libraries, Jan '98*

SEE ALSO Breast Cancer Sourcebook, Cancer Sourcebook for Women, Healthy Heart Sourcebook for Women, Osteoporosis Sourcebook

■

Workplace Health & Safety Sourcebook

Basic Consumer Health Information about Workplace Health and Safety, Including the Effect of Workplace Hazards on the Lungs, Skin, Heart, Ears, Eyes, Brain,

Reproductive Organs, Musculoskeletal System, and Other Organs and Body Parts

Along with Information about Occupational Cancer, Personal Protective Equipment, Toxic and Hazardous Chemicals, Child Labor, Stress, and Workplace Violence

Edited by Chad T. Kimball. 626 pages. 2000. 0-7808-0231-4.

"As a reference for the general public, this would be useful in any library." —*E-Streams, Jun '01*

"Provides helpful information for primary care physicians and other caregivers interested in occupational medicine. . . . General readers; professionals."
— *Choice, Association of College & Research Libraries, May '01*

"Recommended reference source."
— *Booklist, American Library Association, Feb '01*

"Highly recommended." — *The Bookwatch, Jan '01*

■

Worldwide Health Sourcebook

Basic Information about Global Health Issues, Including Malnutrition, Reproductive Health, Disease Dispersion and Prevention, Emerging Diseases, Risky Health Behaviors, and the Leading Causes of Death

Along with Global Health Concerns for Children, Women, and the Elderly, Mental Health Issues, Research and Technology Advancements, and Economic, Environmental, and Political Health Implications, a Glossary, and a Resource Listing for Additional Help and Information

Edited by Joyce Brennfleck Shannon. 614 pages. 2001. 0-7808-0330-2.

"Named an Outstanding Academic Title." —*Choice, Association of College & Research Libraries, Jan '02*

"Yet another handy but also unique compilation in the extensive Health Reference Series, this is a useful work because many of the international publications reprinted or excerpted are not readily available. Highly recommended." —*Choice, Association of College & Research Libraries, Nov '01*

"Recommended reference source."
—*Booklist, American Library Association, Oct '01*

Teen Health Series

Helping Young Adults Understand, Manage, and Avoid Serious Illness

List price $65 per volume. **School and library price $58 per volume.**

Alcohol Information for Teens

Health Tips about Alcohol and Alcoholism

Including Facts about Underage Drinking, Preventing Teen Alcohol Use, Alcohol's Effects on the Brain and the Body, Alcohol Abuse Treatment, Help for Children of Alcoholics, and More

Edited by Joyce Brennfleck Shannon. 370 pages. 2005. 0-7808-0741-3.

Allergy Information for Teens

Health Tips about Allergic Reactions Such as Anaphylaxis, Respiratory Problems, and Rashes

Including Facts about Identifying and Managing Allergies to Food, Pollen, Mold, Animals, Chemicals, Drugs, and Other Substances

Edited by Karen Bellenir. 400 pages. 2006. 0-7808-0799-5.

Asthma Information for Teens

Health Tips about Managing Asthma and Related Concerns

Including Facts about Asthma Causes, Triggers, Symptoms, Diagnosis, and Treatment

Edited by Karen Bellenir. 386 pages. 2005. 0-7808-0770-7.

"It is so clearly written and well organized that even hesitant readers will be able to find the facts they need, whether for reports or personal information. . . . A succinct but complete resource."

— School Library Journal, Sep '05

Cancer Information for Teens

Health Tips about Cancer Awareness, Prevention, Diagnosis, and Treatment

Including Facts about Frequently Occurring Cancers, Cancer Risk Factors, and Coping Strategies for Teens Fighting Cancer or Dealing with Cancer in Friends or Family Members

Edited by Wilma R. Caldwell. 428 pages. 2004. 0-7808-0678-6.

"Recommended for school libraries, or consumer libraries that see a lot of use by teens."

— E-Streams, May 2005

"A valuable educational tool."

— American Reference Books Annual, 2005

"Young adults and their parents alike will find this new addition to the *Teen Health Series* an important reference to cancer in teens."

— Children's Bookwatch, February 2005

Diet Information for Teens

Health Tips about Diet and Nutrition

Including Facts about Nutrients, Dietary Guidelines, Breakfasts, School Lunches, Snacks, Party Food, Weight Control, Eating Disorders, and More

Edited by Karen Bellenir. 399 pages. 2001. 0-7808-0441-4.

"Full of helpful insights and facts throughout the book. . . . An excellent resource to be placed in public libraries or even in personal collections."

— American Reference Books Annual 2002

"Recommended for middle and high school libraries and media centers as well as academic libraries that educate future teachers of teenagers. It is also a suitable addition to health science libraries that serve patrons who are interested in teen health promotion and education."

— E-Streams, Oct '01

"This comprehensive book would be beneficial to collections that need information about nutrition, dietary guidelines, meal planning, and weight control. . . . This reference is so easy to use that its purchase is recommended."

— The Book Report, Sep-Oct '01

"This book is written in an easy to understand format describing issues that many teens face every day, and then provides thoughtful explanations so that teens can make informed decisions. This is an interesting book that provides important facts and information for today's teens."

— Doody's Health Sciences Book Review Journal, Jul-Aug '01

"A comprehensive compendium of diet and nutrition. The information is presented in a straightforward, plain-spoken manner. This title will be useful to those working on reports on a variety of topics, as well as to general readers concerned about their dietary health."

— School Library Journal, Jun '01

Drug Information for Teens

Health Tips about the Physical and Mental Effects of Substance Abuse

Including Facts about Alcohol, Anabolic Steroids, Club Drugs, Cocaine, Depressants, Hallucinogens, Herbal Products, Inhalants, Marijuana, Narcotics, Stimulants, Tobacco, and More

Edited by Karen Bellenir. 452 pages. 2002. 0-7808-0444-9.

"A clearly written resource for general readers and researchers alike." *—School Library Journal*

"The chapters are quick to make a connection to their teenage reading audience. The prose is straightforward and the book lends itself to spot reading. It should be useful both for practical information and for research, and it is suitable for public and school libraries."
—American Reference Books Annual, 2003

"Recommended reference source."
—Booklist, American Library Association, Feb '03

"This is an excellent resource for teens and their parents. Education about drugs and substances is key to discouraging teen drug abuse and this book provides this much needed information in a way that is interesting and factual." *—Doody's Review Service, Dec '02*

■

Eating Disorders Information for Teens

Health Tips about Anorexia, Bulimia, Binge Eating, and Other Eating Disorders

Including Information on the Causes, Prevention, and Treatment of Eating Disorders, and Such Other Issues as Maintaining Healthy Eating and Exercise Habits

Edited by Sandra Augustyn Lawton. 337 pages. 2005. 0-7808-0783-9.

■

Fitness Information for Teens

Health Tips about Exercise, Physical Well-Being, and Health Maintenance

Including Facts about Aerobic and Anaerobic Conditioning, Stretching, Body Shape and Body Image, Sports Training, Nutrition, and Activities for Non-Athletes

Edited by Karen Bellenir. 425 pages. 2004. 0-7808-0679-4.

"This book will be a great addition to any public, junior high, senior high, or secondary school library."
—American Reference Books Annual, 2005

■

Learning Disabilities Information for Teens

Health Tips about Academic Skills Disorders and Other Disabilities That Affect Learning

Including Information about Common Signs of Learning Disabilities, School Issues, Learning to Live with a Learning Disability, and Other Related Issues

Edited by Sandra Augustyn Lawton. 337 pages. 2005. 0-7808-0796-0.

■

Mental Health Information for Teens

Health Tips about Mental Health and Mental Illness

Including Facts about Anxiety, Depression, Suicide, Eating Disorders, Obsessive-Compulsive Disorders, Panic Attacks, Phobias, Schizophrenia, and More

Edited by Karen Bellenir. 406 pages. 2001. 0-7808-0442-2.

"In both language and approach, this user-friendly entry in the *Teen Health Series* is on target for teens needing information on mental health concerns." *—Booklist, American Library Association, Jan '02*

"Readers will find the material accessible and informative, with the shaded notes, facts, and embedded glossary insets adding appropriately to the already interesting and succinct presentation."
—School Library Journal, Jan '02

"This title is highly recommended for any library that serves adolescents and parents/caregivers of adolescents." *—E-Streams, Jan '02*

"Recommended for high school libraries and young adult collections in public libraries. Both health professionals and teenagers will find this book useful."
—American Reference Books Annual 2002

"This is a nice book written to enlighten the society, primarily teenagers, about common teen mental health issues. It is highly recommended to teachers and parents as well as adolescents."
—Doody's Review Service, Dec '01

■

Sexual Health Information for Teens

Health Tips about Sexual Development, Human Reproduction, and Sexually Transmitted Diseases

Including Facts about Puberty, Reproductive Health, Chlamydia, Human Papillomavirus, Pelvic Inflammatory Disease, Herpes, AIDS, Contraception, Pregnancy, and More

Edited by Deborah A. Stanley. 391 pages. 2003. 0-7808-0445-7.

"This work should be included in all high school libraries and many larger public libraries. . . . highly recommended."
—American Reference Books Annual 2004

"Sexual Health approaches its subject with appropriate seriousness and offers easily accessible advice and information." *—School Library Journal, Feb. 2004*

Skin Health
Information for Teens

*Health Tips about Dermatological Concerns
and Skin Cancer Risks*

Including Facts about Acne, Warts, Hives, and Other
Conditions and Lifestyle Choices, Such as Tanning,
Tattooing, and Piercing, That Affect the Skin, Nails,
Scalp, and Hair

Edited by Robert Aquinas McNally. 429 pages. 2003.
0-7808-0446-5.

"This volume, as with others in the series, will be a
useful addition to school and public library collections."
                    —*American Reference Books Annual 2004*

"This volume serves as a one-stop source and should be
a necessity for any health collection."
                    —*Library Media Connection*

Sports Injuries
Information for Teens

*Health Tips about Sports Injuries and Injury
Protection*

Including Facts about Specific Injuries, Emergency
Treatment, Rehabilitation, Sports Safety, Competition
Stress, Fitness, Sports Nutrition, Steroid Risks, and
More

Edited by Joyce Brennfleck Shannon. 405 pages. 2003.
0-7808-0447-3.

"This work will be useful in the young adult collections of public libraries as well as high school libraries."
                    —*American Reference Books Annual 2004*

Suicide Information for Teens

*Health Tips about Suicide Causes and
Prevention*

Including Facts about Depression, Risk Factors, Getting Help, Survivor Support, and More

Edited by Joyce Brennfleck Shannon. 368 pages. 2005.
0-7808-0737-5.

Health Reference Series